Pediatric Gender Identity

Michelle Forcier
Gerrit Van Schalkwyk • Jack L. Turban
Editors

Pediatric Gender Identity

Gender-affirming Care for Transgender & Gender Diverse Youth

Springer

Editors
Michelle Forcier
Department of Pediatrics
Brown University
Providence, RI
USA

Gerrit Van Schalkwyk
Department of Psychiatry
and Human Behavior
Brown University
Providence, RI
USA

Jack L. Turban
Division of Child & Adolescent Psychiatry
Massachusetts General Hospital
Boston, MA
USA

ISBN 978-3-030-38908-6 ISBN 978-3-030-38909-3 (eBook)
https://doi.org/10.1007/978-3-030-38909-3

This Springer imprint is published by the registered company Springer Nature Switzerland AG
The registered company address is: Gewerbestrasse 11, 6330 Cham, Switzerland

Preface

We welcome our readers – medical and mental healthcare professionals, health and human service experts, as well as parents and patients who wish to learn more – to our multidisciplinary, collaborative textbook *Pediatric Gender Identity*. This text offers a broad overview of the latest research, clinical recommendations, and conceptual frameworks in the field. We hope that it will help readers develop a practical understanding regarding affirmative care for transgender and gender diverse (TGD) youth. Inherent in this approach is an understanding that gender identity development is just that – a developmental process, not a disease or a pathology. Our approach is grounded in the importance of thoughtfully listening to and respecting TGD youth who are undergoing the process of gender identity development during a time of ever-evolving understanding for the adults who seek to care for them.

We recognize that pediatric gender identity research and clinical care are constantly advancing. We are continuously learning from new research, language, concepts, and clinical options as they relate to our understanding of gender identity. We are excited by the growing body of evidence that supports affirmative care and resources for a population that has long suffered from health disparities and social injustice – often at the hands of health and human services providers. We hope this text will highlight for you new opportunities we have to provide patient-centered, consent-based care to TGD youth, working to fight against the historical maltreatment of these young people and striving to listen to and affirm the variety of authentic gendered selves these patients share with us.

We appreciate the time and efforts contributed by our authors, national and international leaders from a variety of health and human services disciplines, including our TGD-identified authors who contributed a combined lens of experts and members of the community. Our goal is that the readers have access to thoughtful, respectful, evidence-based options both for direct clinical services and for new ways to advocate for positive sociocultural changes in our communities.

Readers are invited to hear more about language and paradigms that acknowledge and support diversity and encourage resiliency. We then move into the epidemiology of pediatric gender identity, followed by overviews of relevant developmental psychology and neurobiology. Discussions of the impact of social stigma, discrimination, and harassment are framed within the minority stress model, offering opportunities and points of intervention to impact future generations of TGD youth and adults. Both primary care and specialty care medical topics are reviewed with a design to improve not just knowledge but practical, on-the-ground, clinical services and program developments. Specific attention to the neurodevelopmental and psychosocial needs of TGD youth has been geared for a wide variety of providers, considering issues of specific developmental periods, neurodiversity, and areas of importance in the realm of mental healthcare for TGD youth. Recognized hormonal and surgical recommendations are reviewed in detail so as to support better communication and education among the varied disciplines in the community of gender care providers. Authors provide practical information and potential applications for advocacy in improving schools, communities, and clinical settings. Authors explicitly overview several legal and cultural considerations that may improve clinical services and frame professional responsibilities as social change agents for these young and resilient youth.

Most of all, we appreciate the trust our patients have placed in us. We will continue to carefully listen and make deliberate efforts to learn more from our gender diverse children, colleagues, and members of the community. Transgender and gender diverse youth are increasingly visible and articulate, refusing to accept the status quo, expanding our understanding of gender and self-identity, and willing to engage with providers to create a culture that creates support and resources for the diverse ways we might grow up healthy and safe in each of our own unique gender identities.

Providence, RI, USA Michelle Forcier
Providence, RI, USA Gerrit Van Schalkwyk
Boston, MA, USA Jack L. Turban

Contents

Contributors

Marijn Arnoldussen, MD Department of Child and Adolescent Psychiatry, Center of Expertise on Gender Dysphoria, Amsterdam UMC, VU University Medical Center, Amsterdam, The Netherlands

Wendy P. Bamatter, PhD McLean Hospital, Belmont, MA, USA

Jonathan P. Brower, MD Department of Plastic Surgery, Rhode Island Hospital, Alpert Medical School of Brown University, Providence, RI, USA

Sarah M. Burke, PhD Brain and Development Research Centre, Department of Developmental & Educational Psychology, Institute of Psychology, Leiden University, Leiden, The Netherlands

Mamatha Challa, MD Department of Psychiatry & Behavioral Sciences, Stanford University School of Medicine, Stanford, CA, USA

Kathleen Chung, BA Warren Alpert Medical School of Brown University, Providence, RI, USA

Micaela Condon, LICSW Butler Hospital, Providence, RI, USA

Teresa Daniels, MD Brown University, Providence, RI, USA

Annelou L. C. de Vries, MD, PhD Department of Child and Adolescent Psychiatry, Center of Expertise on Gender Dysphoria, Amsterdam UMC, VU University Medical Center, Amsterdam, The Netherlands

Diane Ehrensaft, PhD University of California, San Francisco, CA, USA

Tony Ferraiolo, CPC Tony Ferraiolo, LLC, North Branford, CT, USA

Transgender Youth and Family Support Groups, North Branford, CT, USA

Jim Collins Foundation, North Branford, CT, USA

Michelle Forcier, MD, MPH Department of Pediatrics, Brown University, Providence, RI, USA

Coralie E. Fuchs, PhD Amsterdam UMC, VU University Medical Center, Department of Medical Psychology, Center of Expertise on Gender Dysphoria, Amsterdam, The Netherlands

Chelsea Graham, DO Thundermist Health Center and Brown Family Medicine Residency, Pawtucket, RI, USA

Agnieszka Janicka, MD Adult Gender and Sexuality Behavioral Health Program at Lifespan, Providence, RI, USA

Alison M. Jost, LICSW Adult Gender and Sexuality Behavioral Health Program at Lifespan, Providence, RI, USA

Alex S. Keuroghlian, MD, MPH National LGBT Health Education Center at the Fenway Institute, Massachusetts General Hospital/Harvard Medical School, Boston, MA, USA

Baudewijntje P. C. Kreukels, PhD Center of Expertise on Gender Dysphoria, Department of Medical Psychology, Amsterdam University Medical Centers, Amsterdam, The Netherlands

Daniel Kwan, MD Department of Plastic Surgery, Rhode Island Hospital, Alpert Medical School of Brown University, Providence, RI, USA

Anusha Lachman, FCPSYCH, MMED, Mphil Department of Psychiatry, Stellenbosch University, Cape Town, South Africa

Naomi Libby, MD Yale Child Study Center, Yale University, New Haven, CT, USA

Aida Manduley, LCSW Women of Color Sexual Health Network, Boston, MA, USA

Kira Manser, LICSW Clinical Social Worker and Sex Educator in Private Practice, Pawtucket, RI, USA

Jenifer K. McGuire, PhD, MPH Department of Family Social Science, University of Minnesota, Twin Cities, MN, USA

Vikram G. Mookerjee, BA Department of Plastic Surgery, Rhode Island Hospital, Alpert Medical School of Brown University, Providence, RI, USA

Quinlyn J. Morrow, MA Department of Family Social Science, University of Minnesota, Twin Cities, MN, USA

Leena Nahata, MD Department of Pediatrics, The Ohio State University College of Medicine/Nationwide Children's Hospital, Columbus, OH, USA

Center for Biobehavioral Health, The Research Institute at Nationwide Children's Hospital, Columbus, OH, USA

Christy L. Olezeski, PhD Yale School of Medicine, Department of Psychiatry, New Haven, CT, USA

Elizabeth S. Perzanowski, MD Department of Pediatrics, Massachusetts General Hospital for Children, Boston, MA, USA

Zheala Qayyum, MD Yale University School of Medicine (Department of Psychiatry), New Haven, CT, USA

Sarah Rhoads, MD Medicine-Pediatrics Residency Program, Brown University, Providence, RI, USA

Alicia Rolin, BA Warren Alpert Medical School of Brown University, Providence, RI, USA

Andrew C. Sackett-Taylor, PMHNP Gándara Mental Health Center, Springfield, MA, USA

Kristen Sayles, RN Butler Hospital, Providence, RI, USA

Caroline Scott, BSPH Washington University School of Medicine, St. Louis, MO, USA

Cynthia J. Telingator, MD Harvard Medical School, Department of Psychiatry, Cambridge Health Alliance, Cambridge, MA, USA

Ryan Thoreson, JD, DPhil Yale Law School, New Haven, CT, USA

Amy C. Tishelman, PhD Departments of Endocrinology and Psychiatry, Harvard Medical School/Boston Children's Hospital, Boston, MA, USA

Maria Trumpler, PhD Office of LGBTQ Resources, Yale University, New Haven, CT, USA

Jack L. Turban, MD, MHS Division of Child & Adolescent Psychiatry, Massachusetts General Hospital, Boston, MA, USA

Erin Ursillo, LMHC Butler Hospital, Providence, RI, USA

Anna Valentine, MD Department of Pediatrics, The Ohio State University College of Medicine/Nationwide Children's Hospital, Columbus, OH, USA

Anna I. R. van der Miesen, MD Amsterdam UMC, VU University Medical Center, Department of Child and Adolescent Psychiatry, Center of Expertise on Gender Dysphoria, Amsterdam, The Netherlands

Gerrit Van Schalkwyk, MB, ChB Warren Alpert School of Medicine, Brown University, Providence, RI, USA

Roy H. T. van Vlerken, MD Amsterdam UMC, VU University Medical Center, Department of Child and Adolescent Psychiatry, Center of Expertise on Gender Dysphoria, Amsterdam, The Netherlands

Jaye Watts, LICSW Thundermist Health Center and Brown Family Medicine Residency, Pawtucket, RI, USA

Cecil R. Webster Jr., MD Harvard Medical School, Department of Psychiatry, McLean Hospital, Boston, MA, USA

1 Overview and Terminology

Elizabeth S. Perzanowski, Tony Ferraiolo, and Alex S. Keuroghlian

Introduction

Imagine you are a pediatric primary care clinician seeing a 3-year-old child for a well visit. You have known this child and family for several years. The parents surprise you by saying, "She keeps telling us she's a boy, even though we've told her over and over again that she's a girl. What does that mean? Is there something wrong with her?"

Maybe, a 7-year-old child presents for a sick visit, and as you reach for the door knob to exit the room, the parent mentions, "By the way, he keeps saying he wants to wear skirts to school. We're ok with him wearing them at home, but what will happen if he wears them to school? Is this normal? Should we let him? When will it stop?"

Perhaps a high school senior walks into your office for a check-in. After navigating a difficult road through high school, including school avoidance and depression, you are proud of this adolescent's perseverance and plans to attend college. After you've excused the parent, the teenager bursts out in tears. "I've got something to tell you. I'm not really a girl, I've been a boy my whole life. Can you help me?"

E. S. Perzanowski (✉)
Department of Pediatrics, Massachusetts General Hospital for Children, Boston, MA, USA
e-mail: elizabeth.perzanowski@childrens.harvard.edu

T. Ferraiolo
Tony Ferraiolo, LLC, North Branford, CT, USA

Transgender Youth and Family Support Groups, North Branford, CT, USA

Jim Collins Foundation, North Branford, CT, USA
e-mail: tony@tonyferraiolo.com

A. S. Keuroghlian
National LGBT Health Education Center at the Fenway Institute, Massachusetts General Hospital/Harvard Medical School, Boston, MA, USA
e-mail: akeuroghlian@partners.org

M. Forcier et al. (eds.), *Pediatric Gender Identity*,
https://doi.org/10.1007/978-3-030-38909-3_1

What do you say to each of these parents and their children? How can you help them? In the course of this text, we hope to guide you toward how to respond and provide affirmative care for both youth and their families.

In recent years, transgender and gender diverse (TGD) youth have gained increased recognition, with concurrent nondiscrimination battles at the local and state level regarding regulations around bathroom use, sports team membership, employment and housing, and harassment [1–5]. This focus has been mirrored in peer-reviewed literature as the medical and mental health communities work to expand our knowledge of this marginalized population and how we as medical and mental health clinicians can best serve these youth, especially given rapid increases in the number of patients seeking gender-affirming care [6, 7]. Several guidelines exist regarding the evaluation and care of TGD youth, though these are largely tailored for subspecialty clinicians, limiting their broader utility [8–11]. Despite the existence of these guidelines, numerous examples in the health literature demonstrate a lack of training, knowledge, and competence regarding care for TGD people of all ages, which is evident to our gender diverse patients [12–24].

A significant barrier for medical and mental health caregivers to providing quality care for patients with gender diverse identities is insufficient education to competently address the unique needs of these patients [25, 26]. Our hope in writing this text is to guide readers to a more expansive, evidence-based understanding of gender through an overview of terminology, gender development, and various aspects of caring for TGD children and adolescents. Intuitively one would expect people who identify along the TGD continuum to seek more care and have more favorable outcomes when they are engaged with clinicians who are fluent in the language and health needs of the TGD population. Indeed, survey data demonstrate this to be true [27].

Clinicians of all disciplines who serve children and adolescents can play a crucial role providing anticipatory guidance about gender identity development and creating space to explore this aspect of a youth's developing identity. Clinicians can help cultivate readiness in families to support and facilitate their children's identity exploration, discovery, and affirmation. As with routine sexual history taking, normalizing conversations about gender identity, expression, and role sets the stage for patients and their families to entrust their clinician with subsequent and potentially more difficult conversations related to gender affirmation.

Pediatric primary care and mental health clinicians are well positioned to reduce many existing barriers to affirming care for patients who are gender diverse. Pediatric primary care clinicians in particular, who see such a wide swath of youth and tend to engage in advocacy related to child and adolescent wellness, are poised to lead as a driving force in the medical community for promoting acceptance and affirmation for this population [28].

Concepts and Terminology

Each of us has a gender identity, though many of us never give it much thought. Gender identity develops early in childhood—preschool children are able to define and declare their own gender and begin to feel pressure to conform to societally supported gender stereotypes [24, 29]. It is important to review the essential concepts and terminology underpinning discussions in this textbook (see Table 1.1 for a summary). With regard

Table 1.1 Essential concepts and terminology [5, 31]

Sex/gender assigned at birth/ natal sex/birth sex	In the traditional trichotomous paradigm, designation of a person as "female," "male," or "intersex" based on anatomy (external genitalia and/ or internal reproductive organs) and/or biology (sex chromosomes and/or hormones)
	"Sex" and "gender" are often used interchangeably, but they are distinct entities. It is best to distinguish between sex, gender identity, and gender expression and to avoid making assumptions about a patient regarding one of these characteristics based on knowledge of the others.
	This is sometimes abbreviated as AFAB (assigned female at birth) or AMAB (assigned male at birth)
Gender identity	A person's inner sense of being a girl/woman, boy/man, some combination of both, or something else, including having no gender at all. This may or may not correspond to the gender assigned at birth.
Gender expression	The outward manifestation of a person's gender, which may or may not reflect their inner gender identity based on traditional expectations. Gender expression incorporates how a person carries themselves, their dress, accessories, grooming, voice/speech patterns and conversational mannerisms, and physical characteristics.
Transgender	An umbrella term describing individuals whose gender identity does not align in a traditional sense with the gender they were assigned at birth. It may also be used to refer to a person whose gender identity is binary and not traditionally associated with that assigned at birth.
	Though this term is commonly used, there are some gender diverse people who do not identify this way. It is important to ask patients how they identify with regard to gender.
	It is best practice to use this term as an adjective rather than a noun. Many find the term "trangendered" to be pejorative as it implies there was an event that made a person transgender.
Transgender girl/ woman	A person who identifies as a girl/woman and was assigned male sex at birth
Transgender boy/ man	A person who identifies as a boy/man and was assigned female sex at birth
Gender diverse	An umbrella term describing individuals with gender identities and/or expressions that vary from expected developmental norms. This includes people who identify as multiple genders or with no gender at all.
Nonbinary	A term used by some individuals whose gender identity is neither girl/ woman nor boy/man
Cisgender	Describes a person whose gender identity aligns in a traditional sense with the sex assigned to them at birth
Gender dysphoria (GD)	A concept defined in the *Diagnostic and Statistical Manual of Mental Disorders, 5th edition* (DSM-5) as clinically significant distress or impairment related to a strong desire to be of another gender, which may include desire to change primary and/or secondary sex characteristics [32]. Not all TGD persons experience dysphoria.
Sexual orientation	Describes the types of individuals toward whom a person has emotional, physical, and/or romantic attachments

(continued)

Table 1.1 (continued)

Lesbian, Gay, Bisexual, Transgender, Queer, plus (LGBTQ+) Or Gender and sexual minoritized persons	An umbrella term attempting to encompass all gender and sexual minority identities that are outside of the cisgender, heterosexual binaries
Intersex	A term encompassing the numerous and varied conditions involving diverse sex chromosomes, gonads, internal reproductive organs, sex hormones, and/or external genitalia. A person can have aspects of both traditionally male and female internal and/or external anatomy, hormonal milieu, and/or sex chromosomes. Some of these conditions are not recognized until puberty, when secondary sex characteristics do not develop as expected or at all.
	In the medical community, the term "disorders of sex development" ("DSD") has been used, though this term is considered stigmatizing by intersex advocates and ought to be avoided. Some have recommended use of the term "differences of sexual development."
	In the past, intersex conditions have been associated with the term "hermaphrodite," which is considered pejorative and should be avoided

to categories of gender, many societies recognize just two: girl/woman and boy/man. This paradigm is recognized as the gender binary, as it is composed of two categories of gender. Some people experience a gender identity which does not fit into these two designations, instead existing as a combination of the two, something else entirely, or as not identifying with any category of gender at all. Access to affirming care is particularly challenging for people whose gender identity falls outside of the traditional gender binary of girl/woman or boy/man. For TGD people who are also members of other traditionally marginalized groups, such as racial or ethnic minorities, the challenges of accessing care are further compounded [30].

In addition, clinicians ought to be aware of the ever-evolving nature of the language used by gender diverse youth to self-identify. As with other aspects of patient-centered care, reflecting the language used by youth is a good place to start. In addition, when a patient uses terms you are unfamiliar with, it is acceptable to ask in a nonjudgmental manner: "I'm not familiar with that term. What does it mean to you?" By actively listening to each patient's description of their gender identity and what it means to them, clinicians have the opportunity to convey respect and communicate that their practice is a safe and welcoming space [31]. It is also important to note that in general the onus of understanding core concepts related to gender identity, including transgender and nonbinary identities, rests not with the patient but with the clinician. This allows the youth to remain in their role of the cared for patient, rather than caring for the provider.

This text espouses a gender-affirmative model of care, wherein children and adolescents are supported in exploring and affirming their gender identity and expression

[28, 33]. In this model, transgender and nonbinary identities are considered to be natural and healthy aspects of gender diversity among humans, rather than diagnostic entities with assigned pathology. The gender-affirmative model of care is supported by major pediatric medical and psychological associations, including the American Academy of Pediatrics (AAP), the American College of Osteopathic Pediatricians (ACOP), the American Academy of Child and Adolescent Psychiatry (AACAP), the American Psychological Association (APA), and the Society for Adolescent Health and Medicine (SAHM) [28, 34, 35]. This framework for care recognizes that mental health problems and health disparities among gender diverse youth often result from (1) distress at having physical sex characteristics misaligned with gender identity and (2) external stigma-related stress on an everyday basis related to gender nonconformity [28]. Put more plainly, health disparities experienced by TGD youth are primarily the result of societal mistreatment rather than gender identity itself.

Creating a Welcoming Care Environment

Transgender youth often have traumatic experiences when seeking medical care, which can contribute to adverse health outcomes for an already socially marginalized population. It is important to remember some of your patients who are TGD have been refused medical treatment by other care teams. In some cases, they may have been told explicitly that their transgender or nonbinary identity is wrong. Outside of explicit bias and acts of harassment or hate, this can be due to a sheer lack of awareness about the importance of language in support of TGD patients on the part of health-care staff. Creating a welcoming environment for patients includes fostering an affirming experience from the first call to your office, to the office visit itself, to any follow-up communication and care that may occur, including referrals to other health-care practices to ensure they too are competent and affirming with TGD patients.

As many as 31% of transgender adults have not disclosed their gender identity to any of their health-care clinicians for fear of maltreatment and in one survey 23–48% delayed needed care for fear of discrimination [36]. Clinician education alone is not enough to create safe, welcoming environments for our TGD patients and their families. The initial call to your office sets the tone for your patient: it is their first impression of whether the health care in your practice is respectful and safe, and the basis for predictions about whether staff they might later encounter will be trained to interact with them in an affirming way. Staff education and training alerts them to affirmative language, policies, and standards of care as well as helping staff reconcile potential differences between their existing personal values and their professional responsibility to provide affirming, inclusive care for all communities. Some staff may have political, cultural, and/or religious objections to TGD identities. Being courteous and professional with TGD patients does not require abandoning those beliefs, but rather being aware of one's own bias in the workplace and preventing this bias from adversely impacting good care and service delivery for our patients.

It is important to be aware that standard diversity training intended to increase affirming behaviors in clinicians and office staff may not be enough to eliminate bias-related marginalizing behaviors. This has been best studied with regard to racially related bias, but we can extrapolate those experiences to other marginalized groups [37]. Understanding this discrepancy requires an appreciation of the concepts of explicit and implicit bias. Explicit bias is related to conscious stereotypes and beliefs, and can be measured by self-report. On the other hand, implicit or automatic bias is related to deeply ingrained beliefs, which act in the unconscious to influence behavior. Various studies have attempted to look at implicit bias with response-latency testing for unconscious associations, which has been found to not necessarily align with explicitly reported beliefs [38]. Evidence demonstrates that standard diversity trainings designed to counter bias against LGB populations may improve explicit bias, which is highly impacted by social desirability, but that implicit biases often persist. What results is a divergence between reported affirmation of LGB populations and the continuation of bias-motivated incidents experienced by LGB people [39]. There are little-to-no data available regarding explicit and implicit bias toward TGD people, but extrapolating these data suggests that despite increasing societal recognition and support, our TGD patients continue suffer from implicit as well as explicit bias. Luckily, implicit bias is elastic and can be reshaped [40]. Overcoming implicit bias requires critical introspection and thoughtful recognition of unconscious thought patterns and the resulting behaviors, in addition to the work of a community to identify incidents of bias committed by one another and working together to restructure the attendant attitudes and beliefs [37].

Another key element of affirmative care is to avoid making assumptions about all patients' gender identities, an important guiding principle to apply in clinical practice even beyond the realm of gender-affirming care specifically [41]. In your first meeting with any new patient, ask about the name they go by and their pronouns. It can be as simple as asking, "What name would you like us to use?" and "What are your pronouns?" Even if a patient does not currently identify as gender diverse or is not ready to disclose this to you, asking the question goes a long way in demonstrating that you are someone they can open up to when they feel ready, setting the stage for possible future conversations about gender identity. It additionally models to persons less familiar with gender diversity how to be expansive and inclusive. It is important to know that "she/her/hers" and "he/him/his" are not the only pronoun series. "They/them/theirs" is now a common pronoun series to refer to a single person, and additional nonbinary pronoun series also exist. You might explain concretely to the patient: "Some people's pronouns are 'she/her/hers,' some people's pronouns are 'he/him/his,' some people's pronouns are 'they/them/theirs,' some people's pronouns are something else. What are yours? Then, once the patient has provided pronouns, ensure you use these and that all others in your practice know to use the patient's asserted name and pronoun set as well. If you accidentally use the wrong pronoun, calmly apologize and correct yourself

Name on legal documents*:				Chosen name:
Sex on legal documents*:	Female	Male	Other_____†	
Pronouns: he/him,	she/her,	they/them,	Other______	
*While we recognize a number of genders/sexes, for insurance and billing purposes we must also use the name listed on your insurance for documents pertaining to insurance, billing, and some correspondence.				

† At the time of publication there are two states (Washington and California) and one city (New York City) that allow gender to be marked with the non-binary designation "X".

Fig. 1.1 Sample intake form header

before moving on. Being called by the wrong name or using the wrong pronoun can be experienced as a painful insult, and may make patients feel shamed for being transgender or nonbinary, or question your office's support of their identity [41]. If a mistake is made, correct it, apologize, and move on as it is not the patient's role to educate and support the provider.

Questions to elicit chosen name and pronouns should be included on intake forms in addition to asking about administrative, legal, or insurance name and sex, which are still required for insurance and billing purposes. Asking these questions upfront and incorporating them into standard operating health records and procedures signals to patients that this practice routinely offers a competent, safe, and welcoming staff and environment. See Fig. 1.1 for an example. For patients you are already caring for, it is key to provide standardized questions about gender identity, which will be discussed later in this text.

In general, information should be recorded such that when patients call or check in, the correct name and pronouns are used. In cases where youth or adults have not disclosed their TGD identity to others, careful documentation and use of requested name/pronoun in different spaces may be required. If documentation of an LGBTQ+ status would be accessed by unsupportive adults with a potential for harm, you may consider avoiding formal documentation of their sexual orientation or gender identity in the accessible medical record. Timing and method of disclosure is based on patient needs and preferences. Some people may never feel comfortable formally disclosing their gender identity in public or other settings.

The physical environment of the office itself should also communicate a safe and welcoming space. Prominently displayed signage identifying the office as an LGBTQ+ safe zone and posting nondiscrimination statements that include protections regarding gender identity and expression in multiple languages demonstrates to your patients your commitment to them even before talking to your office's staff. Consider offering and adding children's books and images that feature protagonists who challenge gender norms and are gender diverse themselves, thus giving all caregivers and youth who frequent your office examples of a more expansive view of gender.

Working with Stigma and Dysphoria

Many gender diverse youth struggle with some degree of body incongruence, which can reach the level of gender dysphoria as defined in the DSM-5. While gender minority stress is a major contributor to the health and mental health issues associated with TGD identities, this dysphoria related to one's own body can itself also be damaging. There is widespread misunderstanding about the realities of the uniqueness of each TGD individual's body and their individual wishes for their body. These knowledge gaps can create a chasm between patient and clinician if assumptions are made [41]. Clinicians should ask rather than assume any individual patient's desired journey with regard to aspects of social, medical, or surgical affirmation. Asking for specific needs, concerns, and goals communicates to patients that you are open, listening, and supportive of their unique identity. Gently reassure patients that if they decide to undergo specific gender-affirming medical or surgical care, they are not alone and you can help support them through whatever process will affirm their authentic self.

TGD youth have a wide range of experiences. Below are just a few examples of how some youth view their bodies and dysphoria when asked the question, "What does body dysphoria feel like?" (Figs. 1.2 and 1.3).

Chest and genital examinations can be uncomfortable and often traumatic for TGD patients. If this type of examination is medically necessary, such as for Tanner staging or to evaluate a symptom related to those organ systems, it is important to have a conversation beforehand to frame why this difficult aspect of the examination is important. Patients benefit from knowing what to expect, what can help them feel more comfortable, and what language they find most affirming [41, 43].

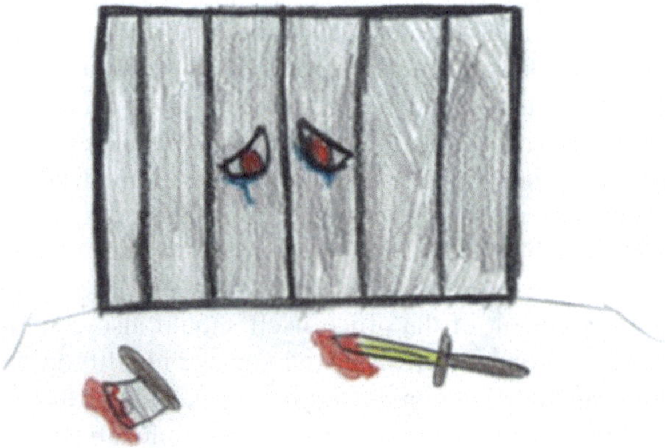

Fig. 1.2 "Body dysphoria feels to me like being locked in a cage (as cliché as that sounds). Sometimes I feel superior, but my 'human form' is keeping me down. There are lots of things I'll never be able to experience because of my body. Even worse, many people think that my aforementioned human form has to define me. I drew weapons around my cage because I feel like I am being tortured for having any confidence, and my body is my punishment." Illustrations are created by gender diverse youth in response to the question, "What does body dysphoria feel like?" [42]

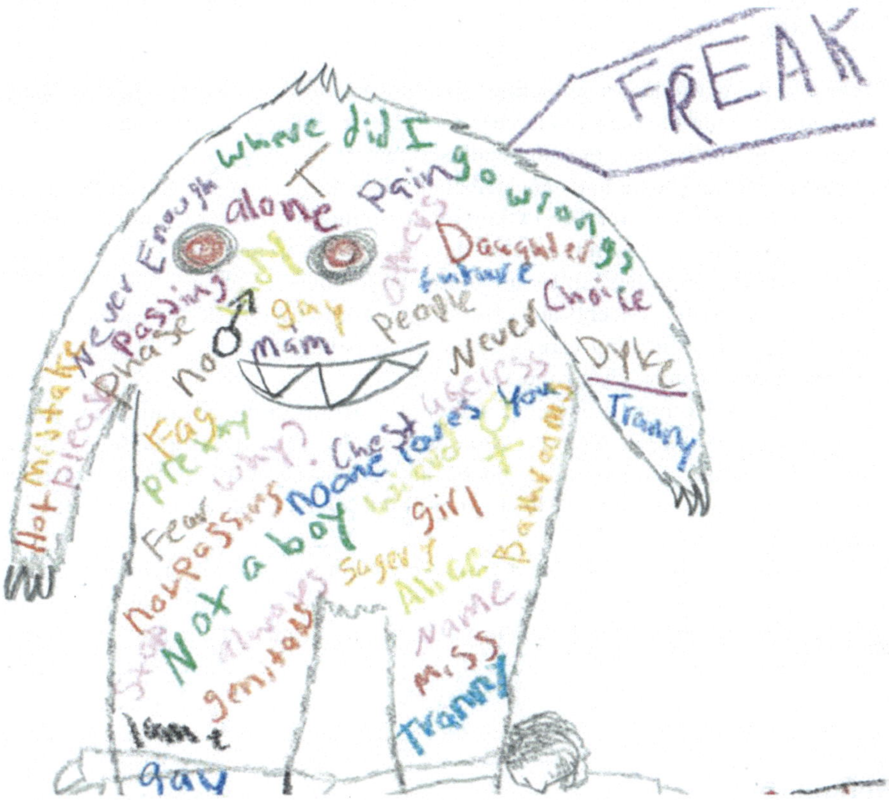

Fig. 1.3 "For me dysphoria comes from the words I hear, from others and from my own mind. Sometimes it seems like the only way to get away from a huge monster on my back is self-harm." Illustrations are created by gender diverse youth in response to the question, "What does body dysphoria feel like?" [42]

Consent and bodily autonomy are important concepts for all children to learn. Patients can defer sensitive examinations or testing or ask to have them done at a future date in a patient-centered, consent-based model of care. Providers can educate patients about consent and about necessary potential steps in care in reassuring and respectful ways.

Difficulty accessing culturally sensitive medical and mental health care is a notable contributing factor to the health disparities that TGD patients face, and are factors that clinicians have the power to change. Pediatric clinicians of all types can play a major role by modeling support and affirmation for TGD youth to families and the community. Listen to your patients when they express their need for gender affirmation by social, psychological, medical, and surgical means. Helping TGD patients feel affirmed in their identities when accessing health-care environments will help save lives [41].

Summary

- Despite the existence of guidelines for the care of TGD youth, clinicians lack adequate training to sensitively care for them, and many TGD youth encounter hostility in medical and mental health settings.
- Pediatric primary care and mental health clinicians are uniquely positioned to support and advocate for TGD youth by instituting routine screening and anticipatory guidance regarding gender development, not just for TGD-identified youth and their families but for all youth and families.
- Understanding the concepts and affirming language used to discuss gender identity and gender-affirming care is essential, as is understanding that language is dynamic and changes over time.
- Creating a welcoming office environment involves training all staff on concepts of gender identity, gender expression, and gender diversity, displaying signage indicating affirmation of all genders, and providing waiting room materials (including children's books) displaying children and adolescents of all gender experiences.
- As a clinician, it is critical not to make assumptions about gender identity but rather to approach the patient with an open, supportive curiosity and listen closely regarding their chosen name, pronouns, and goals for gender affirmation.

References

1. Schuster MA, Reisner SL, Onorato SE. Beyond bathrooms – meeting the health needs of transgender people. N Engl J Med. 2016;375:101–3. https://doi.org/10.1056/NEJMp1605912.
2. American Civil Liberties Union. Transgender people and the law [Internet]. American Civil Liberties Union; 2019 [cited 2019 Mar 5]. Available from: https://www.aclu.org/know-your-rights/transgender-people-and-law.
3. National Scholastic Athletics Foundation. National scholastic athletics foundation transgender participation policy & procedure [Internet]. National Scholastic Athletics Foundation; 2019 [cited 2019 Mar 5]. Available from: https://www.nationalscholastic.org/nbin/transgender/.
4. Griffin P, Carroll H. NCAA inclusion of transgender student-athletes [Internet]. NCAA Office of Inclusion; 2011 [cited 2019 Mar 5]. Available from: https://www.ncaa.org/sites/default/files/Transgender_Handbook_2011_Final.pdf.
5. Turban JL, de Vries ALC, Zucker K. Gender dysphoria and gender incongruence. In: Martin A, Bloch MH, Volkmar FR, editors. Lewis's child and adolescent psychiatry: a comprehensive textbook. 5th ed. Philadelphia: Lippincott Williams & Wilkins; 2018.
6. Turban JL, van Schalkwyk GI. "Gender dysphoria" and autism spectrum disorder: is the link real? J Am Acad Child Adolesc Psychiatry. 2018;57(1):8–9.e2. https://doi.org/10.1016/j.jaac.2017.08.017.
7. Chen M, Fuqua J, Eugster EA. Characteristics of referrals for gender dysphoria over a 13-year period. J Adolesc Health. 2016;58(3):369–71. https://doi.org/10.1016/j.jadohealth.2015.11.010.

8. Hembree WC, Cohen-Kettenis PT, Gooren L, Hannema SE, Meyer WJ, Murad MH, et al. Endocrine treatment of gender-dysphoric/gender-incongruent persons: an endocrine society clinical practice guideline. Endocr Pract. 2017;23(12):1437. https://doi.org/10.4158/1934-2403-23.12.1437.
9. World Professional Association for Transgender Health. Standards of care for the health of transsexual, transgender, and gender-nonconforming people. 7th ed. Minneapolis: World Professional Association for Transgender Health; 2012.
10. American Psychological Association. Guidelines for psychological practice with transgender and gender nonconforming people. Am Psychol. 2015;70(9):832–64. https://doi.org/10.1037/a0039906.
11. American Academy of Child and Adolescent Psychiatry. Practice parameters on gay, lesbian, or bisexual sexual orientation, gender nonconformity, and gender discordance in children and adolescents. J Am Acad Child Adolesc Psychiatry. 2012;51(9):957–74. https://doi.org/10.1016/j.jaac.2012.07.004.
12. Gruschow S, Kinsman S, Dowshen N. Pediatric primary care provider knowledge, attitudes, and skills in caring for gender non-conforming youth. J Adolesc Health. 2018;62(2):S29. https://doi.org/10.1016/j.jadohealth.2017.11.058.
13. Mehta PK, Easter SR, Potter J, Castleberry N, Schulkin J, Robinson JN. Lesbian, gay, bisexual and transgender health: obstetrician-gynecologists' training, attitudes, knowledge, and practice. J Women's Health. 2018;27(12):1459–95. https://doi.org/10.1089/jwh.2017.6912.
14. Puckett JA, Cleary P, Rossman K, Mustanski B, Newcomb ME. Barriers to gender-affirming care for transgender and gender nonconforming individuals. Sex Res Social Policy. 2017;15(1):48–59. https://doi.org/10.1007/s13178-017-0295-8.
15. Chisolm-Straker M, Jardine L, Bennouna C, Morency-Brassard N, Coy L, Egemba MO, et al. Transgender and gender nonconforming in emergency departments: a qualitative report of patient experiences. Transgend Health. 2017;2(1):8–16. https://doi.org/10.1089/trgh.2016.0026.
16. Samuels EA, Tape C, Garber N, Bowman S, Choo EK. "Sometimes you feel like the freak show": a qualitative assessment of emergency care experiences among transgender and gender-nonconforming patients. Ann Emerg Med. 2018;71(2):170–82.e1. https://doi.org/10.1016/j.annemergmed.2017.05.002.
17. Moll J, Krieger P, Moreno-Walton L, Lee B, Slaven E, James T, et al. The prevalence of lesbian, gay, bisexual, and transgender health education and training in emergency medicine residency programs: what do we know? Acad Emerg Med. 2014;21(5):608–11. https://doi.org/10.1111/acem.12368.
18. Dubin SN, Nolan IT, Streed CG, Greene RE, Radix AE, Morrison SD. Transgender health care: improving medical students' and residents' training and awareness. Adv Med Educ Pract. 2018;9:377–91. https://doi.org/10.2147/AMEP.S147183.
19. Mcdowell M, Bower KM. Transgender health care for nurses: an innovative approach to diversifying nursing curricula to address health inequities. J Nurs Educ. 2016;55(8):476–9. https://doi.org/10.3928/01484834-20160715-11.
20. Jaffee KD, Shires DA, Stroumsa D. Discrimination and delayed health care among transgender women and men: implications for improving medical education and health care delivery. Med Care. 2016;54(11):1010–6. https://doi.org/10.1097/MLR.0000000000000583.
21. Lelutiu-Weinberger C, Pollard-Thomas P, Pagano W, Levitt N, Lopez EI, Golub SA, et al. Implementation and evaluation of a pilot training to improve transgender competency among medical staff in an urban clinic. Transgend Health. 2016;1(1):45–53. https://doi.org/10.1089/trgh.2015.0009.
22. Rutherford K, McIntyre J, Daley A, Ross LE. Development of expertise in mental health service provision for lesbian, gay, bisexual and transgender communities. Med Educ. 2012;46(9):903–13. https://doi.org/10.1111/j.1365-2923.2012.04272.x.

23. Obedin-Maliver J, Goldsmith E, Stewart L, White W, Tran E, Brenman S, et al. Lesbian, gay, bisexual, and transgender-related content in undergraduate medical education. JAMA. 2011;306(9):971–7. https://doi.org/10.1001/jama.2011.1255.
24. Stoddard J, Leibowitz SF, Ton H, Snowdon S. Improving medical education about gender-variant youth and transgender adolescents. Child Adolesc Psychiatr Clin N Am. 2011;20(4):779–91. https://doi.org/10.1016/j.chc.2011.07.008.
25. Ard KL, Keuroghlian AS. Training in sexual and gender minority health – expanding education to reach all clinicians. N Engl J Med. 2018;379(25):2388–91.
26. Keuroghlian AS, Ard KL, Makadon HJ. Advancing health equity for lesbian, gay, bisexual and transgender (LGBT) people through sexual health education and LGBT-affirming health care environments. Sex Health. 2017;14:119–22. https://doi.org/10.1071/SH16145.
27. Christian R, Mellies AA, Bui AG, Lee R, Kattari L, Gray C. Measuring the health of an invisible population: lessons from the Colorado Transgender Health Survey. J Gen Intern Med. 2018;33(10):1654–60. https://doi.org/10.1007/s11606-018-4450-6.
28. Rafferty J, AAP Committee on Psychosocial Aspects of Child and Family Health, AAP Committee on Adolescence, AAP Section on Lesbian, Gay, Bisexual, and Transgender Health and Wellness. Ensuring comprehensive care and support for transgender and gender diverse children and adolescents. Pediatrics. 2018;142(4):e20182162.
29. Toomey RB, Ryan C, Diaz RM, Card NA, Russell ST. Gender-nonconforming lesbian, gay, bisexual, and transgender youth: school victimization and young adult psychosocial adjustment. Dev Psychol. 2010;46(6):1580–9. https://doi.org/10.1037/a0020705.
30. Dowshen N, Lee S, Franklin J, Castillo M, Barg F. Access to medical and mental health services across the HIV care continuum among young transgender women: a qualitative study. Transgend Health. 2017;2(1):81–90. https://doi.org/10.1089/trgh.2016.0046.
31. National LGBT Health Education Center. Glossary of LGBT terms for health care teams [Internet]. Boston: National LGBT Health Education Center; 2017 [cited 2018 Dec 5]. Available from: https://www.lgbthealtheducation.org/wp-content/uploads/2018/03/Glossary-2018-English-update-1.pdf.
32. American Psychiatric Association. Diagnostic and statistical manual of mental disorders. 5th ed. Arlington: American Psychiatric Association; 2013.
33. Hidalgo MA, Ehrensaft D, Tishelman AC, Clark LF, Garofalo R, Rosenthal SM, et al. The gender affirmative model: what we know and what we aim to learn. Hum Dev. 2013;56:285–90. https://doi.org/10.1159/000355235.
34. Murchison G. Supporting & caring for transgender children [Internet]. Washington, DC: Human Rights Campaign; 2016 [cited 2018 Oct 11]. 24 p. Available from: https://assets2.hrc.org/files/documents/SupportingCaringforTransChildren.pdf.
35. Tishelman AC, Kaufman R, Edwards-Leeper L, Mandel FH, Shumer DE, Spack NP. Serving transgender youth: challenges, dilemmas and clinical examples. Prof Psychol Res Pr. 2015;46(1):37–45. https://doi.org/10.1037/a0037490.
36. James SE, Herman JL, Rankin S, Keisling M, Mottet L, Anafi M. The report of the 2015 U.S. transgender survey. Washington, DC: National Center for Transgender Equality; 2016.
37. Staats C, Capatosto K, Mamo S. State of the science: implicit bias review. Columbus: Kirwan Institute; 2017 [cited 2018 Dec 12]. 88 p. Available from: http://kirwaninstitute.osu.edu/wp-content/uploads/2017/11/2017-SOTS-final-draft-02.pdf.
38. Burke SE, et al. Do contact and empathy mitigate bias against gay and lesbian people among heterosexual medical students? A report from Medical Student CHANGE study. Acad Med. 2015;90(5):645–51. https://doi.org/10.1097/ACM.0000000000000661.
39. Dean MA, Victor E, Guidry-Grimes L. Inhospitable healthcare spaces: why diversity training on LGBTQIA issues is not enough. J Bioeth Inq. 2016;13:557–70. https://doi.org/10.1007/s11673-016-9738-9.

40. Staats C. State of the science: implicit bias review. Columbus: Kirwan Institute; 2014 [cited 2018 Dec 12]. 90 p. Available from: http://kirwaninstitute.osu.edu/wp-content/uploads/2014/03/2014-implicit-bias.pdf.
41. Turban J, Ferraiolo T, Martin A, Olezeski C. Ten things transgender and gender nonconforming youth want their doctors to know. J Am Acad Child Adolesc Psychiatry. 2017;56(4):275–7. https://doi.org/10.1016/j.jaac.2016.12.015.
42. Ferraiolo T. Artistic expressions of transgender youth: volume 1. 1st ed: Tony Ferraiolo, LLC; United States of America, 2015.
43. Goldhammer H, Malina S, Keuroghlian A. Communicating with patients who have nonbinary gender identities. Ann Fam Med. 2018;16:559–62. https://doi.org/10.1370/afm.2321.

Epidemiology of Pediatric Gender Identity

2

Mamatha Challa, Caroline Scott, and Jack L. Turban

Introduction

Transgender and gender diverse (TGD) individuals are increasingly visible in politics, popular culture, and clinical practice [1–5]; thus, providers must be prepared to meet their health care needs [6]. In parallel, there has been an exponential increase in published medical literature about this vulnerable population (Fig. 2.1).

Childhood and adolescence are vital periods of self-discovery for all youth. However, these can also be times of significant stress for TGD youth as they begin to feel a misalignment between their gender assigned at birth and gender identity. This understanding often comes with additional stress as patients encounter societal constructs that are nonaffirming of TGD identities. Due to these factors, these young people face dramatic mental health disparities.

To understand the health care needs of these youth, it is crucial to start with basic epidemiology. How many TGD people are there? How many of these individuals are youth? Where are they located? How have these demographics changed over time? What are their disparities, and how do these disparities interact?

Unfortunately, existing literature is limited in power and generalizability. Estimating the prevalence of TGD youth is particularly difficult when it comes to definitions of gender diversity, especially regarding individuals who identify outside of the gender binary [7]. Fortunately, research in this area has been growing

M. Challa
Department of Psychiatry & Behavioral Sciences, Stanford University School of Medicine, Stanford, CA, USA

C. Scott
Washington University School of Medicine, St. Louis, MO, USA

J. L. Turban (✉)
Division of Child & Adolescent Psychiatry, Massachusetts General Hospital, Boston, MA, USA
e-mail: Jack.Turban@mgh.harvard.edu

M. Forcier et al. (eds.), *Pediatric Gender Identity*,
https://doi.org/10.1007/978-3-030-38909-3_2

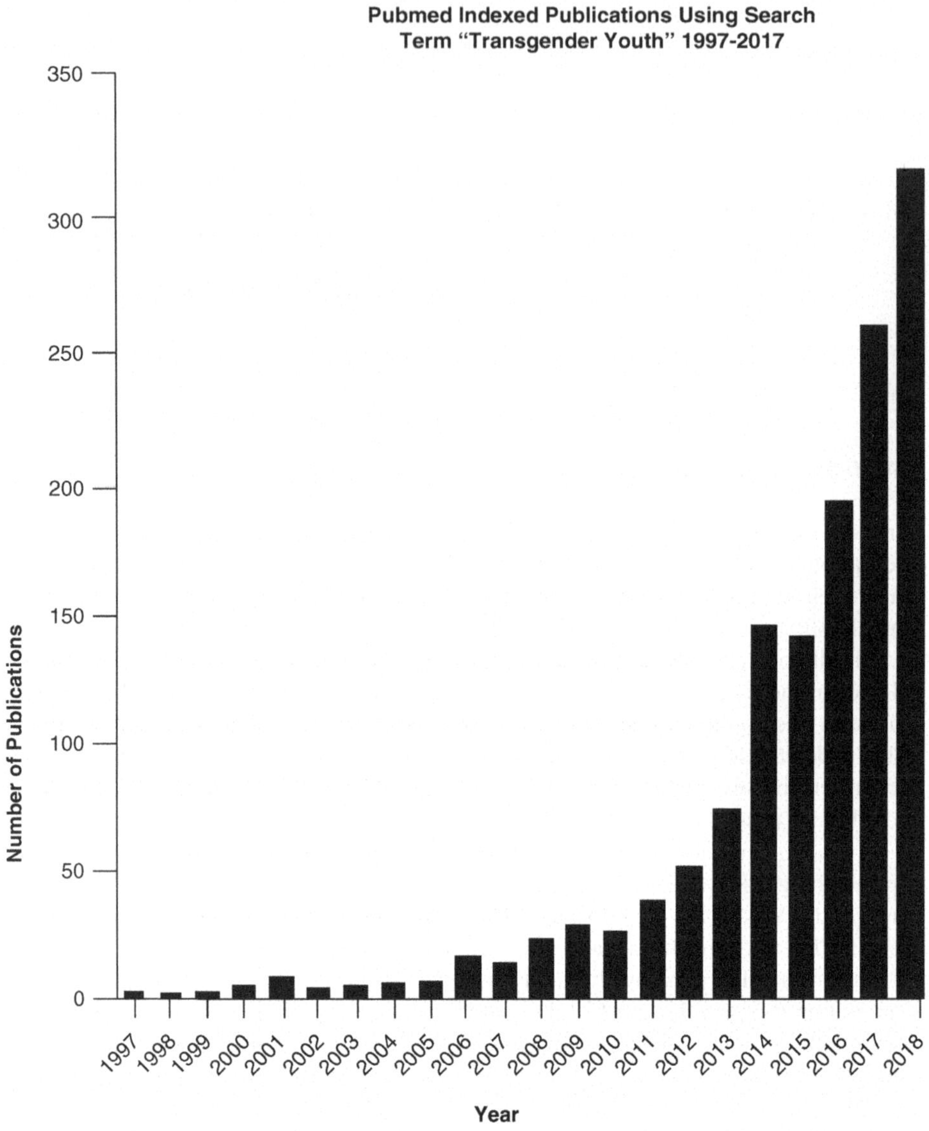

Fig. 2.1 Number of PubMed indexed manuscripts using the search term transgender youth from the year 1997 to the year 2018. There has been an exponential increase in research about this vulnerable population

steadily over the last decade, and we are beginning to have a greater understanding of the needs of TGD youth. In this chapter, we examine the existing literature with the hope of providing a general epidemiologic foundation for providers serving this vulnerable population.

Prevalence

According to the UCLA Williams Institute report in 2017, "Age of Individuals Who Identify as Transgender in the United States," the answer to their posed question is not so simple [8]. Large federal population-based surveys rarely ask questions regarding gender identity; thus, we rely on smaller, state-based surveys for estimation. For many years, our best estimate came from the 2011 Williams Institute report that estimated that there were 700,000 transgender adults in the United States; however, this study only included surveys from California and Massachusetts. More state-level surveys have since emerged, and the newer Williams Institute's 2017 report uses the 2014 CDC's Behavioral Risk Factor Surveillance System (BRFSS) survey of adults to estimate that 0.6% of US adults identify as transgender, or approximately 1.4 million individuals (nearly double the previous estimate). Notably, there appears to be a skew toward younger adults; approximately 0.7% of 13–24-year-olds identify as transgender, as compared to 0.58% of 25–64-year-olds and 0.50% of people 65 and older [8]. Notably, the Williams Institute report estimates the percentage of youth based on estimates in the adult population.

It is unlikely that the prevalence of transgender identification doubled over 5 years. One potential explanation, rather, is that increased societal discourse around gender has provided a larger number of people with the language necessary to describe their identity. As the United States becomes more accepting of TGD people, we may also be seeing more people willing to identify openly instead of hiding their identities. Regardless, the reality is that we are just now starting to ask the right questions to measure the basic demographics of this population, and it will take time to have enough data to assess for true changes in population size.

Data on youth are much more limited. Though the BRFSS only surveys adults, the Williams Institute 2017 report extrapolated from these data to estimate that roughly 150,000 adolescents in the United States identity as transgender. Other surveys of middle-school- and high-school-aged youth have yielded estimates of TGD identity ranging from 1.3% to 3.2% [9]. The primary sources for these estimates have been local studies. The Boston Youth Survey (BYS) was a probability survey that used a single-item question to measure transgender identities within the city school district. The study found that approximately 1.7% of the 908 youth surveyed (13–19 years old) identified as TGD [10]. Similarly, in 2011, the San Francisco United School District included a question about gender identity on their middle and high school Youth Risk Behavior Surveillance System (YRBSS) instruments, and within 36 schools' reports, found that 1.3% of middle school and 1.6% of high school students identified as transgender [11, 40]. Data from the 2016 Minnesota Student Survey (n = 80,929) found that 2.7% of high school students identified as TGD [88]. On a national level, unpublished data presented by Greytak in 2013 used a nationally representative online survey of adolescents distributed over 2 years to find that 1.4% of the year 1 and 3.2% of the year 2 respondents identified as TGD [12]. A study of 8166 high school students in New Zealand found that 1.2% of participants identified as transgender and 2.5% reported being not sure about their gender [87].

Rhode Island's 2017 Youth Risk Behavior Survey similarly asked students if they identify as transgender; however, it also asked them to rate their gender expression, with response options ranging from "very feminine" to "very masculine" [91]. Whereas only 2.3% of students identified as transgender, 19% were found to be gender expansive – that is, they identified as either androgynous ("equally feminine and masculine"), masculine if assigned female at birth, or feminine if assigned male at birth [92]. As language around gender expansive identities evolves, the methods used to study individuals who identify as such must evolve, as well.

The CDC recently released a report based on population-based survey data of high school students from 10 states that estimated that 1.8% of high school students identify as transgender [93].

Geographic Trends

According to the 2017 Williams Institute report, the largest gross populations of transgender individuals are estimated to be in California (22,200), Texas (13,800), and New York (9750), mirroring relative population sizes of US states [8]. The smallest gross populations of trans people are estimated to be equally small in North Dakota, Vermont, and Wyoming (200). If you examine the percentages of the population that identifies as transgender, the results are not consistent with perspectives that suggest TGD identities are tied to a progressive political environment; the highest relative percentages of transgender people are estimated to be in West Virginia (1.04%), Hawaii (1.01%), and New Mexico (0.88%). The smallest percentages are estimated to be in Montana (0.49%), Connecticut, and Iowa (both 0.39%) [8]. These findings refute claims that TGD youth identities are somehow a product of any particular local political environment. These data also suggest that our current approach to pediatric gender clinics (which tend to be in largely populated cities) may not adequately provide access to gender-comprehensive care for TGD youth in more rural and sparsely populated states [13].

Birth-Assigned Gender Ratios Across Age Groups

Ratios of gender assigned at birth for TGD individuals are typically reported based on the profiles of patients referred to gender clinics. These ratios differ by developmental stage. Many of these estimates are from the early 1980s to 2000s, and ratios may change over time.

Children

Birth-assigned female children are more likely than birth-assigned male children to exhibit cross-gender behaviors in the general population [14, 15]. However, birth-assigned boys are more frequently referred to gender clinics than birth-assigned girls for cross-gender behavior, with ratios of birth-assigned boys to girls ranging from 2:1 to 5.75:1 [16, 17].

Cross-gender behavior in birth-assigned boys is tolerated significantly less by peers, teachers, and parents than such behavior in birth-assigned girls [17–21]. This disparate sensitivity to cross-gender behavior may result in higher rates of clinical referrals for birth-assigned boys, whereas these behaviors in birth-assigned girls may not raise such concern. Two studies support this theory, as they found that birth-assigned girls were referred significantly later than birth-assigned boys to gender clinics, although they also demonstrated a higher average level of cross-gender behavior [17, 22]. In both studies, however, there were no significant differences between the genders assigned at birth for rates of children who met the prior DSM criteria for gender identity disorder (GID).

There are also cultural factors at play. Internationally, gender diverse behavior appears consistently more tolerated for birth-assigned girls than boys, as demonstrated in the studies of the United States, India, China, and Belgium [23]. It has been noted that the skewed birth-assigned gender ratio for TGD children is more dramatic in North America compared to The Netherlands, suggesting a cultural component in which North American parents may be more alarmed by gender diverse behavior and thus more likely to bring youth to a gender clinic [24–26]. It is important to note that many of these children referred to gender clinics may have gender diverse expressions but continue to identify with their gender assigned at birth.

Adolescents

For gender clinic-referred adolescents, the birth-assigned gender ratio is closer to 1:1 [16]; two studies have reported ratios of birth-assigned males to females of 1.32:1 and 1.20:1, respectively [27, 28]. More recent studies have found a slight inversion of this ratio to favor birth-assigned females [25, 29, 30].

Whether this is a result of actual changes in transgender identity prevalence versus other factors is unknown, though several theories have been proposed. For example, for many TGD youth, concerns about physical sex characteristics tend to intensify during adolescence and puberty [31, 32]. While individuals of both birth-assigned genders are more likely to seek clinical services around puberty, we may see higher rates of birth-assigned girls newly presenting in adolescence who did not present earlier because gender diverse behavior is more socially acceptable among birth-assigned females than birth-assigned males.

As with childhood, cross-gender behavior in adolescence has also been found to elicit significantly harsher reactions in birth-assigned males than birth-assigned females, especially from peers [33]. Indeed, adolescent birth-assigned males with gender dysphoria (GD) have reported significantly more "bullying" than adolescent birth-assigned females with GD [25]. Given these reports, it has been argued that it may be easier for birth-assigned females to "come out" in adolescence as transgender and request gender specialist treatment, than adolescent birth-assigned males who face increased social sanctions against feminine behavior [25].

Adults

As with children, birth-assigned males are more heavily represented in studies of adults diagnosed with GD, with ratios that range from 1:1 to 6.1:1 [16, 34–39]. The reason for this remains unknown; some propose that the narrower definitions of masculinity compared to femininity provide birth-assigned females with greater flexibility to express cross-gender behavior without seeking clinical interventions [41–43]. This has also been attributed to other factors including the increased availability of gender affirmation surgery – specifically genital reconstruction – for birth-assigned males, and thus increased rates of birth-assigned males seeking interventions from gender clinics [42].

However, in Japan and Poland, the ratio of adults seeking clinical assistance from gender specialists appears to favor birth-assigned females, with ratios of 2.2:1 and 5.5:1, respectively [16, 44, 45]. Additionally, birth-assigned gender ratios have shifted in different ways in different locations. In Sweden, the ratio shifted from 1:1 in the 1960s to 2:1 (favoring birth-assigned males) in the 1990s [38]. In Germany, gender clinic referral rates between 1970 and 1994 favored birth-assigned males at a ratio of 2:1, but from 1996 to 2000, the rate dropped to 1.2:1 [37]. These disparate results, and changes over time and across location, further support likely societal rather than intrinsic factors influencing birth-assigned gender ratios of adults seeking gender-affirming medical care, though more research is needed.

Natural History of Cross-Gender Identification

One of the most common questions that parents ask providers regarding their TGD children is whether or not childhood gender diverse identities "persist" into adulthood. The literature remains a subject of academic debate.

There have been several attempts to measure the proportion of cross-gender-identifying prepubertal children who continue to identify this way over time. However, nearly all studies of this type have been methodologically flawed. For example, several included cases that would likely not meet the criteria for GD as it is defined today; many of the children may not have identified as transgender [46, 47]. Rather, many of these children may have expressed cross-gender behavior (i.e., boys with traditionally feminine behavior and "tomboys") but continued to identify with their gender assigned at birth.

Additionally, children who identify as transgender may report later that they are not in order to avoid stigma, not necessarily because of a change in gender identity. This theory is supported when evaluating studies of identity persistence temporally. Such studies conducted before the year 2000 estimated persistence rates between 2% and 9% [48, 49]. However, those conducted after 2000 – in a more accepting environment for TGD individuals – estimate rates of persistence ranging from 12% to 39% [47, 50–53].

Whereas some TGD prepubertal youth will persist in their gender identity into adolescence, it appears that some will not. The current literature does not offer ways to definitively distinguish between these two groups. One study examined predictors of cross-gender identification persistence from childhood into adolescence using multivariate analysis. The following characteristics were associated with persistence: female gender assigned at birth, older age at gender clinic assessment, lower socioeconomic status, and early social transition. This study also replicated previous studies linking persistence with higher intensity of childhood GD [50–53], as well as being assigned female at birth [53].

Due to research limitations regarding both cohort size and design, the natural history of the persistence of cross-gender identification from childhood into adolescence cannot be definitively characterized. However, observations of clinicians treating TGD children reveal that there exists a population of young children who are able to communicate TGD identities that remain stable into and beyond adolescence [54]. These developmental trajectories are currently being investigated with improved methodology through the TransYouth project [55–57].

Research is also limited regarding persistence from adolescence into adulthood. One study of patients treated at a Netherlands gender clinic from 1972 to 2015 found that 1.9% of adolescents who began pubertal suppression eventually ceased suppression and did not pursue cross-sex hormonal replacement [58]. A study of 55 adolescents who received cross-sex hormonal interventions from the same clinic found that 100% of them still identified as transgender in young adulthood [59]. These data align with published clinical observations that suggest that gender identity tends to be stable after puberty for most TGD people [28]. Unfortunately, there is currently no research on rates of adolescent cessation of estrogen or testosterone, although one case study has been published about this scenario [60].

Several studies have linked childhood gender variance with "same-sex" sexual orientation in adulthood [53, 61]. One study found that gender variant individuals were 8.4–15.8 times more likely to have some type of sexual orientation toward their gender assigned at birth in adulthood, depending on the type of orientation (attraction, fantasy, behavior, and identity) [61].

The majority of adolescents and adults with symptoms of GD report exhibiting extensive cross-gender behavior in childhood [7, 41, 62–64]. These findings are largely based on self-report, which may be considered unreliable for determining the specific age of onset of their childhood cross-gender behavior [65]. However, for gender clinic-referred children, the onset of such behavior is often between the ages of 2 and 4 years, which aligns with the time period when many children begin to express gendered interests and behaviors [16].

When discussing this literature, we must recognize that these studies have been quite limited in power and generalizability and should not be misused to create barriers for TGD youth seeking gender-affirming care. The most relevant conclusions from these studies are that insistent cross-gender identification in adolescence most often correlates with persistent TGD identities in adulthood, and that cross-gender identification in prepubescent youth may not always persist into adulthood. However, the reality is that TGD youth have a wide variety of trajectories in their gender development.

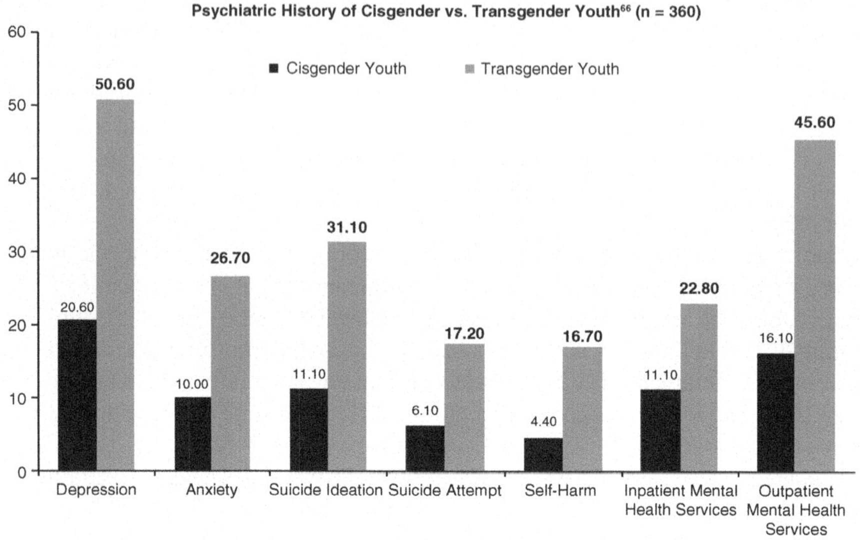

Fig. 2.2 Graphical representation of data published by Reisner et al. showing between-group differences of mental health disparities, comparing transgender youth with cisgender controls [66]

Mental Health and Suicidality

TGD youth are at an increased risk for a variety of mental health concerns, which will be explored in detail in Chap. 9. One illustrative example is a study comparing the mental health of transgender youth in Boston with cisgender controls (Fig. 2.2). This high risk of mental health concerns is often conceptualized as being secondary to the minority stress model, which will be further discussed in Chap. 5.

Transgender youth report an alarming rate of suicidality, with nearly 50% of transgender youth reporting a history of suicidal ideation and 25% reporting a history of suicide attempts [67]. Research stratifying these data by gender identity has noted that 50.8% of adolescent transgender males have attempted suicide, followed by 41.8% of nonbinary teenagers and 29.9% of transgender female teens [68]. These rates escalate by adulthood, with 41% of transgender adults reporting suicide attempts, compared to 4.6% of the general population [69]. Figure 2.3 highlights the estimated elevated risk of suicide attempts among transgender people across the lifespan.

Importantly, recent cross-sectional research demonstrated that prepubescent children who are supported and affirmed in their gender identities by being allowed to "socially transition" – that is, to live and express themselves as their identified gender without necessarily undergoing medical interventions (which are, by clinical guidelines, not provided until after puberty begins) – reported depression and self-worth comparable to siblings and nontransgender control groups [55, 56]. They reported marginally higher anxiety; however, their mean symptoms were not in the

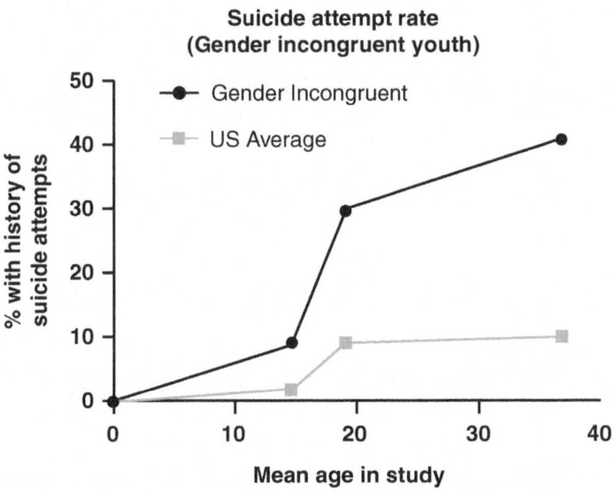

Fig. 2.3 Suicide attempt rates among gender incongruent youth. Gender incongruent youth suffer dramatically higher suicide attempt rates compared with national averages. Examining populations of gender incongruent youth seeking endocrine care, investigators have found a 9.3% suicide attempt rate by a mean age of 14.8 [30], a 30% suicide attempt rate by a mean age of 19.2 [89], and a 41% suicide attempt rate among transgender adults with a mean age of 37.0 [74]. Estimates of US average suicide attempts by age were derived from the American Foundation for Suicide Prevention, as described in previous reports [90]

preclinical or clinical ranges [55, 56]. Of note, all participants held binary identities, and both studies were cross-sectional and do not necessarily provide insight into the children's future mental health. However, these notably suggest that TGD youth who have early affirmation of their identity may be able to avoid the highly increased risk for mental health problems that typically affect TGD adolescents and adults.

Health and Social Vulnerabilities

TGD youth face enormous social vulnerabilities compared to their cisgender peers, particularly in areas related to socioeconomic status, physical and sexual safety, and health. These risk factors often persist into adulthood. Providers should be aware of the many risks that their young TGD patients may face so that they may provide early interventions to improve outcomes and quality of life.

Homelessness

TGD youth are overrepresented in the homeless youth population, with approximately 4% of all homeless youth identifying as transgender or nonbinary [71, 72]. 67.1% of transgender homeless youth report that their primary reason for homelessness was being forced out or having to run away from home due to their identity [72]. TGD homeless youth are noted to have longer durations of homelessness compared to their non-LGBTQ+ homeless counterparts [73]. This TGD youth data corroborates that of adults, as 19% of transgender people reporting being homeless at some point in their life, with 55% reporting harassment when they sought housing and 29% being outright rejected [74].

Safety

Transgender youth experience high rates of physical violence, verbal harassment, and economic discrimination, both at home and at school [41]. Close to three-quarters (73.6%) of transgender youth report ever experiencing verbal harassment, 32.5% report being physically harassed, and 16.2% report being physically assaulted [75]. In a study exploring childhood gender atypicality and trauma in LGBTQ+ youth, 9% reported a history of sexual victimization [76]. These safety concerns can be particularly prominent in the school setting.

In the 2015 GLSEN National School Climate Survey, 75.1% of transgender students reported feeling unsafe at school because of their gender, compared to 61.6% of nonbinary students, 32.2% of cisgender males, and 22.5% of cisgender females. 64.5% of transgender youth reported verbal harassment at school due to their gender expression, 24.9% experienced physical harassment at school, and 12% reported physical assault [75]. Notably, transgender youth of color tend to have higher rates of victimization than their white counterparts, including at school [75]. Hostile school climate can dissuade TGD students from future educational pursuits, which may further socioeconomic disparities.

Health Disparities

There are a number of unique health care disparities that TGD youth experience in the areas of health care access, substance use disorders, sexually transmitted infections, and related sequelae. These disparities are undoubtedly influenced and compounded by other vulnerabilities common in this demographic, including low socioeconomic status, homelessness, and high rates of physical and sexual abuse.

Health Care Access

TGD youth consistently report inadequate access to health care, particularly mental health care. Barriers to access include fear of discrimination and stigma from providers, lack of transgender health-educated providers, increased homelessness, and lack of financial supports [77]. Research exploring utilization of histrelin acetate ("puberty blocking") implants has also suggested racial disparities limiting minority youth access to gender affirmative care [78].

Studies such as the Canadian Trans Youth Health Survey have corroborated these results; a third of transgender respondents note forgoing needed physical health care in the last year, commonly due to fear of how a provider may react to their gender identity [79]. Participants who were out as transgender to their providers reported better physical and mental health, highlighting the importance of creating a safe and gender-affirming clinical environment [79].

Sexually Transmitted Infections

Approximately 25% of transgender individuals report being fired from a job due to their gender identity, and transgender people experience double the rate of unemployment of the general population. Subsequently, about 16% of transgender people report feeling compelled to work in an underground economy for income, with 11% of transgender individuals engaging in sex work [74]. These rates are even higher for transfeminine individuals as well as TGD people of color. Sex work has drastically increased the risk for sexually transmitted infections in this population, particularly HIV. When it comes to adults, approximately 1.2% of nationally interviewed transgender non-sex workers report being HIV positive, compared to 15.3% who engaged in sex work, and 40.6% of black and black multiracial respondents who have engaged in sex work [80]. In terms of youth, research in the area of STIs and HIV has largely been limited to transfeminine youth. One study of transgender female youth of color (age 16–25) found increased risk factors for HIV, including sex in exchange for money, drugs, or shelter, forced sexual intercourse, and unprotected oral or anal sex. Among youth surveyed, 22% were HIV positive, and 12% were diagnosed with an STI within the last year [70]. It is imperative that providers recognize these important vulnerabilities when engaging TGD youth in their health care needs.

Race and Cultural Identity

Research on the experiences of TGD youth of color remains limited, but it is clear that they experience unique societal and personal challenges due to the intersection of their gender and cultural identity; these will be further explored in Chap. 18 [81]. These experiences cannot be understood by simply adding the effects of transphobia and racism; the intersections of these and other identities create oppression that is both unique and further amplified [82], and can result in many increased vulnerabilities [83].

The intersectionality between TGD identities and cultural factors may place TGD youth of color at higher risk for receiving greater discrimination and harassment from teachers and peers at school [84]. In a national study of transgender youth, the majority of respondents felt unsafe at school, but most respondents of color also experienced hearing school staff use racist language [85]. Feeling unsafe at school can result in significant academic difficulties with increased school absences and dropout rates. This can further increase risk for being funneled into the school-to-prison pipeline, particularly for TGD youth who are African-American and Latin-American [84]. TGD youth of color may also face increased discrimination in these systems via police and community harassment [86].

In addition, TGD youth of color may be at a particularly elevated risk for parental harassment and familial rejection, which is in line with an overrepresentation of TGD youth of color among homeless youth [70, 84]. Homelessness further inhibits TGD youth of color from maintaining access to education, employment, community, and health care, which increases vulnerability for exploitation and abuse [70, 84].

Conclusion

The purpose of this chapter was to provide health care providers with a foundation regarding the epidemiology of transgender youth. While the literature appears limited at the surface, there are a number of clear trends.

We know that approximately 1 in 100 young people in the United States identify as TGD, that the population of openly identifying TGD youth is growing in size and visibility, that TGD youth can be found across the entire United States, and undoubtedly, that societal marginalization (particularly for TGD youth of color) places this demographic at high risk for medical and mental health conditions.

The natural history of TGD identities remains an area of active research, and existing data is limited. Though it is unclear how many prepubescent TGD youth will continue to identify as such in adulthood, it appears that the majority of TGD youth who identify this way after puberty will maintain TGD identities in adulthood.

Future directions for epidemiological research with this demographic include increasing large-scale, national surveys of TGD youth, examining the natural history of TGD identities through methodologically rigorous longitudinal studies, and exploring the potential benefits of preventative health care for this vulnerable population.

References

1. Turban J. Hannah is a girl. Doctors finally treat her like one. New York Times [Internet]. 2017 Apr 8 [cited 2018 Oct 7]. Available from: https://www.nytimes.com/2017/04/08/opinion/sunday/hannah-is-a-girl-doctors-finally-treat-her-like-one.html.
2. Donnelly L. Rise in child transgender referrals. The Telegraph (London Ed.) [Internet]. 2015 Apr 7 [cited 2018 Oct 7]. Available from: https://www.telegraph.co.uk/news/health/news/11519603/Rise-in-child-transgender-referrals.html.
3. Grinberg E. Why transgender teen Jazz Jennings is everywhere. CNN [Internet]. 2015 Mar 19 [cited 2018 Oct 7]. Available from: https://www.cnn.com/2015/03/16/living/feat-transgender-teen-jazz-jennings/index.html.
4. Moi CS. Nikki, 13 ans, née Niko [Me, Nikki, 13 years old, born Niko]. Le Monde. 2014 Dec 10 [cited 2018 Oct 7]. Available from: https://www.lemonde.fr/m-actu/article/2014/12/10/moi-nikki-13-ans-nee-niko_4534297_4497186.html.
5. Steensma TD, Cohen-Kettenis PT. Gender transitioning before puberty? Arch Sex Behav. 2011;40(4):649–50.
6. Olson-Kennedy J. Mental health disparities among transgender youth: rethinking the role of professionals. JAMA Pediatr. 2016;170(5):423–4.
7. Olson J, Forbes C, Belzer M. Management of the transgender adolescent. Arch Pediatr Adolesc Med. 2011;165(2):171–6.
8. Herman JL, Flores AR, Brown TN, Wilson BD, Conron KJ. Age of individuals who identify as transgender in the United States [Internet]. Los Angeles: The Williams Institute; 2017 Jan

[cited 2018 Oct 7]. 13 p. Available from: https://williamsinstitute.law.ucla.edu/wp-content/uploads/TransAgeReport.pdf.
9. Wilson BDM, Kastanis AA. Sexual and gender minority disproportionality and disparities in child welfare: a population-based study. Child Youth Serv Rev. 2015;58:11–7.
10. Almeida J, Johnson RM, Corliss HL, Molnar BE, Azrael D. Emotional distress among LGBT youth: the influence of perceived discrimination based on sexual orientation. J Youth Adolesc. 2009;38(7):1001–14.
11. San Francisco Unified School District (SFUSD). Keeping our LGBTQ youth safe and in school. San Francisco: Student, Family, and Community Support Department of SFUSD; 2012 [cited 2018 Oct 7]. Available from: https://www.healthiersf.org/LGBTQ/GetTheFacts/docs/LGBTQ_websiteHealthSurvey1011.pdf.
12. Greytak E. How do you ask the question? Assessing sex and gender in a national sample of adolescents. Paper presented at: Evaluation practice in the early 21st century. 27th Annual Conference of the American Evaluation Association; 2013 Oct 16–19; Washington, D.C.
13. Horvath KJK, Iantaffi A, Swinburne-Romine R, Bockting W. A comparison of mental health, substance use, and sexual risk behaviors between rural and non-rural transgender persons. J Homosex. 2014;61(8):1117–30.
14. Cole HJ, Zucker KJ, Bradley SJ. Patterns of gender-role behaviour in children attending traditional and non-traditional day-care centers. Can J Psychiatr. 1982;27(5):410–4.
15. Sandberg DE, Meyer-Bahlburg HF, Ehrhardt AA, Yager TJ. The prevalence of gender-atypical behavior in elementary school children. J Am Acad Child Adolesc Psychiatry. 1993;32(2):306–14.
16. American Psychiatric Association. Diagnostic and statistical manual of mental disorders. 5th ed. Arlington: American Psychiatric Association; 2013.
17. Cohen-Kettenis PT, Owen A, Kaijser VG, Bradley SJ, Zucker KJ. Demographic characteristics, social competence, and behavior problems in children with gender identity disorder: a cross-national, cross-clinic comparative analysis. J Abnorm Child Psychol. 2003;31(1):41–53.
18. Wallien MS, Veenstra R, Kreukels BP, Cohen-Kettenis PT. Peer group status of gender dysphoric children: a sociometric study. Arch Sex Behav. 2010;39(2):553–60.
19. Zucker KJ, Wilson-Smith DN, Kurita JA, Stern A. Children's appraisals of sex-typed behavior in their peers. Sex Roles. 1995;33(11–12):703–25.
20. Fagot BI. Beyond the reinforcement principle: another step toward understanding sex role development. Dev Psychol. 1985;21(6):1097–104.
21. Sandnabba NK, Ahlberg C. Parents' attitudes and expectations about children's cross-gender behavior. Sex Roles. 1999;40(3–4):249–63.
22. Zucker KJ, Bradley SJ, Sanikhani M. Sex differences in referral rates of children with gender identity disorder: some hypotheses. J Abnorm Child Psychol. 1997;25(3):217–27.
23. Yu C, Zuo X, Blum RW, Tolman DL, Kågesten A, Mmari K, De Meyer S, Michielsen K, Basu S, Acharya R, Lian Q, Lou C. Marching to a different drummer: a cross-cultural comparison of young adolescents who challenge gender norms. J Adolesc Health. 2017;61(4):S48–54.
24. Turban JL, DeVries ALC, Zucker K. Gender incongruence & gender dysphoria. In: Martin A, Bloch MH, Volkmar FR, editors. Lewis's child and adolescent psychiatry: a comprehensive textbook. 5th ed. Philadelphia: Wolters Kluwer; 2018.
25. Aitken M, Steensma TD, Blanchard R, Vander Laan DP, Wood H, Fuentes A, Spegg C, Wasserman L, Ames M, Fitzsimmons CL, Leef JH, Lishak V, Reim E, Takagi A, Vinik J, Wreford J, Cohen-Kettenis PT, de Vries AL, Kreukels BP, Zucker KJ. Evidence for an altered sex ratio in clinic-referred adolescents with gender dysphoria. J Sex Med. 2015;12(3):756–63.
26. Wood H, Sasaki S, Bradley SJ, Singh D, Fantus S, Owen-Anderson A, Di Giacomo A, Bain J, Zucker KJ. Patterns of referral to a gender identity service for children and adolescents (1976–2011): age, sex ratio, and sexual orientation. J Sex Marital Ther. 2013;39(1):1–6.
27. Zucker KJ, Owen A, Bradley SJ, Ameeriar L. Gender-dysphoric children and adolescents: a comparative analysis of demographic characteristics and behavioral problems. Clin Child Psychol Psychiatry. 2002;7(3):398–411.

28. Cohen-Kettenis PT, Pfäfflin F. Transgenderism and intersexuality in childhood and adolescence: making choices. Thousand Oaks: Sage; 2003.
29. Becker I, Gjerji-Lama V, Romer G, Möller B. Merkmale von Kindern und Jugendlichen mit Geschlechtsdysphorie in der Hamburger Spezialsprechstunde [Characteristics of children and adolescents with gender dysphoria referred to the Hamburg Gender Identity Clinic]. Prax Kinderpsychol Kinderpsychiatr. 2014;63(6):486–509. German.
30. Spack NP, Edwards-Leeper L, Feldman HA, Leibowitz S, Mandel F, Diamond DA, Vance SR. Children and adolescents with gender identity disorder referred to a pediatric medical center. Pediatrics. 2012;129(3):418–25.
31. Streitmatter JL. Cross-sectional investigation of adolescent perceptions of gender roles. J Adolesc. 1985;8(2):183–93.
32. Cohen-Kettenis PT, Everaerd W. Gender role problems in adolescence. Adv Adolesc Ment Health. 1986;1(Pt. B):1–28.
33. Young R, Sweeting H. Adolescent bullying, relationships, psychological well-being, and gender-atypical behavior: a gender diagnosticity approach. Sex Roles. 2004;50(7–8):525–37.
34. Zucker KJ, Lawrence AA. Epidemiology of gender identity disorder: recommendations for the Standards of Care of the World Professional Association for Transgender Health. Int J Transgend. 2009;11(1):8–18.
35. Becerra-Fernandez A, Rodriguez-Molina JM, Asenjo-Araque N, Lucio-Perez MJ, Cuchi-Alfaro M, Garcia-Camba E, Perez-Lopez G, Penacho-Roman M, Berrocal-Sertucha MC, Ly-Pen D, Aguilar-Vilas MV. Prevalence, incidence, and sex ratio of transsexualism in the autonomous region of Madrid (Spain) according to healthcare demand. Arch Sex Behav. 2017;46(5):1307–12.
36. Bakker A, van Kesteren PJ, Gooren LJ, Bezemer PD. The prevalence of transsexualism in The Netherlands. Acta Psychiatr Scand. 1993;87(4):237–8.
37. Garrels L, Kockott G, Michael N, Preuss W, Renter K, Schmidt G, Sigusch V, Windgassen K. Sex ratio of transsexuals in Germany: the development over three decades. Acta Psychiatr Scand. 2000;102(6):445–8.
38. Olsson SE, Moller AR. On the incidence and sex ratio of transsexualism in Sweden, 1972–2002. Arch Sex Behav. 2003;32(4):381–6.
39. Wilson P, Sharp C, Carr S. The prevalence of gender dysphoria in Scotland: a primary care study. Br J Gen Pract. 1999;49(449):991–2.
40. Shields JP, Cohen R, Glassman JR, Whitaker K, Franks H, Bertolini I. Estimating population size and demographic characteristics of lesbian, gay, bisexual, and transgender youth in middle school. J Adolesc Health. 2013;52(2):248–50.
41. American Psychological Association. Task force on gender identity and gender variance. Report of the APA task force on gender identity and gender variance [Internet]. Washington, DC: American Psychological Association; 2009 [cited 2018 Aug 5]. Available from: http://www.apa.org/pi/lgbt/resources/policy/gender-identity-report.pdf.
42. De Cuypere G, Van Hemelrijck M, Michel A, Carael B, Heylens G, Rubens R, Hoebeke P, Monstrey S. Prevalence and demography of transsexualism in Belgium. Eur Psychiatry. 2007;22(3):137–41.
43. Hiestand KR, Levitt HM. Butch identity development: the formation of an authentic gender. Fem Psychol. 2005;15(1):61–85.
44. Baba T, Endo T, Ikeda K, Shimizu A, Honnma H, Ikeda H, Masumori N, Ohmura T, Kiya T, Fujimoto T, Koizumi M, Saito T. Distinctive features of female-to-male transsexualism and prevalence of gender identity disorder in Japan. J Sex Med. 2011;8(6):1686–93.
45. Godlewski J. Transsexualism and anatomic sex ratio reversal in Poland. Arch Sex Behav. 1988;17(6):547–8.
46. Olson KR. Prepubescent transgender children: what we do and do not know. J Am Acad Child Adolesc Psychiatry. 2016;55(3):155–6.e3.
47. Ristori J, Steensma TD. Gender dysphoria in childhood. Int Rev Psychiatry. 2016;28(1):13–20.
48. Green R. The "sissy boy syndrome" and the development of homosexuality. New Haven: Yale University Press; 1987.

49. Zuger B. Early effeminate behavior in boys: outcome and significance for homosexuality. J Nerv Ment Dis. 1984;172(2):90–7.
50. Steensma TD, McGuire JK, Kreukels BP, Beekman AJ, Cohen-Kettenis PT. Factors associated with desistence and persistence of childhood gender dysphoria: a quantitative follow-up study. J Am Acad Child Adolesc Psychiatry. 2013;52(6):582–90.
51. Singh D. A follow-up study of boys with gender dysphoria. Toronto: University of Toronto; 2012.
52. Drummond KD, Bradley SJ, Peterson-Badali M, Zucker KJ. A follow-up study of girls with gender identity disorder. Dev Psychol. 2008;44(1):34–45.
53. Wallien MS, Cohen-Kettenis PT. Psychosexual outcome of gender-dysphoric children. J Am Acad Child Adolesc Psychiatry. 2008;47(12):1413–23.
54. Ehrensaft D. The gender creative child: pathways for nurturing and supporting children who live outside gender boxes. New York: The Experiment; 2016.
55. Durwood L, McLaughlin KA, Olson KR. Mental health and self-worth in socially transitioned transgender youth. J Am Acad Child Adolesc Psychiatry. 2017;56(2):116–123.e2.
56. Olson KR, Durwood L, DeMeules M, McLaughlin KA. Mental health of transgender children who are supported in their identities. Pediatrics. 2016;137(3):e20153223.
57. Olson KR, Key AC, Eaton NR. Gender cognition in transgender children. Psychol Sci. 2015;26(4):467–74.
58. Wiepjes CM, Nota NM, de Blok CJM, Klaver M, de Vries ALC, Wensing-Kruger SA, de Jongh RT, Bouman MB, Steensma TD, Cohen-Kettenis P, Gooren LJG, Kreukels BPC, den Heijer M. The Amsterdam cohort of gender dysphoria study (1972–2015): trends in prevalence, treatment, and regrets. J Sex Med. 2018;15(4):582–90.
59. de Vries AL, McGuire JK, Steensma TD, Wagenaar EC, Doreleijers TA, Cohen-Kettenis PT. Young adult psychological outcome after puberty suppression and gender reassignment. Pediatrics. 2014;134(4):696–704.
60. Turban JL, Carswell J, Keuroghlian AS. Understanding pediatric patients who discontinue gender-affirming hormonal interventions. JAMA Pediatr. 2018;172(10):903–4.
61. Steensma TD, van der Ende J, Verhulst FC, Cohen-Kettenis PT. Gender variance in childhood and sexual orientation in adulthood: a prospective study. J Sex Med. 2013;10(11):2723–33.
62. de Vries AL, Cohen-Kettenis PT. Clinical management of gender dysphoria in children and adolescents: the Dutch approach. J Homosex. 2012;59(3):301–20.
63. Smith YL, Van Goozen SH, Kuiper AJ, Cohen-Kettenis PT. Sex reassignment: outcomes and predictors of treatment for adolescent and adult transsexuals. Psychol Med. 2005;35(1):89–99.
64. Doorn CD, Portinga J, Verschoor AM. Cross-gender identity in transvestites and male transsexuals. Arch Sex Behav. 1994;23(2):185–201.
65. Lawrence AA. Sexual orientation versus age of onset as bases for typologies (subtypes) for gender identity disorder in adolescents and adults. Arch Sex Behav. 2010;39(2):514–45.
66. Reisner SL, Vetters R, Leclerc M, Zaslow S, Wolfrum S, Shumer D, Mimiaga MJ. Mental health of transgender youth in care at an adolescent urban community health center: a matched retrospective cohort study. J Adolesc Health. 2015;56(3):274–9.
67. Grossman AH, D'augelli AR. Transgender youth and life-threatening behaviors. Suicide Life Threat Behav. 2007;37(5):527–37.
68. Toomey RB, Syvertsen AK, Shramko M. Transgender adolescent suicide behavior. Pediatrics. 2018;142(4):e20174218.
69. Haas AP, Rodgers PL, Herman JL. Suicide attempts among transgender and gender nonconforming adults [Internet]. Los Angeles: The Williams Institute; 2014 Jan [cited 2018 Oct 7]. 18 p. Available from: https://williamsinstitute.law.ucla.edu/wp-content/uploads/AFSP-Williams-Suicide-Report-Final.pdf.
70. Garofalo R, Deleon J, Osmer E, Doll M, Harper GW. Overlooked, misunderstood and at-risk: exploring the lives and HIV risk of ethnic minority male-to-female transgender youth. J Adolesc Health. 2006;38(3):230–6.
71. Morton MH, Dworsky A, Samuels GM. Missed opportunities: youth homeless in America, national estimates. Chicago: Chapin Hall at the University of Chicago; 2017.

72. Choi SK, Wilson BDM, Shelton J, Gates G. Serving our youth 2015: the needs and experiences of lesbian, gay, bisexual, transgender, and questioning youth experiencing homelessness [Internet]. Los Angeles: The Williams Institute; 2015 Jun [cited 2018 Oct 7]. 22 p. Available from: https://williamsinstitute.law.ucla.edu/wp-content/uploads/Serving-Our-Youth-June-2015.pdf.
73. Morton MH, Dworsky A, Matjasko JL, Curry SR, Schlueter D, Chavez R, Farrell AF. Prevalence and correlates of youth homelessness in the United States. J Adolesc Health. 2018;62(1):14–21.
74. Grant JM, Mottet LA, Tanis J, Harrison J, Herman JL, Keisling M. Injustice at every turn: a report of the National Transgender Discrimination Survey. Washington, DC: National Center for Transgender Equality and National Gay and Lesbian Task Force; 2011.
75. Kosciw JG, Greytak EA, Giga NM, Villenas C, Danischewski DJ. The 2015 National School Climate Survey: the experiences of lesbian, gay, bisexual, transgender, and queer youth in our nation's schools [Internet]. New York: GLSEN; 2016 [cited 2018 Oct 7]. Available from: https://www.glsen.org/sites/default/files/2015%20National%20GLSEN%202015%20National%20School%20Climate%20Survey%20%28NSCS%29%20-%20Full%20Report_0.pdf.
76. D'augelli AR, Grossman AH, Starks MT. Childhood gender atypicality, victimization, and PTSD among lesbian, gay, and bisexual youth. J Interpers Violence. 2006;21(11):1462–82.
77. Grossman AH, D'augelli AR. Transgender youth: invisible and vulnerable. J Homosex. 2006;51(1):111–28.
78. Lopez CM, Solomon D, Boulware SD, Christison-Lagay ER. Trends in the use of puberty blockers among transgender children in the United States. J Pediatr Endocrinol Metab. 2018;31(6):665–70.
79. Clark BA, Veale JF, Greyson D, Saewyc E. Primary care access and foregone care: a survey of transgender adolescents and young adults. Fam Pract. 2018;35(3):302–6.
80. Fitzgerald E, Elspeth S, Hickey D, Biko C, Tobin, HJ. Meaningful work: transgender experiences in the sex trade [Internet]. Washington, DC: National Center for Transgender Equality; 2015 Dec 9 [cited 2018 Oct 7]. Available from: https://www.transequality.org/sites/default/files/Meaningful%20Work-Full%20Report_FINAL_3.pdf.
81. Singh AA. Transgender youth of color and resilience: negotiating oppression and finding support. Sex Roles. 2013;68(11–12):690–702.
82. Crenshaw K. Mapping the margins: intersectionality, identity politics, and violence against women of color. Stanford: Stanford Law Review; 1991.
83. Collins PH. Black feminist thought: knowledge, consciousness, and the politics of empowerment. London: Psychology Press; 2000.
84. Singh A, Eaker R, Hughes K. Transgender and gender-nonconforming youth of color. Thousand Oaks: Sage Publications; 2016. p. 1212–4. (Goldberg A, editor. The SAGE encyclopedia of LGBTQ studies).
85. Greytak EA, Kosciw JG, Diaz EM. Harsh realities: the experiences of transgender youth in our nation's schools. New York: GLSEN; 2009.
86. Reck J. Homeless gay and transgender youth of color in San Francisco: "no one likes street kids" – even in the Castro. J LGBT Youth. 2009;6(2–3):223–42.
87. Clark TC, Lucassen MF, Bullen P, Denny SJ, Fleming TM, Robinson EM, Rossen FV. The health and well-being of transgender high school students: results from the New Zealand adolescent health survey (Youth'12). J Adolesc Health. 2014;55(1):93–9.
88. Rider GN, McMorris BJ, Gower AL, Coleman E, Eisenberg ME. Health and care utilization of transgender and gender nonconforming youth: a population-based study. Pediatrics. 2018;141(3):e20171683.
89. Olson J, Schrager SM, Belzer M, Simons LK, Clark LF. Baseline physiologic and psychosocial characteristics of transgender youth seeking care for gender dysphoria. J Adolesc Health. 2015;57(4):374–80.
90. Turban JL, Ehrensaft D. Research review: gender identity in youth: treatment paradigms and controversies. J Child Psychol Psychiatry. 2018;59(12):1228–43.

91. Rhode Island Department of Health. 2017 Youth Risk Behavior Survey: Rhode Island high school codebook [Internet]. Providence: Rhode Island Department of Health; 2018 [cited 2018 Dec 9]. Available from: http://www.health.ri.gov/materialbyothers/yrbs/2017HighSchoolCodebook.pdf.
92. Rhode Island Department of Health, Sexual Orientation and Gender Identity (SOGI) Equity Workgroup. Rhode Island data brief: supporting and caring for gender-expansive youth. Providence: Rhode Island Department of Health; 2018.
93. Johns MM, Lowry R, Andrzejewski J, Barrios LC, Demissie Z, McManus T, Underwood JM. Transgender identity and experiences of violence victimization, substance use, suicide risk, and sexual risk behaviors among high school students—19 states and large urban school districts, 2017. Morbidity and Mortality Weekly Report. 2019;68(3):67.

Pathways of Gender Development

3

Jenifer K. McGuire and Quinlyn J. Morrow

Variance in Gender Differentiation

Studies of childhood gender development focus on two distinct, yet related, concepts: *gender identity* (one's identification as a girl, a boy, or another gender) and *gender role* (behaviors, attitudes, or characteristics that are usually attributed to, expected from, or preferred in people of a particular gender identity). Early works that established the developmental paradigm of gender identity treated gender as a proxy for assigned sex at birth, and did not consider variance in identity broadly enough to consider developmental pathways that included identification with a gender that differed from the sex assigned at birth [14]. Instead, focus was on gender differentiation, or how male and female bodies come to be, and how they contributed to corresponding gender identities.

Explanations for why gender differentiation occurs can be grouped into three main categories based on what processes are primarily emphasized: gender essentialism, gender environmentalism, and gender constructivism [28], (see also Table 3.1). Gender essentialist theories describe gender differences as being primarily based in inherent, biologically driven sex differences, although these theories can also recognize the moderating effects of environmental factors (e.g., [24]). Gender environmentalism or constructionism emphasizes the role of societal practices in generating and maintaining gender differentiation via social conditioning, observational learning, and gendered language and social ordering (e.g., [7]). Finally, gender constructivist theories posit that children receive biological and environmental cues about gender and then internalize those cues by developing gender schemas about the self and others that underlie their gender beliefs and behavior (e.g., [3]).

J. K. McGuire (✉) · Q. J. Morrow
Department of Family Social Science, University of Minnesota,
Twin Cities, MN, USA
e-mail: jmcguire@umn.edu; morro214@umn.edu

M. Forcier et al. (eds.), *Pediatric Gender Identity*,
https://doi.org/10.1007/978-3-030-38909-3_3

Table 3.1 Essentialist, environmentalist, and constructivist views of gender differentiation

Perspective	Mechanism	Domains of evidence	Relevance for TGD
Essentialist	Biological differences	Height, size, brain structures	Medical intervention, pubertal suppression
Environmentalist	Societal practices	Gendered clothing, athletic opportunity	Challenging norms, social transition
Constructivist	Cognitive schemas	Appearance appraisals, language	Nonbinary pronouns, reclassifying people

Importantly, gender roles manifest differently depending on culture and historical context [28]. Additionally, gender differentiation is not monolithic within gender groups; although research has found evidence of gender differences with predictive power, this research also consistently finds greater variation *within* genders rather than *between* genders [28]. In other words, gender is an important part of identity for many people, but is not deterministic of ability or interests. Finally, gender differentiation may or may not be consistent within individuals: a person may be highly gender differentiated in one domain (e.g., personality) but not in another domain (e.g., occupation; [28]). Together, these factors suggest that gender differentiation is likely a reciprocal process between biological, social, and psychological factors, and that gender essentialist, environmentalist/constructionist, and constructivist theories may each have their place in fully describing gender development processes [14].

Essential Versus Social Construction of Gender

In the area of gender dysphoria or gender incongruence, considerations of essentialist versus social constructionist contributions to identity development are particularly important. Families, and especially parents, are generally thought to be the earliest socializing agents when it comes to teaching children about societal expectations regarding gender [25]. Although some gender socialization occurs directly, such as by telling children that certain objects or activities are only for boys or for girls, most gender socialization occurs indirectly, such as through behavior modeling or parents' reactions to gender stereotypical behavior as compared to gender nonconforming behavior [33]. The twenty-first century has seen increased societal valuing of gender egalitarianism, and in response, some parents avoid cultural stereotypes for gender, and some purposefully align themselves with gender-neutral or feminist parenting strategies. LGBTQ parents in particular may choose to resist gender stereotypes in raising their children by providing a variety of gendered options for toys, clothing, and activities [1, 21]. The vast majority of transgender and gender nonconforming children, however, will be born to parents who are cisgender, and more likely than not, heterosexual, and most parents still have a cisnormative identity expectation for their children. At this point, there is no data to suggest that transgender children become TGD because of the sexuality, gender identity, psychological functioning, or behavior of parents or peers or become *not* transgender because of the sexuality, gender identity, psychological functioning, or behavior of parents or peers [48].

Efforts to promote parental and societal acceptance of TGD persons have often focused on biological correlates of gender variance, using a "Born This Way" philosophy as the basis for a social justice model of inclusion. The aligning research has focused specifically on examining correlates and explaining the origins of gender variance among youth, such as gender dysphoria or differences of sex development (DSD; [13]). Some studies have compared TGD individuals with typically developing children and adults, with the idea that documentation of physiological correlates of gender dysphoria, especially those present in very early childhood, would give some evidence for a biological contribution to gender identity. Thus far, the study of correlates of gender dysphoria includes certain brain structures, otoacoustic emissions (OAE), body structures, and hormone levels (e.g., [5, 6, 9, 12]). This developing line of research suggests that there is some evidence for biological and social influence on the individual's experienced identity and expression [14].

Conceptual conflicts regarding essentialist versus social constructionist beliefs about gender development have led to sometimes strained relationships among social groups that might be assumed to be aligned, with some clinging tightly to socially constructed views of gender, and others focused singularly on the biological contribution to gender dysphoria. Early theoretical beliefs about a complete social construction of gender identity were refuted by cruel and failed attempts of early gender clinicians (e.g., [34]) to impose alternate gender roles on otherwise internally typically developing children with cosmetic injuries. For example, under the advice of psychologist John Money at Johns Hopkins University, the parents of David Reimer agreed to raise David as a girl in response to a failed circumcision. The gender reassignment was hidden from David (who ultimately returned to a male role) and his identical twin brother until age 15 with devastating consequences for everyone [37].

Further evidence against a completely social construction of gender exists in the many failed efforts of clinicians and parents to reverse or deny gender dysphoria, a practice now widely evaluated as unethical [52]. Reparative or conversion therapy is a process that attempts to change sexual orientation or gender identity through cognitive, psychological, neurological, behavioral, or other forms of therapy. All major medical and psychological organizations have rejected conversion therapy as unnecessary and dangerous; 15 states and DC have laws limiting conversion therapy for youth [35].

Multiple Contributors to Gender

Extant research has begun to define multiple contributors to gender identity and to explore gender identity as a complex construct with natural shifts over time [4, 15]. Direct reports from TGD youth reveal distinct components of gender experience that are not typically measured in current clinical environments [44]. The most longstanding gender assessment measures focus on "yes–no" binaries of *male* versus *female* and *nondysphoric* versus *gender dysphoric* identities [2]. The field has grown to the point of accepting the value of early intervention, supporting youth self-expression and evaluating the positive impact of early intervention and support on short- and long-term psychological outcomes [42]. Unfortunately, the continuing

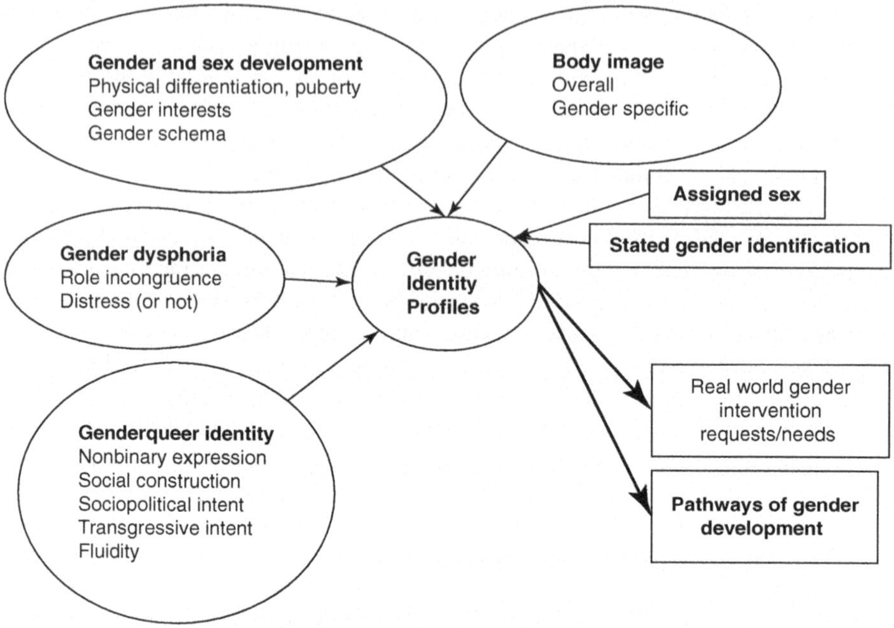

Fig. 3.1 Conceptual model of gender identity predicting dysphoria and intervention requests

reliance on a predominately gender-binary approach to long-term follow-up has limited understanding of gender, and the true impact that affirmative gender interventions may have in the lives of young people's development. A variety of contributors to gender identity have been independently proposed or validated in empirical research, and taken together create a multidimensional picture of gender as a complex and dynamic system (Fig. 3.1).

Several major constructs have been identified and investigated as contributors to gender identity, including gender development, body image, gender dysphoria/euphoria, and genderqueer or nonbinary identity. Gender development includes childhood interests, gender expression and congruence, and nonconformity [39]. This construct also includes other developmental concepts such as pubertal development, sex differentiation, and gender schema [28]. Body image as a construct includes both concern for specific body parts and generalized body image and sense of self as healthy. Body image is most often associated with disordered eating, including anorexia, but might also include gendered concerns about the body, such as concerns with menstruation, curvature, or other body characteristics that are aligned with one's assigned birth sex [30]. Gender dysphoria has long been measured to examine need for gender services but has suffered significant limitations due to the binary nature of longstanding measures (e.g., UGDS, [53]). Historically, measurement of gender dysphoria focused on the individual's distress with role incongruence, body hatred, or longing to transition genders in a relatively binary way. Newer nonbinary measures allow for a full spectrum of identity measurement, assess both dysphoria and comfort in affirmed gender (sometimes called gender euphoria), and meet assumptions of longitudinal measurement, meaning TGD clients can take the same measure multiple times, regardless of where they may be in a transition process [32]. Finally, genderqueer/nonbinary identity describes an individual's sense of self as any gender that is not exclusively masculine or feminine in nature, or even that challenges or transgresses the concept of gender altogether. Nonbinary identity can manifest in physical expression, social roles, and sociopolitical/theoretical ways [31]. Taken together, these concepts form the basis of a multidimensional conceptualization of gender identity that begins to approximate the internal complexity of gender, externally expressed verbally and physically in the lives of TGD persons.

Pathways of Development

Medical interventions to affirmatively support adolescents with gender variance are relatively new from a historical perspective, initiating in the late 1990s with the first uses of puberty-blocking hormones in the Netherlands. From that time for 15–20 years, discussions about how clinicians, families, and communities could most supportively respond to childhood and adolescent gender variance and gender dysphoria were largely centered on binary conceptualizations of gender identity and transgender status. Specifically, clinical interventions have historically focused on diagnosing gender dysphoria (formerly gender identity disorder) with an intent to determine who should be supported to transition from one sex to the other, including pubertal suppression, gender affirmative hormone therapy (GAHT), and later surgeries as necessary. The earliest longitudinal studies of gender dysphoria came from this (then ubiquitous) predominantly binary perspective, and introduced the language of persistence and desistance to describe youth who transitioned medically (persisters) and those who did not (desisters) often by a fairly young age (between the ages of 16 and 23, depending on study; [16, 47, 49, 51]). Fundamentally, such a perspective is limiting because it is focused on the idea that a person either is or is not transgender rather than holding a perspective that multiple developmental pathways exist, with no particular pathway being inherently superior to another.

Continuing research has revealed a much broader range of developmental pathways than these early studies assumed. The time when a person first expresses a TGD identity can be influenced by many factors that are independent of identity, such as stigma, lack of knowledge about TGD identities, general developmental timing, or family support. Some children will begin asserting a transgender identity as early as toddlerhood [20] and will consistently identify as that gender throughout their lives; other children may not obviously express any discomfort with their assigned sex until they begin experiencing gender dysphoria at puberty because of the development of secondary sex characteristics [10]; still other people will not come to identify as a gender other than the one they were assigned at birth until adulthood [10], or even later in life [43]. Importantly, gender-affirming interventions may be pursued at any of these points (with medical interventions only being pursued after puberty onset). Additionally, some people are genderfluid, meaning they may fluctuate between genders and/or may experience multiple genders simultaneously [29].

Genderfluidity is distinct from gender development in that it is a stable gender identity that expects variance in experienced gender (i.e., one is consistently genderfluid but may feel more or less identified with masculinity, femininity, androgyny, or another gender spectrum at any given moment). Genderfluid individuals may not ever "settle" on a masculine, feminine, or androgynous identity, but that does not mean that there are not any stable components of their gender (e.g., they may always feel dysphoric about their chest, shoulders, hands, etc.). Given the many contributing factors to developmental pathways, timing should not be considered diagnostic.

Delineating gender expression from gender identity can help to identify and clarify TGD developmental pathways – just because a child is behaving in gender nonconforming ways does not necessarily mean they are experiencing gender dysphoria or identify as a gender other than the one they were assigned at birth. In fact, many cisgender lesbian, gay, bisexual, and queer people behave in gender nonconforming ways [8], and gender play (i.e., trying on roles, affectations, clothing, or other attributes typically associated with a different gender) can be an important part of gender development for all people, regardless of gender or sexual identity [50]. Early longitudinal studies of gender clinic referrals found that some children were referred for gender assessment and later identified as cisgender LGB, suggesting social influences in referral patterns particularly for assigned male children who behaved in feminine ways and later identified as gay males [49]. This same study and another [47, 49] were able to delineate *behavioral* indicators of identity in children from *verbal* identity indicators in children. Some children will clearly state "I am a different gender," and others will engage behavioral indicators (name changes, clothing changes, and body preferences) that may require time, observation and conversation to fully interpret.

With now 20 years of adolescent gender affirmative medical experience, the shortcomings of the early longitudinal studies, and how they have influenced language and thinking about gender development pathways have become clearer. Newhook et al. [36] recently reviewed four longitudinal studies of gender dysphoria that used persistence versus desistence language to predict either probability of group membership, characteristics of group membership, or in one qualitative study, description of experiences within each group [16, 47, 49, 51]. Together, these studies and some others have been used [improperly] to suggest that about 80% of gender nonconforming prepubescent children will not seek gender affirmative care as adolescents or young adults, and to make a case against childhood social transitions [36]. There are many methodological and conceptual limitations of those longitudinal studies (addressed by [36], and responded to by [46]). The studies were essentially limited by changing diagnostic criteria for gender dysphoria over time, meaning that youth who were subthreshold for current standards of gender dysphoria would of course be unlikely to seek transition services [16]. Referral patterns across countries and over time also vary, and the persistence studies mostly included the entire pool of clinical referrals, even those who may not have been gender dysphoric at intake (e.g., had other nonconforming behavior, parental concerns, or sexual acting out), thus creating an overinflated estimate of people who "desisted" in gender dysphoria. Most importantly, because those studies focused on a binary, transnormative model of gender transition, illustrated by the phrase "persistence versus desistence," they contributed to a developing narrative of binary transgender transition for children and adolescents. Taken together, the framing of these studies whose designs were originally meant to predict later need for services limited discussion of multiple pathways or developmental trajectories.

Ongoing research with TGD children has consolidated around broader more complex models of affirmative care (see Rider et al., 2019, for the Gender Affirmative Lifespan Approach GALA), which support young peoples' developing identities across a full spectrum. In prevailing affirmative care approaches, children are given space to explore their gender at their own pace, and with no expectations from parents or clinicians about the trajectory that their gender development might follow [18, 23]. In accordance with studies showing that the most reliable way to know a child's gender identity is to ask them [49]; in gender affirmative care models, the individual is the strongest authority on their own gender [39]. Fundamental to gender affirmative care models is the recognition that there is nothing inherently unhealthy or lesser about a transgender identity.

Transgender Prepubertal Development

When they grow up in a supportive environment, TGD children's gender development typically mirrors that of cisgender children. As compared to gender-matched peers (based on expressed gender, not sex assigned at birth), preschool-aged, socially transitioned children demonstrate similar preferences for same-gender peers, toys, and clothing; express similar gender stereotypes about how boys and girls act; consistently identify as their expressed gender; and report feeling similar to other children of their expressed gender [20, 40]. See Table 3.2 for a general timeline of gender development and suggestions for supporting TGD through typical gender milestones.

TGD youth do differ from their cisgender peers in that their understanding of gender is more likely to encompass the potential for gender nonconformity and a

Table 3.2 Gender development milestones and needs

Age	Milestone	Needs	TGD specific
18 months	Begin to categorize people by gender	Broad exposures	N/A
3–4 years	Develop a more-stable gender identity	Teach anatomy labels Allow clothing choices Degender objects	Destigmatize Do not correct Advocate for safe spaces Watch
School age	Experience and enforce increased social pressure to be gender conforming Desire to fit in Loss of magical thinking	Educate children to recognize gender bias and to be open to gender nonconformity Create environments that celebrate and respect differences	Monitor social identity choices Support with responding to bullying from peers and stigma from important adults Plan for safe bathroom access Educate about transition processes

(continued)

Table 3.2 (continued)

Age	Milestone	Needs	TGD specific
Prepuberty/ preteen	Preparing for puberty and associated body changes Greater desires for independence	Explain upcoming pubertal changes Educate about sexual orientation	Screen for body dysphoria, eating disorders
Puberty onset/ early adolescence	Begins to demonstrate ability for logic and abstract thought Begins to question authority and societal standards Begins to develop stronger sense of self	Discuss relationship needs and desires LGBTQ-inclusive, comprehensive sexual health Hygiene	Understand pubertal suppression – discuss what pubertal suppression will and will not do
Midadolescence	Questions and analyzes more extensively Begins to form own code of ethics Considers possible future goals more systematically, thinks more long-term	Ethical sexual interactions Pregnancy prevention Body image	Understand gender-affirming hormonal interventions – discuss potential implications for reproduction Understand future fertility preservation choices
Late adolescence/ early adulthood	Independent living/ education or work Long-term planning	Intimate partnerships Healthy sexuality	Preparation for surgical care needs
Launching	Financial independence	Family formation	Reproductive support Support with navigating potential stigma in adult life, including employment and housing

Note. Needs at each stage of development are cumulative. For example, it is important to advocate for safe spaces for TGD youth starting in toddlerhood and then throughout their childhood and adolescence. Similarly, discussions of relationship needs and sexual safety should not end during early adolescence, but instead continue into early adulthood

transgender identity. Specifically, TGD youth are less likely than age-matched cisgender peers to believe that their past gender was stable, although trans youth did see their own future gender as matching their current expressed gender [39]. In other words, when TGD children settle into their authentic gender, most don't expect it to continue to change [20]. Additionally, TGD children see gender diversity as more acceptable and are more willing to befriend TGD children than are their cisgender peers [38].

Regarding mental health, TGD youth who socially transition report depression and self-worth similar to cisgender peers, but slightly higher anxiety [17, 41]. This is notable in that TGD youth who are not allowed to socially transition demonstrate significantly higher rates of depression and anxiety than their cisgender peers, suggesting that social transition can be fundamental for the healthy development of TGD children [17, 41].

Despite the benefits of social transition, TGD youth can encounter a lack of support from family members, other important adults (e.g., teachers), and peers. For example, TGD children and their family members report several areas of conflict related to gender affirmation planning. Specifically, family members reported feelings of loss and grief in response to their TGD relations' transition, which can come across to TGD children as a lack of affirmation from their families [19]. Additionally, in a study investigating peer-group contexts, cisgender children preferred cisgender peers over socially transitioned peers; however, they also liked peers of their own gender better than the other gender, meaning that cisgender girls liked other cisgender girls the best, followed by transgender girls and cisgender boys liked other cisgender boys the best, followed by transgender boys [22]. Additionally, cisgender children who recognized socially transitioned children as their affirmed gender were more accepting of transgender peers than were cisgender children who persisted in identifying socially transitioned children by their assigned sex [22], suggesting that creating a TGD-accepting peer environment requires that all children be taught basic gender literacy (see Table 3.3 for a list of TGD-affirming children's books to begin conversations).

Table 3.3 TGD-affirming children's books

Title and author	Summary
Red: A Crayon's Story by Michael Hall	This book follows Red, a crayon with a bright red label, who is in fact blue. Red's teacher, mother, and classmates all try to help him be red. But Red is miserable. He just can not be red, no matter how hard he tries! Finally, a brand-new friend offers a new perspective, and Red discovers what readers have known all along. He's blue!
Introducing Teddy by Jessica Walton	Errol and his teddy, Thomas, are best friends who do everything together. One sunny day, Errol finds that Thomas the Teddy is sad, and Errol can't figure out why. Then, Thomas the Teddy finally tells Errol what Teddy has been afraid to say: "In my heart, I've always known that I'm a girl Teddy, not a boy Teddy. I wish my name was Tilly." And Errol replies, "I don't care if you're a girl teddy or a boy teddy! What matters is that you are my friend."
Julián Is a Mermaid by Jessica Love	While riding the subway home from the pool with his abuela one day, Julián notices three people spectacularly dressed up. Their hair billows in brilliant hues, their dresses end in fishtails, and their joy fills the train car. When Julián gets home, daydreaming of the magic he's seen, all he can think about is dressing up in his own fabulous mermaid costume. But what will Abuela think about how Julián sees himself? *Julián Is a Mermaid* provides a role model of a grandmother who loves and affirms her grandson and his exploration of his interests.
Backwards Day by S. Bear Bergman	Set on the planet Tenalp, a world where there is a single day each year when everything everywhere is backwards. Andrea looks forward to Backwards Day eagerly every year, so she can turn into a boy for the day. But one year she doesn't turn along with everyone else. She's miserable. The very next day, however, she turns into a boy – and stays that way! He's delighted, but his parents are distressed and take him to the big city to consult with Backwardsologists. When they finally figure out what's happened, the miracles of Backwards Day are fully revealed to the reader.

Note. For a more-expansive list of potential books to develop gender literacy in children, visit WelcomingSchools.org and click on the "Resources" tab [27]

Gender Affirmative Care and Informed Assent

Gender affirmative approaches to clinical care are characterized by the following perspectives: "(a) gender variations are not disorders; (b) gender presentations are diverse and varied across cultures, therefore requiring our cultural sensitivity; (c) to the best of our knowledge at present, gender involves an interweaving of biology, development and socialization, and culture and context, with all three bearing on any individual's gender self; (d) gender may be fluid, and is not binary, both at a particular time and if and when it changes within an individual across time; (e) if there is pathology, it more often stems from cultural reactions (e.g., transphobia, homophobia, sexism) rather than from within the child" [23]. Given this foundational perspective, treatment approaches have developed that include medical intervention (i.e., pubertal suppression, gender-affirming hormones, surgical interventions) but also psychosocial supports such as gender literacy education, family relationship support, parent gender socialization support, contextual interventions with schools and community groups, and individual education and therapy to support identity development as well as build resiliency to face minority stress (Rider et al., 2019). Children and adolescents have unique developmental needs from adults that require consideration regarding their understanding of interventions, desire to participate in them, and capacity to anticipate probable consequences.

The American Academy of Pediatrics provides guidelines for pediatricians to seek informed parental permission and adolescent assent for medical procedures [26]. According to these guidelines, "Informed consent incorporates three duties: disclosure of information to patients and their surrogates, assessment of patient and surrogate understanding of the information and their capacity for medical decision-making, and obtaining informed consent before treatments and interventions." A complete examination of the duty of informed consent given the unique developmental trajectories of gender variant youth is outside the range of this chapter. However, we will pose some questions for consideration at various developmental phases, as well as draw attention to some others who have begun to dissect this issue with more detail [45, 54].

Prior to puberty, medical interventions are not indicated specifically for gender variance. Children and parents may come to a clinic and choose to join psychoeducation programs on gender literacy, parent–child support groups, gender affirmative play groups or camps or other sorts of social interventions, or individual or family therapy. A prepubertal child should be able to understand the basic content of a course or program before entering the program and should be able to understand whether or not that program or activity is necessary for any desired outcome (e.g., to later receive any treatment). Children may bring up questions about things like name changes, using different bathrooms, or other social transition concerns. Cognitively preparing a child for how others may react to such social changes and determining if the child is able to understand this level of contingency thinking can ease the process and improve the child's ability to respond if faced with negative reactions from others.

Shumer and Tishelman [45] specifically address the issue of capacity to provide informed assent for puberty suppression by an adolescent with reduced cognitive functioning. They focus on three factors: developmentally appropriate awareness of condition, what to expect with treatment, and assessment of patients' understanding and sense of pressure. At the point of pubertal suppression, a child would need to understand that their identity as TGD was distinct from most other youth, and that the pubertal suppression would stop the progression of puberty. Some distinct cognitive factors that can also be relevant include an understanding of what puberty blockers will *not* do, including stimulate cross-sex changes, or influence the way peers or family members experience the client. Finally, youth need to understand that they can discontinue blockers and are not in any way expected to continue with a treatment they don't want. Disclosure of potential side effects of pubertal suppression is part of informed consent.

At the time of gender-affirming hormone initiation, issues of informed consent become more involved, as interventions become less reversible. By this age, adolescents have developed more advanced cognitive skills as well as more consolidated identities. Adolescents should be able to understand the irreversible nature of some bodily changes that will occur with gender-affirming hormones. Additionally, conversations about reproductive capacity and fertility preservation are important at this point (see Chap. 15, Fertility Considerations). Research about the decision process for gender-affirming hormone initiation is just beginning [11], and has found that families view decisions as predominately something to be decided internally with limited support from health-care providers. Pathways of development have become increasingly diverse. With medical advances, technologies to support gender affirmation and modification are refined regularly, making gender identity congruence available for more people than was ever possible before. In this increasingly complex arena, health-care providers play an important role for children and families as they interface with complex developmental needs and medical considerations. Framing around developmentally appropriate informed assent and consent can provide a lens to ensure that children and parents have information they need, in a way they understand that is relevant to their specific developmental concerns.

Concluding Thoughts

In this chapter, we've shared a brief overview of how scientific understandings of gender identity and development have changed over time to be more inclusive of a greater array of gender experiences, with specific considerations for supporting the healthy development of TGD youth. In particular, we described how biological, environmental, and psychological factors interact to explain the development of gender identity. We emphasized the importance of giving children and adolescents space to explore and develop their own identities, rather than attempting to force any particular identity, role, or developmental pathway upon them. We discussed limitations of binary conceptualizations of gender that only account for male and female genders, and described more recent research that uses nonbinary measurements of gender components to better capture the full spectrum of gender experience. Finally, we introduced some considerations for clinicians regarding informed assent in gender affirmative care models.

References

1. Averett KH. The gender buffet: LGBTQ parents resisting heteronormativity. Gend Soc. 2016;30(2):189–212. https://doi.org/10.1177/0891243215611370.
2. Bauer GR, Hammond R, Travers R, Kaay M, Hohenadel KM, Boyce M. "I don't think this is theoretical; this is our lives": how erasure impacts health care for transgender people. J Assoc Nurses AIDS Care. 2009;20(5):348–61. https://doi.org/10.1016/j.jana.2009.07.004.
3. Bem SL. Gender schema theory: a cognitive account of sex typing. Psychol Rev. 1981;88:354–64.
4. Bockting WO. Transgender identity development. In: Tolman DL, Diamond L, editors. APA handbook of sexuality and psychology, vol. 1: person-based approaches. Washington, DC: American Psychological Association; 2014. p. 739–58. https://doi.org/10.1037/14193-024.
5. Burke SM, Menks WM, Cohen-Kettenis PT, Klink DT, Bakker J. Click-evoked otoacoustic emissions in children and adolescents with gender identity disorder. Arch Sex Behav. 2014;43(8):1515–23. https://doi.org/10.1007/s10508-014-0278-2.
6. Burke SM, Manzouri AH, Savic I. Structural connections in the brain in relation to gender identity and sexual orientation. Sci Rep. 2017;7(November):1–12. https://doi.org/10.1038/s41598-017-17352-8.
7. Bussey K, Bandura A. Social cognitive theory of gender development and differentiation. Psychol Rev. 1999;106:676–713.
8. Catalpa JM, McGuire JK, Berg DR, Fish JN, Rider GN, Bradford NJ. Predictive validity of the Genderqueer Identity Scale (GQI): differences between genderqueer, transgender and cisgender sexual minority individuals. Int J Transgend. 2019;20:305. https://doi.org/10.1080/15532739.2018.1528196.
9. Cohen-Kettenis PT, Veltman DJ, Burke SM, Schagen SEE, Wouters FM, Delemarre-van de Waal HA, Bakker J. Puberty suppression and executive functioning: an fMRI-study in adolescents with gender dysphoria. Psychoneuroendocrinology. 2015;56:190–9. https://doi.org/10.1016/j.psyneuen.2015.03.007.
10. Coleman E, Bockting W, Botzer M, Cohen-Kettenis P, DeCuypere G, Feldman J, et al. Standards of care for the health of transsexual, transgender, and gender-nonconforming people, version 7. Int J Transgend. 2011;13(4):165–232. https://doi.org/10.1080/15532739.2011.700873.
11. Daley T, Grossoehme D, McGuire JK, Corathers S, Conard L, Lipstien E. "I couldn't see a downside": decision-making about gender-affirming hormone therapy. J Adolesc Health. 2019;65:274–9. https://doi.org/10.1016/j.jadohealth.2019.02.018.
12. Davis SN, Risman BJ. Feminists wrestle with testosterone: hormones, socialization and cultural interactionism as predictors of women's gendered selves. Soc Sci Res. 2015;49:110–25. https://doi.org/10.1016/j.ssresearch.2014.07.012.
13. de Vries ALC, Doreleijers TAH, Cohen-Kettenis PT. Disorders of sex development and gender identity outcome in adolescence and adulthood: understanding gender identity development and its clinical implications. Pediatr Endocrinol Rev. 2007;4(4):343–51. Retrieved from http://www.ncbi.nlm.nih.gov/pubmed/17643082
14. de Vries ALC, Kreukels BPC, Steensma TD, McGuire JK. Gender identity development: a biopsychosocial perspective. In: Kreukels BPC, Steensma TD, De Vries ALC, editors. Gender dysphoria and disorders of sex development: progress in care and knowledge. New York: Springer; 2014. https://doi.org/10.1007/978-1-4614-7441-8_3.
15. Diamond LM, Pardo ST, Butterworth MR. Transgender experience and identity. In: Shwartz SJ, Luyckx K, Vignoles VL, editors. Handbook of identity theory and research. New York: Springer; 2011. p. 629–47. https://doi.org/10.1007/978-1-4419-7988-9.
16. Drummond K, Bradley S, Peterson-Badali M, Zucker K. A follow-up study of girls with gender identity disorder. Dev Psychol. 2008;44:34–45. https://doi.org/10.1037/0012-1649.44.1.34.

17. Durwood L, McLaughlin KA, Olson KR. Mental health and self-worth in socially transitioned transgender youth. J Am Acad Child Adolesc Psychiatry. 2017;56(2):116–123.e2. https://doi.org/10.1016/j.jaac.2016.10.016.Mental.
18. Ehrensaft D. The gender creative child. New York: The Experiment Publishing; 2016.
19. Ehrensaft D, Simons L, Schrager SM, Clark LF, Belzer M, Olson J, et al. Transitioning meanings? Family members' communicative struggles surrounding transgender identity. Clin Child Psychol Psychiatry. 2013;7(4):9–28. https://doi.org/10.1177/1359104502007003035.
20. Fast AA, Olson KR. Gender development in transgender preschool children. Child Dev. 2018;89(2):620–37. https://doi.org/10.1111/cdev.12758.
21. Flanders CE, Legge MM, Plante I, Goldberg AE, Ross LE. Gender socialization practices among bisexual and other nonmonosexual mothers: a longitudinal qualitative examination. J GLBT Fam Stud. 2019;15(2):105–26. https://doi.org/10.1080/1550428X.2018.1461583.
22. Gülgöz S, Gomez EM, Demeules MR, Olson KR, Gülgöz S, Gomez EM, et al. Children's evaluation and categorization of transgender children. J Cogn Dev. 2018;19(4):325–44. https://doi.org/10.1080/15248372.2018.1498338.
23. Hidalgo M, Ehrensaft D, Tishelman A, Clark L, Garofalo R, Rosenthal S, et al. The gender affirmative model: what we know and what we aim to learn. Hum Dev. 2013;56:285–90. https://doi.org/10.1159/000355235.
24. Hines M. Gonadal hormones and sexual differentiation of human behavior: effects on psychosocial and cognitive development. In: Matsumoto A, editor. Sexual differentiation of the brain. Boca Raton: CRC Press; 2000. p. 257–78.
25. Kane EW. The gender trap: parents and the pitfalls of raising boys and girls. New York: NYU Press; 2012.
26. Katz AL, Webb SA. Informed consent in decision-making in pediatric practice. Pediatrics. 2016;138(2):e20161485. https://doi.org/10.1542/peds.2016-1485.
27. Lesson plans to help students understand gender and to support transgender and non-binary children, 2019. Retrieved June 2, 2019, from http://www.welcomingschools.org/resources/lesson-plans/transgender-youth/transgender-with-books/.
28. Liben LS, Bigler RS. In: Overton WF, editor. The developmental course of gender differentiation. Boston: Blackwell Publishing; 2002.
29. Mardell A. The ABC's of LGBT+. Miami: Mango; 2016.
30. McGuire JK, Doty JL, Catalpa JM, Ola C. Body image in transgender young people: findings from a qualitative, community based study. Body Image. 2016;18:96–107. https://doi.org/10.1016/j.bodyim.2016.06.004.
31. McGuire JK, Beek TF, Catalpa JM, Steensma TD. The Genderqueer Identity (GQI) scale: measurement and validation of four distinct subscales with trans and LGBQ clinical and community samples in two countries. Int J Transgend. 2018;20:289. https://doi.org/10.1080/15532739.2018.1460735.
32. McGuire JK, Rider GN, Catalpa JM, Steensma TD, Cohen-Kettenis PT, Berg DR. Utrecht Gender Dysphoria Scale-Gender Spectrum (UDGS-GS). In: Milhausen R, Sakaluk J, Fisher T, Davis C, Yarber W, editors. Handbook of sexuality-related measures. New York: Routledge; 2019. https://doi.org/10.4324/9781315183169.
33. Mesman J, Groeneveld MG. Gendered parenting in early childhood: subtle but unmistakable if you know where to look. Child Dev Perspect. 2018;12(1):22–7. https://doi.org/10.1111/cdep.12250.
34. Money J. Ablatio penis: normal male infant sex-reassigned as a girl. Arch Sex Behav. 1975;4(1):65–71. https://doi.org/10.1007/BF01541887.
35. NCLR: National Center for Lesbian Rights 2019. http://www.nclrights.org/bornperfect-the-facts-about-conversion-therapy/#q1. Accessed 14 January 2020.
36. Newhook JT, Pyne J, Winters K, Feder S, Holmes C, Tosh J, et al. A critical commentary on follow-up studies and "desistance" theories about transgender and gender-nonconforming children. Int J Transgend. 2018;19(2):212–24. https://doi.org/10.1080/15532739.2018.1456390.

37. Okami P. Chapter 16: Sex, gender, and sexual behavior. In: Psychology: contemporary perspectives. New York: Oxford University Press; 2014. Retrieved from http://oxfordpresents.com/okami/david-reimer/.
38. Olson KR, Enright EA. Do transgender children (gender) stereotype less than their peers and siblings? Dev Sci. 2018;21:e12606. https://doi.org/10.1111/desc.12606.
39. Olson KR, Selin G. Early findings from the transyouth project: gender development in transgender children. Child Dev Perspect. 2018;12(2):93–7. https://doi.org/10.1111/cdep.12268.
40. Olson KR, Key AC, Eaton NR. Gender cognition in transgender children. Psychol Sci. 2015;26(4):467–74. https://doi.org/10.1177/0956797614568156.
41. Olson KR, Durwood L, DeMeules M, McLaughlin KA. Mental health of transgender children who are supported in their identities. Pediatrics. 2016;137(3):e20153223. https://doi.org/10.1542/peds.2015-3223.
42. Rafferty J, AAP Committee on Psychosocial Aspects of Child and Family Health, AAP Committee on Adolescence, AAP Section on Lesbian, Gay, Bisexual, and Transgender Health and Wellness. Ensuring comprehensive care and support for transgender and gender diverse children and adolescents. Pediatrics. 2018;142(4):e20182162.
43. Reed B, Rhodes S, Schofield P, Wylie K. Gender variance in the UK. Prevalence, incidence, growth and geographic distribution. London: GIRES – the Gender Identity Research and Education Society; 2009. Retrieved from http://www.gires.org.uk/assets/Medpro-Assets/GenderVarianceUK-report.pdf.
44. Richards C, Bouman WP, Seal L, Barker MJ, Nieder TO, Tsjoen G. Non-binary or genderqueer genders. Int Rev Psychiatry. 2016;28(1):95–102. https://doi.org/10.3109/09540261.2015.1106446.
45. Shumer DE, Tishelman AC. The role of assent in the treatment of transgender adolescents. Int J Transgend. 2015;16:97–102. https://doi.org/10.1080/15532739.2015.1075929.
46. Steensma TD, Cohen-Kettenis PT. A critical commentary on "A critical commentary on follow-up studies and 'desistence' theories about transgender and gender non-conforming children". Int J Transgend. 2018;19(2):225–30. https://doi.org/10.1080/15532739.2018.1468292.
47. Steensma TD, Biemond R, de Boer F, Cohen-Kettenis PT. Desisting and persisting gender dysphoria after childhood: a qualitative follow-up study. Clin Child Psychol Psychiatry. 2011;16(4):499–516. https://doi.org/10.1177/1359104510378303.
48. Steensma T, Kreukels B, de Vries A, Cohen-Kettenis P. Gender identity development in adolescence. Horm Behav. 2013a;64(2):288–97.
49. Steensma TD, McGuire JK, Kreukels BPC, Beekman AJ, Cohen-Kettenis PT. Factors associated with desistence and persistence of childhood gender dysphoria: a quantitative follow-up study. J Am Acad Child Adolesc Psychiatry. 2013b;52(6):582–90. https://doi.org/10.1016/j.jaac.2013.03.016.
50. Thorne B. Gender play: girls and boys in school. New Brunswick: Rutgers University Press; 1993.
51. Wallien MSC, Cohen-Kettenis PT. Psychosexual outcome of gender-dysphoric children. J Am Acad Child Adolesc Psychiatry. 2008;47(12):1413–23. https://doi.org/10.1097/CHI.0b013e31818956b9.
52. Drescher J. Queer diagnoses revisited: the past and future of homosexuality and gender diagnoses in DSM and ICD. Int Rev Psychiatry. 2015;5:386–95.
53. Cohen-Kettenis PT, van Goozen SHM. Sex reassignment of adolescent transsexuals: a follow-up study. J Am Acad Child Adolesc Psychiatry. 1997;36:263–71.
54. Ashley F. Thinking an ethics of gender exploration: against delaying transition for transgender and gender creative youth. Clin Child Psychol Psychiatry. 2019;24:223–36. https://doi.org/10.1177/1359104519836462.

Neurobiology of Pediatric Gender Identity

4

Baudewijntje P. C. Kreukels and Sarah M. Burke

Introduction

Sex assigned at birth is usually based on the new born's physical sex characteristics, whereas gender identity refers to the thoughts and feelings someone has of belonging to a certain gender (male, female, among other non-binary possibilities). There are two main reasons for studying the neurobiology of gender diversity in youth. First, identifying the neurobiological correlates of gender identity in relation to sex assigned at birth will inform our understanding of the development of gender diversity. Second, because youth diagnosed with gender incongruence (GI) [1], a marked incongruence between one's experienced gender and sex assigned at birth, may be treated with puberty-suppression and cross-sex hormones, it is important to know the effects of these interventions on the development of the brain.

In this chapter, we review the literature investigating mechanisms that may underlie gender diversity from a neurobiological perspective. We specifically focus on the genetic aspects that may contribute to gender diversity and summarize the brain imaging research that included children and adolescents with GI.

B. P. C. Kreukels (✉)
Center of Expertise on Gender Dysphoria, Department of Medical Psychology, Amsterdam University Medical Centers, Amsterdam, The Netherlands
e-mail: b.kreukels@amsterdamumc.nl

S. M. Burke
Brain and Development Research Centre, Department of Developmental & Educational Psychology, Institute of Psychology, Leiden University, Leiden, The Netherlands

M. Forcier et al. (eds.), *Pediatric Gender Identity*,
https://doi.org/10.1007/978-3-030-38909-3_4

Genetic Effects

One area of interest in examining the biological mechanisms behind gender diversity and gender incongruence is to study if genetic factors influence the development of gender role (behavior interests and traits) and gender identity (the feeling of being a boy, girl or some alternative gender).

The contribution of genetic, shared and non-shared environmental factors can be studied in monozygotic (MZ) and dizygotic (DZ) twins. These studies can give an estimate of the heritability of a certain trait by examining the concordance and discordance of this trait in monozygotic (MZ) twins (100% genetically identical) compared to dizygotic (DZ) twins (share 50% of their genes). Discordance of a certain trait in MZ twins suggests the influence of environmental factors, whereas concordance would suggest genetic influence. One study summarized case studies of twins with GI and added their own clinical series, resulting in a total of 23 MZ and 21 DZ twin pairs [2]. None of the DZ twins were concordant for GI, whereas 39% of the MZ twins were, which was deemed to show that genetic factors play a considerable role in the development of GI.

Several studies in transgender and gender diverse (TGD) individuals have investigated polymorphisms in genes, mainly genes that are involved in the biosynthesis or action of sex steroids. The findings of these studies are fairly inconsistent. In TGD males (female assigned at birth, male gender identity), polymorphisms were found in the oestrogen receptor β (ERβ) [3] and CYP-17 gene in a Spanish cohort, but Ujike et al. [4] did not observe polymorphisms in these genes in a Japanese cohort. In TGD females (male assigned at birth, female gender identity), one study observed a polymorphism of CAG repeat length [5] which was not replicated by another study [6]. Another finding in TGD females was an increased prevalence of a long CA repeat in ERβ compared to control men [7]. These findings may be inconsistent due to small and heterogeneous samples. Interestingly, a recent study examined associations and interactions of the androgen receptor (AR), oestrogen receptor α (ERα), ERβ and aromatase in a large and more homogeneous population with regard to the onset of gender dysphoria and sexual orientation [8]. In androphilic (attracted to men) TGD females with an early onset of GI, an inverse allele interaction was found between ERβ and AR. In TGD males, ERα and ERβ were involved, but no interaction between the polymorphisms was observed. They thus seem to affect the development of gender dysphoria independently. Because all TGD females in this cohort were attracted to men and all TGD males were attracted to women, findings may also be explained by sexual orientation, which warrants further study.

Gender role, gender identity and related concepts have been examined in heritability studies in twins during childhood and adolescence (for a recent overview, see [9]). Masculinity and femininity were measured by the Pre-School Activities Inventory (PSAI) in 3–4-year-old twins in two related studies [10, 11]. The PSAI measures the gender role behavior in young children. For birth-assigned boys, they found that heritability accounted for 34% of the variation in PSAI scores, for birth-assigned girls this was 57%. For the femininity score in birth-assigned boys, the heritability was 17% and for the masculinity score in birth-assigned girls 40% [11]. Heritability was thus observed to be higher for birth-assigned girls.

A study in somewhat older (7- and 10-year-old) twins examined the heritability of gender diversity in role and identity by two items of the Child Behavior Checklist (i.e. 'behaves like opposite sex' and 'wishes to be of opposite sex') [12]. Using a composite score of both items, heritability was estimated to be 77% at age 7 and 71% at age 10. No differences were observed between the sexes. In twins with a wider age range (4–17 years old), Coolidge and colleagues [13] presented items derived from the DSM-IV criteria for then-termed gender identity disorder (GID) to their parents. The study lacked statistical power to distinguish between genetic and environmental effects [9].

A study in a large sample of Japanese twins with an even wider age range (3–27 years old) examined items that were also based on the DSM-IV criteria for GID [14, 15]. For birth-assigned males, the majority of the variance was explained by environmental factors among children, adolescents and adults. For birth-assigned females, however, the estimate for heritability was considerable for children and adolescents. It is important to be aware that the DSM-IV criteria were more focused on gender role as compared to the current DSM-5 criteria for gender dysphoria [16].

It is also of interest to mention that studies in adult twins show that gender-related measures can predominantly be explained by genetic and unique environmental effects, whereas shared environmental effects (cultural factors) are negligible [9]. Shared environmental effects refer to aspects of the home environment for which siblings are perfectly correlated. In children and adolescents, shared environmental effects seem to be more important than in adults.

Based on the data of these heritability studies, the hypothesis is formulated that gender identity is a complex trait that results from a combination of multiple genetic and environmental factors with a heritable polygenic component [9]. This means, there is not one single gene that accounts for the development of gender identity, but many genes are asserted to contribute to the trait, in addition to other factors that are non-genetic.

Early Sexual Differentiation

Another area of interest in the study of biological contributions to the development of gender identity is to examine the role of sex hormones. Animal studies have shown that sex hormones drive the sexual differentiation of the brain by affecting the organization of the brain from prenatal development onwards (organizing effects) and by the influence of circulating hormones on brain and behavior later during life (activating effects) [17, 18]. For example, exposure to high levels of testosterone during prenatal development in female animals results in more 'masculine' animal behaviour [19]. In humans, similar processes are thought to occur, but are obviously difficult to study by experimental manipulation. However, studies in people with differences of sexual development (DSD, also referred to as intersex conditions) have increased our understanding of the effects of sex hormones on behaviour. In one study, birth-assigned females with congenital adrenal hyperplasia, a condition in which they are exposed to elevated androgen levels prenatally, prefer masculine toys and display more male-typical play behaviour [20]. Individuals with Complete Androgen Insensitivity Syndrome (CAIS), who have an XY karyotype but are insensitive to the effects of androgens, are phenotypically female with regard to behavioural and external physical characteristics.

In addition, studies in individuals with various DSDs have mainly found evidence for effects of sex hormones on gender-typical behaviour and interests (gender role), but the effects on the development of gender identity are less clear. Gender dysphoria appears to be more prevalent in these groups [21], but other factors, such as medical interventions and social context, have been suggested to play a role in this respect as well [22]. Recent studies have observed that women with CAIS predominantly show female-typical brain structure and function, but also some male-typical neural characteristics [23]. In such studies, it is difficult to disentangle the effects of exposure to hormones, chromosomes and social factors.

A series of post-mortem studies observed a sex reversal in volume and neuron number of the central portion of the bed nucleus of the stria terminalis [24, 25], the interstitial nuclei 3 and 4 of the anterior hypothalamus [26] and kisspeptin expression [27] in TGD females. These findings were critical for the formulation of a sexual differentiation hypothesis for development of a transgender identity [28, 29]. Time windows for prenatal development of genitals (first trimester) and sexual differentiation of the brain (2nd and 3rd trimester) are different. Therefore, the findings of these post-mortem studies, which were sex-atypical for their sex assigned at birth but in line with their experienced gender identity, were hypothesized to be a result of exposure to atypical levels of prenatal sex hormones during a certain gestational period [30]. This has been the key hypothesis in many of the neuroimaging studies that evaluated if brain measures in TGD individuals showed more resemblance to those of people with whom they share their gender identity or with whom they share the sex assigned at birth [18, 31]. However, the findings of the post-mortem studies were all coming from one laboratory and have not been replicated thus far, and further work is needed to determine the strength of this hypothesis.

Adolescent Brain Development

In addition to the prenatal developmental period, adolescence has been recognized as sensitive period for brain development in terms of further neural sexual differentiation [32–38], and in terms of cognitive and social–emotional maturation [39–42], which includes the process of (gender) identity formation [43, 44].

Interestingly, in the case of gender incongruence, it has been suggested that early adolescence (ages 10–13 years) forms a critical period in the development of gender dysphoric feelings. Three factors in this period may be particularly important: (1) the physical changes due to puberty, (2) the changing social environment (in which one is treated according to one's gender more explicitly) and (3) the discovery of sexuality [45, 46]. In those adolescents in whom GI continues into adolescence, feelings of discomfort and distress around their bodies usually worsen after the onset of puberty, which often triggers symptoms of social anxiety, depression, suicidal ideation and self-harming behaviours [47–49]. For a discussion with regard to developmental trajectories of gender dysphoria, see [50–52].

Pubertal suppression with gonadotropin-releasing hormone analogues (GnRHa) can be a great relief for those with persistent feelings of GI and provides extra time to make a balanced decision on further treatment steps without the distress of puberty [53]. The effects of this treatment are reversible in the sense that if treatment is discontinued, endogenous puberty will proceed. Subsequently, adolescents often benefit from gender-affirming hormonal treatment and later gender-affirming surgery in terms of psychological well-being [54–56]. However, these interventions induce changes that are only partly reversible. Moreover, longitudinal studies describing the impact of these hormonal interventions on adolescent brain development are currently lacking.

Two large-scale functional magnetic resonance imaging (fMRI) studies including gender-incongruent youth have been conducted at the Centre of Expertise on Gender Dysphoria, Amsterdam, the Netherlands. The first fMRI study initiated in 2007 (referred to as Cohort 1) includes a total of 93 TGD and 96 age-matched cisgender (i.e. not trans, when gender identity and sex assigned at birth align) participants between 11 and 23 years of age. This study looks at brain activations during verbal-fluency and executive functions. A second 2009 (f)MRI study with prospective longitudinal design also included pre-pubertal youth. This younger, ages 7–12 years, subsample compares 43 TGD youth with 41 cisgender controls. We will discuss the findings from these cohorts in subsequent sections.

Whereas a fair amount of magnetic resonance imaging (MRI) research comparing trans- and cisgender adults has focused on structural brain differences in terms of white matter microstructure [57–59], cortical thickness [60, 61], and white and grey matter volume [62–66], only one study (of Cohort 1) thus far has described morphological brain characteristics in TGD youth [67]. TGD participants (54 trans boys, 37 trans girls), as a combined sample of different treatment conditions, on a whole-brain level, showed no signs of any sex-atypical grey matter volumes and were thus comparable with the cisgender groups of the same sex assigned at birth. However, more focused analyses in only the sexually dimorphic regions (hypothalamus, cerebellum, superior mPFC) revealed subtle sex-atypical deviations in volume.

Interestingly, more recent studies in adults suggested differences between trans- and cisgender participants in the superior medial prefrontal cortex (mPFC) region [65]. Manzouri et al. [68] found smaller mPFC cortical thickness in trans men compared to *both* cisgender males and females, and Spizzirí et al. [65] reported on *sex-typical* volumes of this region in oestradiol-treated TGD women. Thus, future studies comparing larger samples of treatment-naïve individuals with GI should investigate how regional grey matter volumes differ as a function of sex and gender identity, and how structural alterations relate to differences in brain function.

One of the first studies investigating differences in *functional* brain sexual differentiation in TGD youth was conducted by Soleman et al. in Cohort 1 [69]. A verbal-fluency fMRI paradigm, for which sex differences in performance favouring birth-assigned females had been reported [70], was used to compare 8 TGD girls (male sex assigned at birth, female gender identity) and 14 TGD boys (female sex assigned at birth, male gender identity), all treatment-naïve, to 25 male and 26 female cisgender controls. Group comparisons revealed significantly stronger brain activation in cis boys than in cis girls in the right rolandic operculum, suggesting increased use of verbalization in cisgender males [71]. Interestingly, in the TGD groups, differences in activation only reached trend level (TGD girls > TGD boys), suggesting less pronounced sexual differentiation of verbal-fluency processes.

Using an innovative olfactory fMRI paradigm, including the participants of Cohort 2, sex differences in neural responses of the hypothalamus were triggered by exposure to the putative human pheromone odour *androstadienone* [72]. The older, adolescent group (receiving GnRHa) was found to respond remarkably like their experienced gender, thus sex-*a*typical. A similar finding was previously reported in adult TGD women [73], suggesting a different, even sex-reversed sexual differentiation of this specific brain function among TGD individuals. However, whereas significant sex differences in activation were observed in the cisgender pre-pubertal children, their TGD peers showed responses that were either sex-typical (TGD girls) or not distinguishable from either of the two control groups (TGD boys).

In the most recent fMRI study, also including the participants of Cohort 2, Nota et al. [74] investigated sex assigned at birth (male versus female) and gender identity (cis- versus transgender) differences in resting state functional brain connectivity, that is, temporal correlations of fluctuations of the blood-oxygen-level-dependent (BOLD) signal among spatially distributed brain regions [71, 72]. Such intrinsic connectivity networks at rest have been found to be associated with behaviour and to represent distinct functional systems [75]. For example, the widely studied *Default Mode Network* (DMN) has been found to be implicated in mind-wandering and self-referential thinking [76–78]. A different processing of self has only recently been suggested as an alternative neurobiological explanation of GI [68, 79–81], and sex differences in functional connectivity networks have been reported [82, 83].

A comparison of the adolescent sub-samples revealed cisgender sex differences in functional connectivity within the sensory motor network (SMN) and the DMN, with sex-atypical (i.e. in line with their gender identity) functional connectivity patterns in these networks in both TGD girls (DMN and SMN) and boys (SMN). Of note, the adolescent TGD girls also showed a singular pattern of activation with stronger intrinsic connectivity within the visual network, compared to the three other groups (TGD boys, cisgender girls, cisgender boys). This finding was interpreted as a first hint towards transgender-specific alterations of brain functions, thus beyond the hypothesized difference from the cisgender sexual dimorphism. Furthermore, in the young sub-sample no significant group differences were found.

These age-specific findings in two different fMRI paradigms (olfactory and resting state) allow for alternative possible explanations. First, in line with the notion that the period of early adolescence seems decisive with regard to gender identity development [45, 46], it may be that (neuro-)developmental processes (including further neural sexual differentiation) during early adolescence are needed for the sex-*a*typical brain activation pattern to be expressed or activated. Second, it is possible that the sex-*a*typical responses in TGD adolescents might be related to their puberty-suppression treatment [84]. However, given that in another study (involving participants of Cohort 1), those receiving GnRHa showed even exaggerated sex-typical brain activations [85], this possibility does not seem very likely. A third explanation may be that the younger, pre-pubertal sample was more pluripotent with regard to future developmental trajectories of their gender identity. The few longitudinal studies that allow estimations on the development of GI found that the majority of children with GI do not continue to experience GI and start puberty suppression in adolescence [86–88]. Future (follow-up) studies should therefore aim to address the unanswered question of what neurobiological mechanisms characterize and explain childhood GI.

Effects of Hormone Treatment

It has been suggested that puberty suppression could interfere with significant developmental brain changes, particularly within the prefrontal cortex, which underlie adolescence-specific changes in behaviour [89]. Examining participants from Cohort 1, investigators assessed the effects of GnRHa on executive function. This study compared TGD youth, receiving GnRHa treatment, with treatment-naïve TGD adolescents [85], and cisgender groups. Participants performed an fMRI version of the Tower of London task, indexing executive functioning. No differences in performance were found between treated and treatment-naïve TGD groups. Whereas the treatment-naïve TGD adolescents showed *sex-atypical* activations, the GnRHa-treated groups showed *sex-typical* patterns of task-related brain activation (in precuneus, dorso-lateral PFC). Though surprising, this finding of, even exaggerated, sex-typical brain functions is in line with a previous study in GnRHa-treated sheep [90].

In a recent case study of an 11-year-old trans girl (male birth-assigned sex), cognitive functions and changes in diffusion measures of white matter microstructure (indexing myelination, axonal diameter and white matter integrity, which all contribute to efficient information transfer) were assessed before initiation of GnRHa treatment and during two follow-up measurements at 13 and 14 years of age, respectively [91]. Performance intelligence quotient and memory deteriorated with treatment, and normative, testosterone-dependent white matter maturation (increase in diffusion parameters) was not observed. This study, although only for a single case, thus suggested long-term adverse effects of GnRHa on neurodevelopment and cognitive capacities. However, these findings require replication in larger samples and warrant special attention in upcoming studies.

Even though neuroimaging studies in TGD individuals have started to accumulate evidence on the effects of cross-sex hormonal treatments on brain functions and structure, knowledge on the effects of these treatments remains limited, especially in

TGD youth. In their study on regional brain volume differences between trans- and cisgender youth (Cohort 1), Hoekzema et al. [67] found that hypothalamus volumes in a mixed sample of treatment-naïve and hormone-treated TGD girls (N = 12 received cross-sex hormones) tended to be sex-*a*typical, thus smaller than in cisgender boys. This finding was in line with a prior study in TGD women, which showed a significant decrease in hypothalamus volume after having received oestradiol and anti-androgen treatment for 3 months [92]. Similarly, another study in TGD women reported on a general decrease of cortical thickness and subcortical volumes with oestradiol plus anti-androgen treatment [60]. Of note, given that the TGD female participants in all three studies had received both anti-androgen *and* oestradiol treatment, it is impossible to discern whether the observed effects on brain structure can be ascribed to the suppression of endogenous hormone production or to the addition of oestradiol. These studies, however, have major limitations of small sample sizes and cross-sectional study design. Furthermore, the clinical significance of these volumetric differences is unclear. Future research is needed in this regard.

Thus far, only one *longitudinal* study investigated cross-sex hormone treatment effects on spatial cognition, measured with an fMRI mental rotation task, in gender-incongruent youth (adolescent sub-sample of Cohort 2) [93]. Previously reported robust sex differences in performance (accuracy, reaction times) favouring birth-assigned males [94, 95] and sex differences in brain activation [96, 97] suggested that birth-assigned males and females use different strategies during mental rotation. Accordingly, cisgender girls were found to show stronger activations in the precuneus and precentral gyrus compared to cisgender boys. Interestingly, TGD boys differed significantly from the cisgender girls, but showed activation patterns comparable to those of the cisgender boys, thus suggesting sex-*a*typical spatial functioning. During a follow-up, 10 months after the TGD boys had initiated testosterone treatment, they showed significantly increased activation during mental rotation (in superior parietal, superior frontal cortex) relative to the previous session (under GnRHa), similar to the cisgender boys, and significantly different from the cisgender girls (who showed no changes between sessions). These findings in youth are generally in line with two fMRI studies in adult TGD men. Sommer et al. [98] found a trend for testosterone-related increases in brain activations during mental rotation, and Burke et al. [81] reported on significant changes in cortical thickness and functional connectivity that were associated with treatment-related changes in self- and own-body perception.

Gaps of Knowledge and Future Directions

First, with regard to the influence of genetic factors in the development of gender incongruence, the hypothesis that gender identity is a complex trait that results from a combination of multiple genetic and environmental factors with a heritable polygenic component [9] deserves further study. An interesting observation was that twin studies on gender role behaviour [11] and GI [15] suggest higher heritability estimates for birth-assigned girls than for birth-assigned boys. On the other hand, a study investigating click-evoked otoacoustic emissions as a retrospective marker of perinatal androgen exposure found sex-typical emission strengths in birth-assigned girls with GI (7–16 years old), but sex-*a*typical in birth-assigned boys with GI (6–14 years old) [99]. These seemingly opposing findings may suggest that genetic factors and early hormonal influences weigh in differently for the two sexes in their contribution of the development of gender identity, gender role behaviour and also GI. Further work is needed to better understand whether and how the developmental trajectories of gender identity are different between TGD boys and girls.

We have seen that the studies in TGD adolescents show indications of sex-*a*typical (with regard to sex assigned at birth) patterns in several neuroimaging measures and demonstrate neurobiological patterns that are more in line with their identified TGD identity. However, for pre-pubertal TGD children this picture is less clear.

Neuroimaging studies in TGD adults point to a difference in neurobiological correlates as a function of sexual orientation (e.g. gynephilic versus androphilic trans women) [18] and for sexual orientation as a contributor to the sex-atypical findings in TGD individuals [100]. In the two large MRI projects in youth with GI thus far, the TGD groups differed from the cisgender comparison group (of the same at birth-assigned sex) not only in terms of gender identity but also in terms of sexual orientation. Given this limitation of the study design, it is possible that some of the differences in MRI findings were related to sexual orientation rather than gender identity. Future studies should therefore include control groups with various sexual orientations to clarify this aspect.

Recent neuroimaging findings provide tentative evidence for different own-body perception and altered underlying neural networks as alternative explanation for the body dysphoria experienced by TGD individuals [68, 79–81, 100, 101]. However, all these studies thus far included adult participants, and no study has examined the 'own-body perception hypothesis' in pre-pubertal and/or post-pubertal TGD youth. Given that the distress resulting from physical changes due to puberty was indicated as one important factor for future continuation of GI [46], it may be worthwhile for future studies to investigate the underlying mechanisms of a different body image development *in interaction* with less pronounced brain sexual differentiation in TGD adolescents.

Although the studies in TGD children and adolescents thus far have revealed some interesting findings, they all originate from one research centre and replication studies from other centres are urgently needed. Also, knowledge on the long-term effects of GnRHa treatment and cross-sex hormones on the brain is very limited, and systematic studies in larger, representative samples are currently lacking, partly due to the relatively recent introduction of these interventions in TGD adolescents.

Despite evidence of improvement in anxiety, depression and self-harm among TGD adolescents who receive these treatments [102, 103], the long-term effects of, in particular, GnRHa treatment in physically healthy young adolescents are unclear. Longitudinal evidence does exist, but only from studies in girls with idiopathic central precocious puberty, studies in healthy adult cisgender women and studies in animal models (sheep). Some of these studies have suggested adverse effects of GnRHa treatment on general intelligence [104, 105], information processing speed [106], emotion regulation [90, 107], reward-processing and associated amygdala reactivity [108], spatial memory performance in sheep [109, 110], sex-specific (stronger in female sheep) effects on structural brain development [111] and regulation of gene expression in the sheep amygdala [112]. However, others found no differences between GnRHa-treated and treatment-naïve comparison groups for measures of spatial orientation [90], cognition and psychosocial functioning [107], but see [105] for a critical commentary.

Importantly, it should be acknowledged that withholding GnRHa treatment would be harmful to the psychological developmental of TGD youth, for example, due to the risk of stigmatization and living with prolonged distress [53]. Because such studies in TGD youth are still lacking, it is therefore critical to continue the study of the effects of puberty suppression in TGD youth on brain development, and to examine the effects on TGD adolescents' cognitive and socio-emotional functioning. Follow-up studies in the two cohorts that have been studied thus far during adulthood are highly recommended.

One should be aware that neuroimaging findings may reflect mechanisms that causally relate to gender incongruence, but may also be a result of the experience of living with an identity that is not typically congruent with their assigned sex at birth. In addition, studies thus far have investigated neurobiological correlates and descriptions of TGD anatomy and brain function on a group level. Therefore, MRI measures are not an appropriate tool to use diagnostically to, for example, confirm or exclude gender incongruence in a specific individual. Nevertheless, MRI has been proven to be informative to clinical and academic communities alike with regard to the existence and the aetiological factors underlying gender identity and -diversity. We are far from revealing a single neurobiological pattern that fully describes TGD neurobiology. Based on the current state of knowledge, it is more conceivable that there is no single distinctive neurobiological signature for gender incongruence at all. It remains an empirical question to what degree gender identity development is 'preprogrammed' (genetic, early hormonal influences) and what the relative contribution of environmental factors is. For understanding how to better serve our TGD youth, we should continue the search for neurobiological correlates of gender identity and gender diversity, as this will ultimately help to better characterize the cognitive and emotional needs of TGD youth and provide them with the best individualized-care approach.

Editorial Disclaimer This chapter describes a summary of the literature in this area by experts in the field, and conclusions drawn reflect the views of the authors, not the editors.

References

1. World Health Organization. International classification of diseases. 11th ed. Geneva: Author; 2018.
2. Heylens G, De Cuypere G, Zucker KJ, Schelfaut C, Elaut E, Vanden Bossche H, De Baere E, T'Sjoen G. Gender identity disorder in twins: a review of the case report literature. J Sex Med. 2012;9:751–7.

3. Fernández R, Esteva I, Gómez-Gil E, Rumbo T, Almaraz MC, Roda E, Haro-Mora J-J, Guillamón A, Pásaro E. The (CA)n polymorphism of ERβ gene is associated with FtM transsexualism. J Sex Med. 2014;11:720–8.
4. Ujike H, Otani K, Nakatsuka M, et al. Association study of gender identity disorder and sex hormone-related genes. Prog Neuro-Psychopharmacol Biol Psychiatry. 2009;33:1241–4.
5. Hare L, Bernard P, Sánchez FJ, Baird PN, Vilain E, Kennedy T, Harley VR. Androgen receptor repeat length polymorphism associated with male-to-female transsexualism. Biol Psychiatry. 2009;65:93–6.
6. Fernández R, Esteva I, Gómez-Gil E, Rumbo T, Almaraz MC, Roda E, Haro-Mora J-J, Guillamón A, Pásaro E. Association study of ERβ, AR, and CYP19A1 genes and MtF transsexualism. J Sex Med. 2014;11:2986–94.
7. Henningsson S, Westberg L, Nilsson S, et al. Sex steroid-related genes and male-to-female transsexualism. Psychoneuroendocrinology. 2005;30:657–64.
8. Fernández R, Guillamon A, Cortés-Cortés J, Gómez-Gil E, Jácome A, Esteva I, Almaraz M, Mora M, Aranda G, Pásaro E. Molecular basis of gender dysphoria: androgen and estrogen receptor interaction. Psychoneuroendocrinology. 2018;98:161–7.
9. Polderman TJC, Kreukels BPC, Irwig MS, et al. The biological contributions to gender identity and gender diversity: bringing data to the table. Behav Genet. 2018;48:95–108.
10. Iervolino AC, Hines M, Golombok SE, Rust J, Plomin R. Genetic and environmental influences on sex-typed behavior during the preschool years. Child Dev. 2005;76:826–40.
11. Knafo A, Iervolino AC, Plomin R. Masculine girls and feminine boys: genetic and environmental contributions to atypical gender development in early childhood. J Pers Soc Psychol. 2005;88:400–12.
12. van Beijsterveldt CEM, Hudziak JJ, Boomsma DI. Genetic and environmental influences on cross-gender behavior and relation to behavior problems: a study of Dutch twins at ages 7 and 10 years. Arch Sex Behav. 2006;35:647–58.
13. Coolidge FL, Thede LL, Young SE. The heritability of gender identity disorder in a child and adolescent twin sample. Behav Genet. 2002;32:251–7.
14. Association AP. Diagnostic and statistical manual of mental disorders. 4th ed., text rev. Washington, DC: Author; 2000.
15. Sasaki S, Ozaki K, Yamagata S, Takahashi Y, Shikishima C, Kornacki T, Nonaka K, Ando J. Genetic and environmental influences on traits of gender identity disorder: a study of Japanese twins across developmental stages. Arch Sex Behav. 2016;45:1681–95.
16. Association AP. Diagnostic and statistical manual of mental disorders. 5th ed. Arlington: American Psychiatric Publishing; 2013.
17. Phoenix CH, Goy RW, Gerall AA, Young WC. Organizing action of prenatally administered testosterone propionate on the tissues mediating mating behavior in the female guinea pig. Endocrinology. 1959;65:369–82.
18. Kreukels BPC, Guillamon A. Neuroimaging studies in people with gender incongruence. Int Rev Psychiatry. 2016;28:120–8.
19. Bakker J. Sex differentiation: organizing effects of sex hormones. Gend Dysphoria Disord Sex Dev. 2014; https://doi.org/10.1007/978-1-4614-7441-8.
20. Hines M. Prenatal endocrine influences on sexual orientation and on sexually differentiated childhood behavior. Front Neuroendocrinol. 2011;32:170–82.
21. de Vries ALC, Doreleijers TAH, Cohen-Kettenis PT. Disorders of sex development and gender identity outcome in adolescence and adulthood: understanding gender identity development and its clinical implications. Pediatr Endocrinol Rev. 2007;4:343–51.
22. Jordan-Young RM. Hormones, context, and 'brain gender': a review of evidence from congenital adrenal hyperplasia. Soc Sci Med. 2012;74:1738–44.
23. Bakker J. The sexual differentiation of the human brain: role of sex hormones versus sex chromosomes. Curr Top Behav Neurosci. 2019; https://doi.org/10.1007/7854_2018_70.
24. Zhou J-NN, Hofman MA, Gooren LJG, Swaab DF. A sex difference in the human brain and its relation to transsexuality. Nature. 1995;378:68–70.

25. Kruijver FPM, Zhou JN, Pool CW, Hofman MA, Gooren LJ, Swaab DF. Male-to-female transsexuals have female neuron numbers in a limbic nucleus. J Clin Endocrinol Metab. 2000;85:2034–41.
26. Garcia-Falgueras A, Swaab DF. A sex difference in the hypothalamic uncinate nucleus: relationship to gender identity. Brain. 2008;131:3132–46.
27. Taziaux M, Swaab DF, Bakker J. Sex differences in the neurokinin B system in the human infundibular nucleus. J Clin Endocrinol Metab. 2012;97:E2210–20.
28. Dörner G. Neuroendocrine response to estrogen and brain differentiation in heterosexuals, homosexuals, and transsexuals. Arch Sex Behav. 1988;17:57–75.
29. Swaab DF, Hofman MA. Sexual differentiation of the human hypothalamus in relation to gender and sexual orientation. Trends Neurosci. 1995;18:264–70.
30. Swaab DF, Garcia-Falgueras A. Sexual differentiation of the human brain in relation to gender identity and sexual orientation. Funct Neurol. 2009;24:17–28.
31. Steensma TD, Kreukels BPC, de Vries ALC, Cohen-Kettenis PT. Gender identity development in adolescence. Horm Behav. 2013;64:288–97.
32. Sisk C, Doncarlos L. Puberty and brain sexual differentiation: getting organized. 2011. https://www.fasebj.org/doi/abs/10.1096/fasebj.25.1_supplement.187.4
33. McCarthy MM, Arnold AP. Reframing sexual differentiation of the brain. Nat Neurosci. 2011;14:677–83.
34. Ahmed EI, Zehr JL, Schulz KM, Lorenz BH, DonCarlos LL, Sisk CL. Pubertal hormones modulate the addition of new cells to sexually dimorphic brain regions. Nat Neurosci. 2008;11:995–7.
35. Schulz KM, Sisk CL. The organizing actions of adolescent gonadal steroid hormones on brain and behavioral development. Neurosci Biobehav Rev. 2016;70:148–58.
36. Vijayakumar N, Allen NB, Youssef G, Dennison M, Yücel M, Simmons JG, Whittle S. Brain development during adolescence: a mixed-longitudinal investigation of cortical thickness, surface area, and volume. Hum Brain Mapp. 2016;37:2027–38.
37. Wierenga LM, Bos MGN, Schreuders E, Vd Kamp F, Peper JS, Tamnes CK, Crone EA. Unraveling age, puberty and testosterone effects on subcortical brain development across adolescence. Psychoneuroendocrinology. 2018;91:105–14.
38. Giedd JN, Raznahan A, Mills K, Lenroot RK. Review: magnetic resonance imaging of male/female differences in human adolescent brain anatomy. Biol Sex Differ. 2012;3:19.
39. Pfeifer JH, Peake SJ. Self-development: integrating cognitive, socioemotional, and neuroimaging perspectives. Dev Cogn Neurosci. 2012;2:55–69.
40. Mills KL, Lalonde F, Clasen LS, Giedd JN, Blakemore SJ. Developmental changes in the structure of the social brain in late childhood and adolescence. Soc Cogn Affect Neurosci. 2014;9:123–31.
41. Blakemore S-J. The social brain in adolescence. Nat Rev Neurosci. 2008;9:267–77.
42. Choudhury S, Blakemore S-J, Charman T. Social cognitive development during adolescence. Soc Cogn Affect Neurosci. 2006;1:165–74.
43. Selman RL. The growth of interpersonal understanding: developmental and clinical analyses. New York: Academic Press; 1980.
44. Harter S. The construction of the self: a developmental perspective. New York: Guilford Press; 1999.
45. Steensma TD, McGuire JK, Kreukels BPC, Beekman AJ, Cohen-Kettenis PT. Factors associated with desistence and persistence of childhood gender dysphoria: a quantitative follow-up study. J Am Acad Child Adolesc Psychiatry. 2013;52:582–90.
46. Steensma TD, Biemond R, de Boer F, Cohen-Kettenis PT. Desisting and persisting gender dysphoria after childhood: a qualitative follow-up study. Clin Child Psychol Psychiatry. 2011;16:499–516.
47. de Graaf NM, Cohen-Kettenis PT, Carmichael P, de Vries ALC, Dhondt K, Laridaen J, Pauli D, Ball J, Steensma TD. Psychological functioning in adolescents referred to specialist gender identity clinics across Europe: a clinical comparison study between four clinics. Eur Child Adolesc Psychiatry. 2018;27:909–19.

48. Kaltiala-Heino R, Sumia M, Työläjärvi M, Lindberg N. Two years of gender identity service for minors: overrepresentation of natal girls with severe problems in adolescent development. Child Adolesc Psychiatry Ment Health. 2015;9:9.
49. Olson J, Schrager SM, Belzer M, Simons LK, Clark LF. Baseline physiologic and psychosocial characteristics of transgender youth seeking care for gender dysphoria. J Adolesc Health. 2015;57:374–80.
50. Temple Newhook J, Pyne J, Winters K, Feder S, Holmes C, Tosh J, Sinnott M-L, Jamieson A, Pickett S. A critical commentary on follow-up studies and 'desistance' theories about transgender and gender-nonconforming children. Int J Transgend. 2018;19:212–24.
51. Zucker KJ. The myth of persistence: response to 'a critical commentary on follow-up studies and 'desistance' theories about transgender and gender non-conforming children' by Temple Newhook et al. (2018). Int J Transgend. 2018;19:231–45.
52. Steensma TD, Cohen-Kettenis PT. A critical commentary on 'a critical commentary on follow-up studies and 'desistence' theories about transgender and gender non-conforming children'. Int J Transgend. 2018;19:225–30.
53. Kreukels BPC, Cohen-Kettenis PT. Puberty suppression in gender identity disorder: the Amsterdam experience. Nat Rev Endocrinol. 2011;7:466–72.
54. Smith KP, Madison CM, Milne NM. Gonadal suppressive and cross-sex hormone therapy for gender dysphoria in adolescents and adults. Pharmacotherapy. 2014;34:1282–97.
55. Dhejne C, Van Vlerken R, Heylens G, Arcelus J. Mental health and gender dysphoria: a review of the literature. Int Rev Psychiatry. 2016;28:44–57.
56. Gómez-Gil E, Zubiaurre-Elorza L, Esteva I, Guillamon A, Godás T, Cruz Almaraz M, Halperin I, Salamero M. Hormone-treated transsexuals report less social distress, anxiety and depression. Psychoneuroendocrinology. 2012;37:662–70.
57. Rametti G, Carrillo B, Gomez-Gil E, Junque C, Segovia S, Gomez A, Guillamon A. White matter microstructure in female to male transsexuals before cross-sex hormonal treatment. A diffusion tensor imaging study. J Psychiatr Res. 2011;45:199–204.
58. Rametti G, Carrillo B, Gómez-Gil E, Junque C, Zubiarre-Elorza L, Segovia S, Gomez Á, Guillamon A. The microstructure of white matter in male to female transsexuals before cross-sex hormonal treatment. A DTI study. J Psychiatr Res. 2011;45:949–54.
59. Hahn A, Kranz GS, Küblböck M, et al. Structural connectivity networks of transgender people. Cereb Cortex. 2015;25:3527–34.
60. Zubiaurre-Elorza L, Junque C, Gómez-Gil E, Guillamon A. Effects of cross-sex hormone treatment on cortical thickness in transsexual individuals. J Sex Med. 2014;11:1248–61.
61. Zubiaurre-Elorza L, Junque C, Gómez-Gil E, Segovia S, Carrillo B, Rametti G, Guillamon A. Cortical thickness in untreated transsexuals. Cereb Cortex. 2013;23:2855–62.
62. Simon L, Kozák LR, Simon V, Czobor P, Unoka Z, Szabó A, Csukly G. Regional grey matter structure differences between transsexuals and healthy controls-a voxel based morphometry study. PLoS One. 2013;8:e83947.
63. Luders E, Sánchez FJ, Gaser C, Toga AW, Narr KL, Hamilton LS, Vilain E. Regional gray matter variation in male-to-female transsexualism. NeuroImage. 2009;46:904–7.
64. Savic I, Arver S. Sex dimorphism of the brain in male-to-female transsexuals. Cereb Cortex. 2011;21:2525–33.
65. Spizzirri G, Duran FLS, Chaim-Avancini TM, et al. Grey and white matter volumes either in treatment-naïve or hormone-treated transgender women: a voxel-based morphometry study. Sci Rep. 2018;8:736.
66. Kim T-H, Kim S-K, Jeong G-W. Cerebral gray matter volume variation in female-to-male transsexuals: a voxel-based morphometric study. Neuroreport. 2015;26:1119–25.
67. Hoekzema E, Schagen SEE, Kreukels BPC, Veltman DJ, Cohen-Kettenis PT, Delemarre-van de Waal H, Bakker J. Regional volumes and spatial volumetric distribution of gray matter in the gender dysphoric brain. Psychoneuroendocrinology. 2015;55:59–71.
68. Manzouri A, Kosidou K, Savic I. Anatomical and functional findings in female-to-male transsexuals: testing a new hypothesis. Cereb Cortex. 2015;27(2):998–1010.

69. Soleman RS, Schagen SEE, Veltman DJ, Kreukels BPC, Cohen-Kettenis PT, Lambalk CB, Wouters F, Delemarre-van de Waal HA. Sex differences in verbal fluency during adolescence: a functional magnetic resonance imaging study in gender dysphoric and control boys and girls. J Sex Med. 2013;10:1969–77.
70. Bolla KI, Lindgren KN, Bonaccorsy C, Bleecker ML. Predictors of verbal fluency (FAS) in the healthy elderly. J Clin Psychol. 1990;46:623–8.
71. Zarnhofer S, Braunstein V, Ebner F, Koschutnig K, Neuper C, Reishofer G, Ischebeck A. The influence of verbalization on the pattern of cortical activation during mental arithmetic. Behav Brain Funct. 2012;8:13.
72. Burke SM, Cohen-Kettenis PT, Veltman DJ, Klink DT, Bakker J. Hypothalamic response to the chemo-signal androstadienone in gender dysphoric children and adolescents. Front Endocrinol (Lausanne). 2014;5:60.
73. Berglund H, Lindström P, Dhejne-Helmy C, Savic I. Male-to-female transsexuals show sex-atypical hypothalamus activation when smelling odorous steroids. Cereb Cortex. 2008;18:1900–8.
74. Nota NM, Kreukels BPC, den Heijer M, Veltman DJ, Cohen-Kettenis PT, Burke SM, Bakker J. Brain functional connectivity patterns in children and adolescents with gender dysphoria: sex-atypical or not? Psychoneuroendocrinology. 2017;86:187–95.
75. Cole MW, Bassett DS, Power JD, Braver TS, Petersen SE. Intrinsic and task-evoked network architectures of the human brain. Neuron. 2014;83:238–51.
76. Fair DA, Cohen AL, Dosenbach NUF, Church JA, Miezin FM, Barch DM, Raichle ME, Petersen SE, Schlaggar BL. The maturing architecture of the brain's default network. Proc Natl Acad Sci U S A. 2008;105:4028–32.
77. Whitfield-Gabrieli S, Moran JM, Nieto-Castañón A, Triantafyllou C, Saxe R, Gabrieli JDE. Associations and dissociations between default and self-reference networks in the human brain. NeuroImage. 2011;55:225–32.
78. Northoff G, Bermpohl F. Cortical midline structures and the self. Trends Cogn Sci. 2004;8:102–7.
79. Feusner JD, Dervisic J, Kosidou K, Dhejne C, Bookheimer S, Savic I. Female-to-male transsexual individuals demonstrate different own body identification. Arch Sex Behav. 2016;45:525–36.
80. Feusner JD, Lidström A, Moody TD, Dhejne C, Bookheimer SY, Savic I. Intrinsic network connectivity and own body perception in gender dysphoria. Brain Imaging Behav. 2016;11:964. https://doi.org/10.1007/s11682-016-9578-6.
81. Burke SM, Manzouri AH, Dhejne C, Bergström K, Arver S, Feusner JD, Savic-Berglund I. Testosterone effects on the brain in transgender men. Cereb Cortex. 2018;28:1582–96.
82. Hjelmervik H, Hausmann M, Osnes B, Westerhausen R, Specht K. Resting states are resting traits–an FMRI study of sex differences and menstrual cycle effects in resting state cognitive control networks. PLoS One. 2014;9:e103492.
83. Scheinost D, Finn ES, Tokoglu F, Shen X, Papademetris X, Hampson M, Constable RT. Sex differences in normal age trajectories of functional brain networks. Hum Brain Mapp. 2015;36:1524–35.
84. Berenbaum SA, Beltz AM. Sexual differentiation of human behavior: effects of prenatal and pubertal organizational hormones. Front Neuroendocrinol. 2011;32:183–200.
85. Staphorsius AS, Kreukels BPC, Cohen-Kettenis PT, Veltman DJ, Burke SM, Schagen SEE, Wouters FM, Delemarre-van de Waal HA, Bakker J. Puberty suppression and executive functioning: an fMRI-study in adolescents with gender dysphoria. Psychoneuroendocrinology. 2015;56:190–9.
86. Wiepjes CM, Nota NM, de Blok CJM, et al. The Amsterdam cohort of gender dysphoria study (1972–2015): trends in prevalence, treatment, and regrets. J Sex Med. 2018;15:582–90.
87. Wallien MSC, Cohen-Kettenis PT. Psychosexual outcome of gender-dysphoric children. J Am Acad Child Adolesc Psychiatry. 2008;47:1413–23.
88. Ristori J, Steensma TD. Gender dysphoria in childhood. Int Rev Psychiatry. 2016;28:13–20.

89. Juraska JM, Willing J. Pubertal onset as a critical transition for neural development and cognition. Brain Res. 2017;1654:87–94.
90. Wojniusz S, Vögele C, Ropstad E, et al. Prepubertal gonadotropin-releasing hormone analog leads to exaggerated behavioral and emotional sex differences in sheep. Horm Behav. 2011;59:22–7.
91. Schneider MA, Spritzer PM, Soll BMB, et al. Brain maturation, cognition and voice pattern in a gender dysphoria case under pubertal suppression. Front Hum Neurosci. 2017;11:528.
92. Hulshoff Pol EH, Cohen-Kettenis PT, Van Haren NEM, Peper JS, Brans RGH, Cahn W, Schnack HG, Gooren LJG, Kahn RS. Changing your sex changes your brain: influences of testosterone and estrogen on adult human brain structure. Eur J Endocrinol. 2006;155:S107–14.
93. Burke SM, Kreukels BPC, Cohen-Kettenis PT, Veltman DJ, Klink DT, Bakker J. Male-typical visuospatial functioning in gynephilic girls with gender dysphoria — organizational and activational effects of testosterone. J Psychiatry Neurosci. 2016;41:395–404.
94. Linn MC, Petersen AC. Emergence and characterization of sex differences in spatial ability: a meta-analysis. Child Dev. 1985;56:1479–98.
95. Voyer D, Voyer S, Bryden MP. Magnitude of sex differences in spatial abilities: a meta-analysis and consideration of critical variables. Psychol Bull. 1995;117:250–70.
96. Jordan K, Wüstenberg T, Heinze HJ, Peters M, Jäncke L. Women and men exhibit different cortical activation patterns during mental rotation tasks. Neuropsychologia. 2002;40:2397–408.
97. Hugdahl K, Thomsen T, Ersland L. Sex differences in visuo-spatial processing: an fMRI study of mental rotation. Neuropsychologia. 2006;44:1575–83.
98. Sommer IEC, Cohen-Kettenis PT, van Raalten T, Vd Veer AJ, Ramsey LE, Gooren LJG, Kahn RS, Ramsey NF. Effects of cross-sex hormones on cerebral activation during language and mental rotation: an fMRI study in transsexuals. Eur Neuropsychopharmacol. 2008;18:215–21.
99. Burke SM, Menks WM, Cohen-Kettenis PT, Klink DT, Bakker J. Click-evoked otoacoustic emissions in children and adolescents with gender identity disorder. Arch Sex Behav. 2014;43:1515–23.
100. Burke SM, Manzouri AH, Savic I. Structural connections in the brain in relation to gender identity and sexual orientation. Sci Rep. 2017;7:17954.
101. Manzouri A, Savic I. Possible neurobiological underpinnings of homosexuality and gender dysphoria. Cereb Cortex. 2019;29(5):2084–101.
102. Cohen-Kettenis PT, Schagen SEE, Steensma TD, de Vries ALC, Delemarre-van de Waal HA. Puberty suppression in a gender-dysphoric adolescent: a 22-year follow-up. Arch Sex Behav. 2011;40:843–7.
103. de Vries ALC, McGuire JK, Steensma TD, Wagenaar ECF, Doreleijers T a H, Cohen-Kettenis PT. Young adult psychological outcome after puberty suppression and gender reassignment. Pediatrics. 2014;134:696–704.
104. Mul D, Versluis-den Bieman H, Slijper F, Oostdijk W, Waelkens J, Drop S. Psychological assessments before and after treatment of early puberty in adopted children. Acta Paediatr. 2007;90:965–71.
105. Hayes P. Commentary: cognitive, emotional, and psychosocial functioning of girls treated with pharmacological puberty blockage for idiopathic central precocious puberty. Front Psychol. 2017;8:44.
106. Stenbæk DS, Fisher PM, Budtz-Jørgensen E, Pinborg A, Hjordt LV, Jensen PS, Knudsen GM, Frokjaer VG. Sex hormone manipulation slows reaction time and increases labile mood in healthy women. Psychoneuroendocrinology. 2016;68:39–46.
107. Wojniusz S, Callens N, Sütterlin S, et al. Cognitive, emotional, and psychosocial functioning of girls treated with pharmacological puberty blockage for idiopathic central precocious puberty. Front Psychol. 2016;7:1053.
108. Macoveanu J, Henningsson S, Pinborg A, Jensen P, Knudsen GM, Frokjaer VG, Siebner HR. Sex-steroid hormone manipulation reduces brain response to reward. Neuropsychopharmacology. 2016;41:1057–65.

109. Hough D, Bellingham M, Haraldsen IR, McLaughlin M, Robinson JE, Solbakk AK, Evans NP. A reduction in long-term spatial memory persists after discontinuation of peripubertal GnRH agonist treatment in sheep. Psychoneuroendocrinology. 2017;77:1–8.
110. Hough D, Bellingham M, Haraldsen IRH, McLaughlin M, Rennie M, Robinson JE, Solbakk AK, Evans NP. Spatial memory is impaired by peripubertal GnRH agonist treatment and testosterone replacement in sheep. Psychoneuroendocrinology. 2017;75:173–82.
111. Nuruddin S, Bruchhage M, Ropstad E, Krogenæs A, Evans NP, Robinson JE, Endestad T, Westlye LT, Madison C, Haraldsen IRH. Effects of peripubertal gonadotropin-releasing hormone agonist on brain development in sheep–a magnetic resonance imaging study. Psychoneuroendocrinology. 2013;38:1994–2002.
112. Nuruddin S, Krogenæs A, Brynildsrud OB, Verhaegen S, Evans NP, Robinson JE, Haraldsen IRH, Ropstad E. Peri-pubertal gonadotropin-releasing hormone agonist treatment affects sex biased gene expression of amygdala in sheep. Psychoneuroendocrinology. 2013;38:3115–27.

Minority Stress and the Impact of Acceptance

5

Christy L. Olezeski and Wendy P. Bamatter

Introduction

The aim of this chapter is to discuss the relationship between the experience of minority stress and acceptance and the health outcomes of transgender and gender diverse (TGD) youth. We discuss the components of a minority stress model, the expansion of this model to include TGD identities, and the risk and protective factors associated with support (or lack thereof) by parents, schools, peers, and medical and mental health providers. We also include strategies to enhance support and related protective factors with regard to each of these subgroups.

Minority Stress

Social stress is a form of stress related to social processes in the environment. Experiences with stigma, prejudice, and discrimination are among the most prominent examples of social stress that disproportionately affect those who fall into a minority group. Scholars have turned to social stress theory to advance collective knowledge regarding the contributing factors impacting elevated rates of psychological distress among lesbian, gay, bisexual, transgender, queer/questioning, plus (LGBTQ+) individuals, as compared to heterosexual and/or cisgender individuals. In 2003, Meyer published a seminal paper in which he introduced a theoretical framework, termed the *minority stress model*, wherein he outlined a number of factors that predict elevated rates of psychological distress among lesbian, gay, and

C. L. Olezeski (✉)
Yale School of Medicine, Department of Psychiatry, New Haven, CT, USA
e-mail: christy.olezeski@yale.edu

W. P. Bamatter
McLean Hospital, Belmont, MA, USA
e-mail: wbamatter@partners.org

M. Forcier et al. (eds.), *Pediatric Gender Identity*,
https://doi.org/10.1007/978-3-030-38909-3_5

bisexual (LGB) communities, all within the context of attending to minority stress processes [1]. The model highlights different types of social stress and coping processes and their impacts on LGB communities. Meyer's model fostered a new narrative that stands in contrast with outdated theories positing that LGB individuals have greater levels of mental illness due to innate qualities associated with *homosexuality* – also an antiquated term.

Minority stress is characterized by at least three factors: (1) it is unique to minority communities and exists above and beyond stressors experienced by most members of society, (2) it is chronic, and (3) it is dictated by social forces [1]. Meyer draws from research to identify both proximal and distal stress processes, as well as coping factors, that can impact mental health outcomes in LGB communities. The distal or external objective events and factors include various forms of discriminatory events (e.g., being called derogatory names, hate crimes). The proximal or subjectively focused factors depend on attention and cognitive appraisal. Since the development of the minority stress model, myriad studies have been published supporting the model and highlighting the positive correlation between the distal and proximal minority stress factors and mental health challenges in the LGB community.

A growing number of researchers and clinicians have begun to explore how the minority stress model can be extended to reflect the experiences of TGD individuals. Perhaps most notably, Henricks, Testa, and colleagues [2, 3] have outlined the many ways in which stress and resilience factors exist specifically with regard to a minority gender identity. Testa and colleagues (2015) [3] developed the Gender Minority Stress and Resilience (GMSR) measure, which is an extension of Meyer's work, aimed at expanding on the theory by attending to stress and resilience factors that are relevant to TGD individuals. The GMSR measure is based on 9 constructs, which include gender-related discrimination, gender-related rejection, gender-related victimization, non-affirmation of gender identity, internalized transphobia, negative expectations for the future, concealment, community connectedness, and pride (see Fig. 5.1). For a more in-depth review of the GMSR measure, see the work of Testa and colleagues [3].

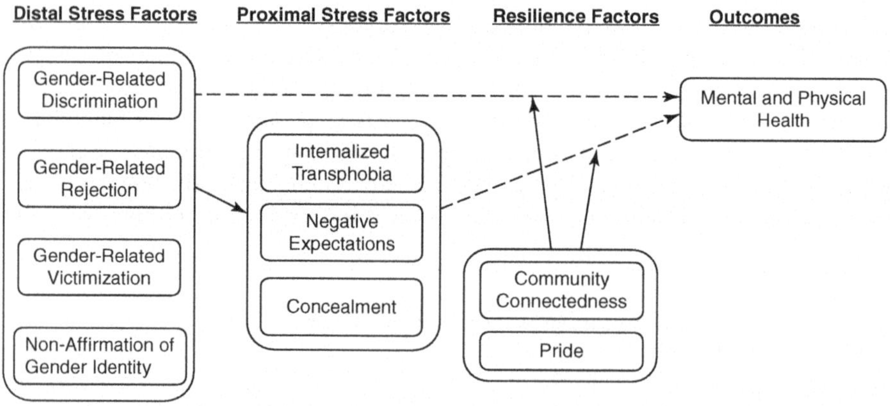

Fig. 5.1 Minority stress and resilience factors in TGD individuals. Dashed lines reflect inverse relationships. (Reprinted with author permission [3])

An explosion of research in the last decade or two has begun to study these distal and proximal stress factors, resilience factors, and their impact on TGD individuals. The negative impact of distal stress factors like discrimination, rejection, victimization, and non-affirmation of gender identity are becoming clearer. For example, stigma and/or perceived discrimination have been correlated with depression, poor overall mental health, suicide attempts, and non-suicidal self-injury (NSSI) [4–6]. Gender-related victimization, which can manifest in bullying, harassment, verbal abuse, stalking, and assault, for example, can predict the use of alcohol and illicit substances, avoidant coping styles, disordered eating, and other maladaptive behaviors in TGD adolescents [7–9]. Liu and Mustanski (2012) [10] found that homelessness, which is related to parents' non-affirmation of their children's gender identity, was predictive of greater NSSI. The increase in attention that the topic of non-affirmation of gender identity has received is highly encouraging, given the significance of this topic. This construct is perhaps most frequently discussed within the context of parents/caregivers; however, it applies to a broad range of individuals who have the chance to affirm (or not affirm) the identity of a TGD individual.

With regard to proximal stress factors, numerous studies have identified the adverse effects of internalized transphobia (negative, internal feelings about being transgender), negative expectations for the future, and non-disclosure. For instance, researchers found that internalized transphobia was predictive of negative mental health outcomes, specifically anxiety and depression [11]. Interestingly, one study found that while the relationships between internalized transphobia and negative psychological outcomes were not significant among participants who engaged in low and mean levels of community activism, there was a significant positive correlation between internalized transphobia and mental health challenges among those involved in a high degree of activism [12]. This is particularly interesting, given that there is often a high degree of community in action-oriented work which, as will be further explained below, appears to be a protective factor in the GMSR model.

Concealment of identity has also been found to predict more psychological distress, especially among transgender women [5]. However, in a study aiming to better understand suicidality in TGD individuals by exploring factors from both the GMSR model as well as Joiner's [13] interpersonal-psychological theory of suicide, non-disclosure of identity explained only a very small percentage of the variance in SI [14]. One proposed hypothesis for this finding was that non-disclosure does not carry the exact meaning of identity concealment (deciding not to disclose your identity is not the same as feeling as though you need to hide it), which may have more pernicious effects. Also of note, concealment can vary across contexts. It is not uncommon for TGD individuals to modify their gender expression depending on the environment, in part to decrease victimization. Having to be hypervigilant regarding one's safety and the chance of being victimized can also act as an added stressor and impact behavioral performance and well-being [15]. While youth can certainly benefit in many ways from disclosing their identity by receiving affirmation and support, they also run the risk of experiencing adverse consequences from disclosing their identity, such as feeling discriminated against and victimized [16].

Finally, the GMSR model also calls attention to resilience factors, which can mediate the relationship between the above-mentioned distal stressors and mental health consequences. Pride in one's identity and community connectedness are the two factors named in the GMSR model [3]. In contrast with internalized transphobia or homophobia, acceptance of, and pride in, one's gender identity and sexual orientation has been connected to reports of fewer depressive symptoms in adolescents and adults [6, 17]. This illustrates one of many reasons why taking an affirmative stance with TGD youth is critical. Other researchers have identified additional factors that appear to increase resiliency in TGD youth. In a qualitative study of resilience among TGD people of color with trauma histories, Singh and McKleroy [18] found six overall common factors among participants leading to resilience in dealing with their traumatic events: (1) having pride in their gender and ethnic/racial identity, (2) recognizing/negotiating gender and racial/ethnic oppression, (3) relationships with one's family, (4) access to health care and financial resources, (5) connecting with an activist trans community of color, and (6) sense of spirituality and hope for the future. Thus, those interested in supporting TGD patients or loved ones will likely benefit from considering the ways in which the above-mentioned resilience factors are being encouraged and built upon over time and across contexts.

Intersection of Identities

It is imperative to acknowledge that TGD individuals make up a highly diverse group of individuals living across the world, and that while some carry with them numerous forms of privilege and social capital, others experience various levels of oppression. TGD people who identify with multiple minority identities may experience violence, harassment, and microaggressions more often than both individuals who do not have a minority identity and those who identify with one minority identity. Thus, TGD individuals who carry multiple minority statuses are commonly at a greater risk of experiencing oppression from a number of different angles [19].

In working with TGD youth and their families, it is important to assess the impact of multiple minority statuses on mental health, as well as the ways in which these individuals can be best supported in their communities. Attending to stigma within certain cultural identities regarding acceptance of transgender identity is also key [15]. Furthermore, it is also well advised to understand how victimization and microaggressions may occur within different circles. Some individuals with multiple minority identities may feel an uncomfortable sense of obligation to "choose" with which identity they would like to most identify in order to have a support system [20]. A series of measures by Balsam and colleagues may be of help in assessing for microaggressions endured by LGBTQ+ people of color [21] and minority stress experiences and their effects among LGB and TQ+ adults [22].

In the literature exploring intersectionality and the impact of multiple marginalized statuses, some of the most highly researched identity statuses among TGD individuals include race, socioeconomic status, sexual orientation, and gender identity. A number of studies have highlighted that transgender women, including those with trauma histories, report higher levels of NSSI, HIV, and discrimination than transgender men, [23–25]. The higher rates of discrimination can in turn lead to higher levels of depression, PTSD symptoms, and overall stress [25]. Increased rates of suicide attempts, NSSI, and victimization have also been identified among those who are younger and have lower incomes and education [7, 21], although more recent research that suggests younger children who are supported in social and medical transitions early show more positive mental health outcomes than older cohorts [26–28]. In addition to transgender women, TGD people of color endorse greater rates of discrimination and victimization [5]. Sexual orientation also plays an important role. One study of TGD youth found that TGD participants who identified as LGB had lower grades than their heterosexual TGD peers, in addition to having more absences from school due to increased depression and/or suspensions [29]. Religious identity can also be highly relevant, given that some individuals who come from religious backgrounds have histories of experiencing prejudice in their communities of worship, to the point of seeking out or being referred to conversion/reparative therapies [30]. Of note, continued research is needed to ensure that the experiences of TGD individuals are being properly assessed and that issues like incidents of violence among different subgroups of the TGD community are being appropriately documented.

Parental Support

A number of studies have pointed to the importance of parental support, as it has been associated with positive health outcomes, higher self-esteem, increased social supports, decreased suicidal ideation and attempts, and a decrease in substance use in LGBTQ+ youth [31]. Parental support has also been associated with lower perceptions of feeling like a burden and higher life satisfaction [32], as well as increased condom use among TGD youth [23]. Some have argued that parental support might be the *most* protective factor against negative mental health outcomes for TGD youth [4, 33], or specifically suicide attempts [34], while others suggest that parental support is as protective against suicidal ideation and attempts as are protections from harassment, gender affirming medical transitions, and documents that reflect an individual's preferred name and gender marker [35]. In addition, while observing family members move from a place of non-acceptance to a place of acceptance is a protective factor against suicidal ideation and attempts [36], it is unclear whether or not the support of one parent acts as a protective factor, or if two parents are needed (if there is a two-parent family) [19]. In addition, positive parenting (authoritative style, positive reinforcement, the ability to engage in open discussions about relationships and intimacy), coupled with parental engagement (measured by time spent together, emotional availability), was found to be a protective factor against substance use in LGBTQ+ youth [37]. Interestingly, research with TGD children suggests that if young children are supported in their TGD identities, they have similar reported symptoms of depression and anxiety as their siblings and age-matched cisgender peers [28, 38]. Though direct comparisons are not possible, this is a stark contrast to past cohorts of transgender youth who were not supported in their gender identities, who had higher rates of internalizing psychopathology [39].

Alternatively, low parental support has been associated with increased rates of depression, suicide attempts, substance abuse, and risky sexual behaviors [40], as well as increased feelings of burdensomeness and lower life satisfaction [32]. However, there is some research that suggests that if parents are able to learn how to support their children in adulthood, there are still protective effects from which to benefit [41].

It is important to note that parents may feel that they are "responsible" for their children's TGD identity, and may worry about the judgments that others place on their parenting [42]. Some parents may also fear that their acceptance of their children's TGD behavior will have a negative impact, leading to an increase in health concerns [43]. This can lead to a struggle where parents experience pressure to abide by societal norms, while also wanting to affirm their children. Supporting parents as they navigate how to best manage different and challenging situations is imperative. If parents feel supported in their decision-making, their children can also feel more supported. Parents may also be pleased to know that emerging research suggests that early social transition does not increase a child's cross-gender identification [44]. Interestingly, in a study exploring parental reactions to their children's coming out process, some parents reported that they had become more flexible and creative in their thinking, which had led to their own individual growth [43].

Other studies have examined the relationship between parental response to their children's identity as TGD and the subsequent effects on the children. For example, youth who reported that their parents had experienced their TGD identity as a loss perceived this as non-acceptance of their identity [23]. Some research has suggested that fathers are less accepting of their transfeminine children, and may pressure their children at greater rates to conform to their birth-assigned gender, which could manifest in the form of verbal harassment and shaming, leading to mental health issues [19].

Parents – Strategies to Help Build Support

Various factors for increasing parental support for TGD youth have been developed to help parents understand the importance of supporting their children's identity. Working from the gender-affirmative model as a framework, parents can learn that gender presentations are varied and the expression of gender can unfold over time, allowing children the space for identity exploration, which is associated with increased confidence and self-acceptance [45]. From this frame, parents can understand how support is associated with higher self-esteem and positive health outcomes. Parents can also learn the importance of modeling appropriate responses to harassment and teasing, while also teaching youth how to use humor to diffuse uncomfortable situations [46].

It is possible that when parenting interventions are modified to include a general understanding of the GMSR model in order to better understand the experiences of TGD youth, additional decreases in symptomatology for youth may result. When targeted in parent management and family-based treatment, it is possible to address worries that parents may have about their children's future relationships, potential victimization, acceptance in society, and medical interventions, while also focusing on normative development (romantic and sexual interests), puberty, fertility, and devices used to mirror normative gendered functioning (e.g., binders, prosthetics) [47]. Parents and youth can also discuss their opinions and fears about medical interventions in a safe setting with an independent observer who can help facilitate communication [48]. Thus, an independent observer can encourage open and productive communication between youth and their parent(s).

One parenting intervention that has been put forward for TGD youth is the Multidimensional Family Approach [49]. According to this approach, parents are guided to move from holding "all or none" viewpoints toward practicing more dialectical "both/and" thinking. For instance, parents learn to hold multiple truths, such that an individual's identity can be affirmed *and* there can be recognition that difficulties will lie ahead. This stands in contrast with a common line of thought that children can *either* be affirmed or safe. Once parents feel more comfortable about affirming their children's identity, they can focus on how to act as advocates for their children, while also promoting their safety. If parents' fears can be decreased, they can better support their children, which can ultimately bolster the children's confidence and lead to increased resilience. While this approach has yet to be empirically validated, it does incorporate discussion of many of the components of the GMSR model and mirrors research that additional support of a child's identity is associated with better health outcomes [28, 31, 38].

It is also important to help parents work through the multiple emotional reactions they might experience while parenting a TGD youth. For example, parents have reported a number of reactions to their children's TGD identity, including perceiving a sense of loss, fear of future victimization, their own non-affirmation by peers and family members for supporting their children, and marital discord if there is disagreement regarding how to proceed with social or medical transitions [50]. A space for the parents to discuss the perceived loss of a child has been deemed important, even though the child is still present. One way to help parents understand this phenomenon is by observing this process as an evolution of the youth [51]. In addition, it may be that parents of youth who are more ambiguous in gender presentation (non-binary) have more difficulty with the idea of a loss [52]. For these parents, time to explore cis-normative culture and personal expectations are imperative. It is also important for the family to be aware of how the child is still present in the family, and explore how the family system can include their identity. In addition, the importance of parent support groups has been noted for parents to discuss the pressures of parenting in general, and to share strategies on how to deal with people who are not supportive of TGD youth [46, 49]. These groups can also help members feel valued and respected by their peers, which might not otherwise occur [46]. In addition to groups, parents may feel more equipped to support their children on their gender journeys by accessing reading materials about gender variance, updated guidelines for affirmative treatment, information on school policies, and guidelines on lobbying for the coverage of affirmative medical treatments [53].

Schools

There has been increased attention to TGD students' experiences in schools. In a recent nationwide survey of students [54], 43% of students reported feeling unsafe in their schools based on their gender expression, 20% reported being physically harassed, and 9% reported being physically assaulted, all due to their gender identity. Sadly, approximately 58% of students reported that they did not report harassment or victimization to school staff, as they did not think either the teachers or administrators would intervene on their behalf. When students disclosed mistreatment to school staff, they reported that nothing was done 64% of the time. Unfortunately, 64% of the students also reported hearing negative homophobic or transphobic comments from teachers and other staff. In addition, TGD youth were also singled out at school; 51% of students reported not being allowed to use their preferred name and pronouns at school; 60% were required to use the bathrooms and locker rooms that corresponded with their birth-assigned gender, and 32% were required to wear clothing congruent with their birth-assigned gender for school photos (36% were required to wear clothing congruent with their birth-assigned gender for graduation). If examining these numbers through the lens of the GMSR model, it is clear that this non-affirmation, victimization, and harassment in school settings could lead to an array of negative health and mental health problems for TGD youth.

Indeed, studies have shown that TGD students who experience harassment and victimization in school have increased days of missed school [29], lower GPAs, fewer plans for post-secondary education [54], higher dropout rates [55, 56], lower self-esteem, increased depressive symptoms, suicidal ideation, problematic drinking, illegal drug use, risky sexual behaviors [57], and more suicide attempts [58, 59]. Students who avoided bathrooms due to feeling unsafe experienced increased incidences of urinary tract infections, kidney infections, and dehydration [55]. Feeling unsafe in restrooms in general has also been associated with missing school field trips, not spending time in public spaces (e.g., malls, stores, and restaurants), and avoiding gyms due to fears of locker rooms [55]. Not only can this fear prevent youth from engaging in normative, developmentally appropriate activities, it can also lead to an increase in isolation and fewer opportunities to create a supportive community of peers – some of the protective factors included in the GMSR model.

Schools – Strategies to Enhance Support

There are a number of protective factors for TGD youth in schools, including a positive connection to school [37], an active Gender and Sexuality Alliance (GSA) [54], school anti-bullying policies that include protections based on gender identity and expression and curricula that are inclusive of LGBTQ+ identities [60]. Students with active GSAs report fewer homophobic or transphobic remarks, and school staff tend to intervene more when negative remarks are made [54]. Conversely, for students without an active GSA, there is an increased risk for the use of cocaine, hallucinogens, and non-prescription drugs [61]. Relatedly, research suggests that having an LGBTQ+-friendly curriculum is associated with youth feeling safer and more supported in school and also feeling more likely to complete high school and pursue post-secondary education [54]. In addition, the use of anti-bullying policies inclusive of gender identity can result in fewer negative remarks by peers and teachers and youth feeling as though their concerns are effectively heard and addressed by administration [54, 62]. Of note, supportive staff appear to have the greatest impact on youth. The more supportive and affirming staff there are in school, the greater the reports of self-esteem, the lower the rates of victimization, the higher the GPAs, and the fewer missed days there are from school [54].

In the 2015 Safe Schools Survey [54], students in middle school reported fewer LGBTQ+ resources – GSAs, LGBTQ+ inclusive curricula, supportive educators, comprehensive policies against bullying – than high school students. Middle school students also reported more homophobic/transphobic remarks and slightly higher experiences of victimization. This points to the importance of having supportive environments and inclusive policies for LGBTQ+ youth in middle as well as high school. When supports are not available in school, it is imperative to help TGD youth find other supportive communities (online or in person) to help them feel more confident and engage in self-advocacy [63].

Schools can also incorporate TGD youth in the creation of school policy to increase self-esteem and feelings of safety, and train advocates in TGD health care, who can follow TGD youth as they progress through the school system [56]. Schools can also host a "Safe Schools Summit" where LGBTQ+ youth can meet with one another, discuss strategies to feel more supported in school, advocate for one another, and model leadership for their school [64].

In addition to supporting TGD youth, schools can build the capacity of their staff. School administration can invest in their staff to become better-trained faculty advisors for the GSAs, and also learn how to effectively intervene when LGBTQ+ harassment occurs [56]. Specifically, teachers can learn to recognize behaviors and statements that are transphobic and homophobic, school psychologists can work with teachers to discuss strategies to decrease bullying, and syllabi can include anti-bullying language with appropriate disciplinary actions laid out [61]. PFLAG [65] also offers guidance for schools to be more inclusive (see Table 5.1). When there are more individuals who are supportive to TGD students, there is higher educational attainment and fewer absences among TGD students, as there is less bullying and victimization, or when there is, staff intervene [60]. Teachers will benefit from acknowledging their potential to have strong, direct impacts. On a broader level, school staff and students can advocate for legislation to protect TGD students. Policies that incorporate anti-bullying and safe school curriculum (curriculum that is supportive and inclusive of LGBTQ+ students) are associated with increased school safety [66]. Additionally, measures of sexual orientation and gender identity can be incorporated into school benchmarks so that inequities of LGBTQ+ students can be identified and properly addressed [66].

Table 5.1 PFLAG's 10 steps to creating inclusive schools

1. Understand the data about discrimination and victimization of LGBTQ youth in schools
2. Learn and use respectful terminology
3. Stop disruptive behavior and model respectful behavior
4. Create effective school policy to protect LGBT students (inclusive of gender identity)
5. Create school-wide opportunities for discussion of respect for all
6. Let youth know you are an ally and advocate
7. Stop cyber-bullying and help the targets
8. Train faculty about bullying and how to intervene
9. Create comprehensive health education that includes LGBTQ identities
10. Have visible and updated resources for individuals to know where to go for help

Courtesy of PFLAG: https://www.pflag.org/publication/toptenwaystomakeschoolssafe

Peers

As noted above, TGD youth are victimized at high rates in school. Lack of peer support is associated with isolation, concealment of one's identity, and negative internalized feelings [67, 68]. Increased bullying and victimization by peers is associated with increased use of alcohol, marijuana, and other illegal drugs, with bullying acting as a mediator for substance abuse [8]. In addition to bullying and verbal and physical harassment, transfeminine youth report increased sexualization and sexual propositioning by peers, which is associated with an increased risk for sexual assault [16]. Interestingly, when divided by identity, non-binary youth reported more symptoms of anxiety and depression than their binary transgender peers did. They also had fewer positive peer relations [38]. This could be due to fewer examples of non-binary people in schools and in society, and only binary choices for restrooms and locker rooms. In addition, pronouns and familial labels can be more complicated, which can make individuals feel more separate and burdensome.

Peers – Strategies to Enhance Peer Support

As peers are an important factor in adolescent development, and belongingness appears to be a protective factor against negative mental health outcomes, it is reasonable that advocating for increased peer support for transgender youth would be beneficial. Promoting group activities (either in person or online) is one way where youth can find support and affirmation from others, while also being able to discuss concerns about transition and general developmental issues. It is in this type of format where youth can question societal and/or cultural norms and expectations and also feel supported in this exploration. Having spaces where youth can feel comfortable being themselves and where they are supported in their identities is associated with less psychological distress [5].

Peer support was found to be a moderator in the relationship between discrimination, harassment and victimization and psychological distress [5]. Relationships with TGD peers has been associated with less anxiety, fewer suicide attempts, less fearfulness, and more comfort in one's identity [69]. Frequent contact with LGBTQ+ peers has been associated with resilience in the face of victimization, as youth are more able to deal with stress and utilize coping skills when they see peers who have shared experiences coping in a positive manner [33]. The creation of lavender graduation (ceremonies to celebrate LGBTQ+ students and allies and their accomplishments), pink (LGBTQ+) proms, media campaigns, and informing administration on policy in schools are all examples of how LGBTQ+ youth can join with peers for support [68]. However, it is important to note that if victimization does not decrease, peer support does not appear to act as a buffer against psychological distress [70].

As peer support is such an important protective factor for TGD youth, it is also important to think about the impact of romantic relationships. Adolescence is a developmental stage where youth experiment with and learn about romantic and sexual relationships. How relationships impact youth is important, as well as how experiences of harassment and victimization affect relationships. In a study looking at the impact of stigma on romantic relationships, researchers found that stigma associated with being in a romantic or sexual relationship with a TGD person not only negatively affected the TGD individual, but also their partner's perception of the relationship quality [71]. It appears that negative messages internalized by TGD individuals also may be internalized by their romantic partners. Therefore, it is important to address the stress and related difficulties associated with general relational issues, as well as the impact of harassment and discrimination on both the TGD individuals and their partners.

While peer support is an important protective factor for TGD youth, supportive peers are not always available in person. The availability of supportive peers online has also been noted as an important protective factor, to connect with others and share positive coping strategies including positive self-talk, the importance of being a role model to other TGD youth, exploring meaningful and creative activities, and exploring reasons for living [34, 36]. Importantly, while online role models have been identified as a positive coping support in order to model resiliency, success, and positive self-worth, youth who reported having online role models reported more negative symptomatology [72]. It is unclear whether it is because having only online role models makes it more apparent that there are no positive role models in the community, or if youth who seek out role models online are doing more poorly in general [72]. This points to the potential importance of having both online supports and also allies and role models in the community.

Mental Health and Medical Settings

Medical and mental health providers also play an important role in either helping TGD youth and their families to feel supported and affirmed, or in more unfortunate circumstances, to feel invalidated, stigmatized, and/or discriminated against. Notably, the largest barrier to care, as identified by TGD individuals, is the lack of knowledgeable providers [73]. Research highlights the clinical importance of supporting individuals align their body with their mind. As such, struggling with barriers such as lack of culturally sensitive professionals, coverage denials from insurance companies, and long wait periods are highly problematic for TGD individuals.

Unhelpful and invalidating experiences with providers cover a wide spectrum of events, from highly unintentional and well-intentioned actions on the providers' part that unfortunately do not feel supportive from the patients' perspective, to more egregious cases. One study [74] of transgender adults captured six themes regarding participants' reports of problematic behaviors experienced while receiving medical care: (1) gender insensitivity, (2) displays of discomfort, (3) denial of services, (4) substandard care, (5) verbal abuse, and (6) forced care (e.g., being involuntarily committed to psychiatric units or undergoing unnecessary medical examinations). Safer and colleagues [73] also reported that financial challenges, discrimination, lack of provider cultural competence, health systems issues, and socioeconomic issues are additional barriers to accessing care among TGD individuals. Trust is also a highly relevant topic, as certain professionals have taken to discussing and writing about issues pertaining to transgender identity from a lens of mistrust, fostering an "us" (providers) versus "them" (TGD patients) dynamic [75].

Mental Health and Medical Settings – Strategies to Enhance Support

While medical and mental health professionals share an overarching goal of providing effective and supportive care to patients in need of services, it is important to also acknowledge our fallibility. Of great importance is our willingness to recognize and correct missteps when they occur. It is arguable that providers may be more prone to missteps with TGD patients, given a number of factors including limited knowledge of the research, minimal exposure to working with TGD individuals, lack of supervision or mentorship on the topic, and personal biases and belief systems. In reflecting on our practice with TGD individuals, it may be helpful to call to mind the ethical principles of beneficence, non-maleficence, autonomy, and justice. For a more detailed explanation of how to attend to each of these principles while working with TGD individuals, see the work of Hann, Ivester, and Denton [76].

Additionally, there are numerous references that providers can consult to foster affirmative, culturally sensitive work with TGD individuals [77–79]. The World Professional Association for Transgender Health (WPATH) provides regularly updated, comprehensive standards of care for working with TGD individuals, including special attention directed to the treatment of TGD youth [79]. Others [80] have also outlined a number of suggestions pertaining to the care of TGD individuals across numerous professional arenas like primary care, mental health interventions, speech and language therapy, surgery, and management of transition care. They also detail the importance of including training on the care of TGD individuals early on in medical training. Additionally, the American Psychological Association has published guidelines for providing psychological services to TGD communities [81]. More recently, factors that TGD youth themselves report they wish their providers would keep in mind when working with them were summarized [82]. This includes language use and communication with TGD patients, education regarding the many ways that TGD youth can experience and express their gender identity, and depathologizing transgender identity, among other topics. Further, other colleagues provide important recommendations for serving LGBTQ+ youth effectively, ensuring to attend to systems-level considerations [83].

With regard to mental health treatment, being apprised of risk and resilience factors is an excellent first step for providers who are new to working with TGD youth and their families. More specifically, it is recommended that while assessing the mental health and safety of TGD youth, clinicians should include questions that assess distal and proximal risk factors as well as resiliency factors noted in the GMSR model. It is also worth noting that clinicians and scholars have begun to develop cultural modifications to standard evidenced-based treatment interventions, such as Cognitive Behavior Therapy. For instance, the Transgender Affirmative Cognitive Behavioral Therapy (TA-CBT) aims to help providers deliver more affirmative CBT interventions to TGD individuals with anxiety, depression, and/or suicide behaviors [84]. The intervention is based on ensuring that the following are addressed in treatment: relevant psychoeducation, thinking styles, social support, and suicide prevention [82]. Thus, among other benefits, therapy can help individuals to attend to their emotional, cognitive, and behavioral responses to experiences with rejection and discrimination, for instance, and subsequently help to reframe unhelpful, biased thoughts that if left unchallenged, could further exacerbate difficulties with shame, internalized transphobia, and hope for the future, among other factors.

Conclusions

TGD youth face a great deal of proximal and distal stress factors that are associated with an increase in health and mental health concerns [4, 5–10, 15]. In addition, there are also noted supports (e.g., parents, schools, peers, and medical providers) whose affirmative approach can mediate these negative health outcomes and boost TGD youth and their families' sense of resilience. It is our hope that providers can utilize the strategies noted above to help affirm TGD youth and inculcate them from environmental stressors. Additionally, it is important for researchers to continue to evaluate the above interventions and use their work to inform future policies aimed at supporting TGD youth.

References

1. Meyer IH. Prejudice, social stress, and mental health in lesbian, gay, and bisexual populations: conceptual issues and research evidence. Psychol Bull. 2003;129(5):674–97.
2. Hendricks ML, Testa RJ. A conceptual framework for clinical work with transgender and gender nonconforming clients: an adaptation of the minority stress model. Prof Psychol Res Pract. 2012;43(5):460–7.

3. Testa RJ, Habarth J, Peta J, Balsam K, Bockting W. Development of the gender minority stress and resilience measure. Psychol Sex Orientat Gend Divers. 2015;2(1):65–77.
4. Veale JF, Peter T, Travers R, Saewyc EM. Enacted stigma, mental health, and protective factors among transgender youth in Canada. Transgend Health. 2017;2(1):207–16.
5. Bockting WO, Miner MH, Swinburne Romine RE, Hamilton A, Coleman E. Stigma, mental health, and resilience in an online sample of the US transgender population. Am J Public Health. 2013;103(5):943–51.
6. McCarthy MA, Fisher CM, Irwin JA, Coleman JD, Pelster AD. Using the minority stress model to understand depression in lesbian, gay, bisexual, and transgender individuals in Nebraska. J Gay Lesbian Ment Health. 2014;18(4):346–60.
7. Lombardi EL, Wilchins RA, Priesing D, Malouf D. Gender violence: transgender experiences with violence and discrimination. J Homosex. 2002;42(1):89–101.
8. Reisner SL, Greytak EA, Parsons JT, Ybarra ML. Gender minority social stress in adolescence: disparities in adolescent bullying and substance use by gender identity. J Sex Res. 2015;52(3):243–56.
9. Watson RJ, Veale JF, Saewyc EM. Disordered eating behaviors among transgender youth: probability profiles from risk and protective factors. Int J Eat Disord. 2017;50(5):515–22.
10. Liu RT, Mustanski B. Suicidal ideation and self-harm in lesbian, gay, bisexual, and transgender youth. Am J Prev Med. 2012;42(3):221–8.
11. Scandurra C, Amodeo AL, Valerio P, Bochicchio V, Frost DM. Minority stress, resilience, and mental health: a study of Italian transgender people. J Soc Issues. 2017;73(3):563–85.
12. Breslow AS, Brewster ME, Velez BL, Wong S, Geiger E, Soderstrom B. Resilience and collective action: exploring buffers against minority stress for transgender individuals. Psychol Sex Orientat Gend Divers. 2015;2(3):253–65.
13. Joiner T. Why people die by suicide. London: Harvard University Press; 2007.
14. Testa RJ, Michaels MS, Bliss W, Rogers ML, Balsam KF, Joiner T. Suicidal ideation in transgender people: gender minority stress and interpersonal theory factors. J Abnorm Psychol. 2017;126(1):125–36.
15. Levitt HM, Ippolito MR. Being transgender: navigating minority stressors and developing authentic self-presentation. Psychol Women Q. 2014;38(1):46–64.
16. Grossman AH, D'Augelli AR. Transgender youth: invisible and vulnerable. J Homosex. 2006;51(1):111–28.
17. Scandurra C, Bochicchio V, Amodeo AL, Esposito C, Valerio P, Maldonato NM, Bacchini D, Vitelli R. Internalized transphobia, resilience, and mental health: applying the psychological mediation framework to Italian transgender individuals. Int J Environ Res Public Health. 2018;15(3):508–26.
18. Singh AA, McKleroy VS. "Just getting out of bed is a revolutionary act" the resilience of transgender people of color who have survived traumatic life events. Traumatology. 2011;17(2):34–44.
19. Ignatavicius S. Stress in female-identified transgender youth: a review of the literature on effects and interventions. J LGBT Youth. 2013;10(4):267–86.
20. Harper GW, Schneider M. Oppression and discrimination among lesbian, gay, bisexual, and transgendered people and communities: a challenge for community psychology. Am J Community Psychol. 2003;31(3–4):243–52.
21. Balsam KF, Molina Y, Beadnell B, Simoni J, Walters K. Measuring multiple minority stress: the LGBT people of color microaggressions scale. Cult Divers Ethn Minor Psychol. 2011;17(2):163–74.
22. Balsam KF, Beadnell B, Molina Y. The daily heterosexist experiences questionnaire: measuring minority stress among lesbian, gay, bisexual, and transgender adults. Meas Eval Couns Dev. 2013;46(1):3–25.
23. Wilson EC, Iverson E, Garofalo R, Belzer M. Parental support and condom use among transgender female youth. J Assoc Nurses AIDS Care. 2012;23(4):306–17.
24. House AS, Van Horn E, Coppeans C, Stepleman LM. Interpersonal trauma and discriminatory events as predictors of suicidal and nonsuicidal self-injury in gay, lesbian, bisexual, and transgender persons. Traumatology. 2011;17(2):75–85.

25. Wilson EC, Chen YH, Arayasirikul S, Raymond HF, McFarland W. The impact of discrimination on the mental health of trans* female youth and the protective effect of parental support. AIDS Behav. 2016;20(10):2203–11.
26. De Vries AL, McGuire JK, Steensma TD, Wagenaar EC, Doreleijers TA, Cohen-Kettenis PT. Young adult psychological outcome after puberty suppression and gender reassignment. Pediatrics. 2014;134(4):696–704.
27. Durwood L, McLaughlin KA, Olson KR. Mental health and self-worth in socially transitioned transgender youth. J Am Acad Child Adolesc Psychiatry. 2017;56(2):116–23.
28. Olson KR, Durwood L, DeMeules M, McLaughlin KA. Mental health of transgender children who are supported in their identities. Pediatrics. 2016;137(3):1–8.
29. Day JK, Perez-Brumer A, Russell ST. Safe schools? Transgender Youth's school experiences and perceptions of school climate. J Youth Adolesc. 2018;1:1–12.
30. Sherry A, Adelman A, Whilde MR, Quick D. Competing selves: negotiating the intersection of spiritual and sexual identities. Prof Psychol Res Pract. 2010;41(2):112–9.
31. Ryan C, Russell ST, Huebner D, Diaz R, Sanchez J. Family acceptance in adolescence and the health of LGBT young adults. J Child Adolesc Psychiatr Nurs. 2010;23(4):205–13.
32. Simons L, Schrager SM, Clark LF, Belzer M, Olson J. Parental support and mental health among transgender adolescents. J Adolesc Health. 2013;53(6):791–3.
33. Bariola E, Lyons A, Leonard W, Pitts M, Badcock P, Couch M. Demographic and psychosocial factors associated with psychological distress and resilience among transgender individuals. Am J Public Health. 2015;105(10):2108–16.
34. Moody C, Smith NG. Suicide protective factors among trans adults. Arch Sex Behav. 2013;42(5):739–52.
35. Bauer GR, Scheim AI, Pyne J, Travers R, Hammond R. Intervenable factors associated with suicide risk in transgender persons: a respondent driven sampling study in Ontario, Canada. BMC Public Health. 2015;15(1):525–39.
36. Moody C, Fuks N, Peláez S, Smith NG. "Without this, I would for sure already be dead": a qualitative inquiry regarding suicide protective factors among trans adults. Psychol Sex Orientat Gend Divers. 2015;2(3):266–80.
37. Aromin RA. Substance abuse prevention, assessment, and treatment for lesbian, gay, bisexual, and transgender youth. Pediatr Clin. 2016;63(6):1057–77.
38. Kuvalanka KA, Weiner JL, Munroe C, Goldberg AE, Gardner M. Trans and gender-nonconforming children and their caregivers: Gender presentations, peer relations, and well-being at baseline. J Fam Psychol. 2017;31(7):889–99.
39. Turban JL. Transgender youth: the building evidence base for early social transition. J Am Acad Child Adolesc Psychiatry. 2017;56(2):101–2.
40. Ryan C. Supportive families, healthy children: helping families with lesbian, gay, bisexual & transgender children. San Francisco: Marian Wright Edelman Institute, San Francisco State University; 2009. Family education booklet available online at http://familyproject.sfsu.edu/publications.
41. McConnell EA, Birkett M, Mustanski B. Families matter: social support and mental health trajectories among lesbian, gay, bisexual, and transgender youth. J Adolesc Health. 2016;59(6):674–80.
42. Dierckx M, Motmans J, Mortelmans D, T'sjoen G. Families in transition: a literature review. Int Rev Psychiatry. 2016;28(1):36–43.
43. Hill DB, Menvielle E. "You have to give them a place where they feel protected and safe and loved": the views of parents who have gender-variant children and adolescents. J LGBT Youth. 2009;6(2–3):243–71.
44. Rae JR, Gulgos S, Durwood L, DeMeules M, Lowe R, Lindquist G, Olson KR. Predicting early childhood gender transitions. Psychol Sci. 2019;30(5):669–81.
45. Hidalgo MA, Ehrensaft D, Tishelman AC, Clark LF, Garofalo R, Rosenthal SM, Spack NP, Olson J. The gender affirmative model: what we know and what we aim to learn. Hum Dev. 2013;56(5):285–90.
46. Menvielle E, Hill DB. An affirmative intervention for families with gender-variant children: a process evaluation. J Gay Lesbian Ment Health. 2010;15(1):94–123.

47. Chen D, Hidalgo MA, Garofalo R. Parental perceptions of emotional and behavioral difficulties among prepubertal gender-nonconforming children. Clin Pract Pediatr Psychol. 2017;5(4):342–52.
48. Wren B. 'I can accept my child is transsexual but if I ever see him in a dress I'll hit him': dilemmas in parenting a transgendered adolescent. Clin Child Psychol Psychiatry. 2002;7(3):377–97.
49. Malpas J. Between pink and blue: a multi-dimensional family approach to gender nonconforming children and their families. Fam Process. 2011;50(4):453–70.
50. Gray SA, Sweeney KK, Randazzo R, Levitt HM. "Am I doing the right thing?": pathways to parenting a gender variant child. Fam Process. 2016;55(1):123–38.
51. Norwood K. Grieving gender: trans-identities, transition, and ambiguous loss. Commun Monogr. 2013;80(1):24–45.
52. Wahlig JL. Losing the child they thought they had: therapeutic suggestions for an ambiguous loss perspective with parents of a transgender child. J GLBT Fam Stud. 2015;11(4):305–26.
53. Riley EA, Sitharthan G, Clemson L, Diamond M. The needs of gender-variant children and their parents: a parent survey. Int J Sex Health. 2011;23(3):181–95.
54. Kosciw JG, Greytak EA, Giga NM, Villenas C, Danischewski DJ. The 2015 national school climate survey: the experiences of lesbian, gay, bisexual, transgender, and queer youth in our nation's schools. New York: Gay, Lesbian and Straight Education Network (GLSEN); 2016.
55. Herman JL. Gendered restrooms and minority stress: The public regulation of gender and its impact on transgender people's lives. J Public Manag Soc Policy. 2013;19(1):65–80.
56. McGuire JK, Anderson CR, Toomey RB, Russell ST. School climate for transgender youth: a mixed method investigation of student experiences and school responses. J Youth Adolesc. 2010;39(10):1175–88.
57. Eisenberg ME, Gower AL, McMorris BJ, Rider GN, Shea G, Coleman E. Risk and protective factors in the lives of transgender/gender nonconforming adolescents. J Adolesc Health. 2017;61(4):521–6.
58. Goldblum P, Testa RJ, Pflum S, Hendricks ML, Bradford J, Bongar B. The relationship between gender-based victimization and suicide attempts in transgender people. Prof Psychol Res Pract. 2012;43(5):468–75.
59. Russell ST, Ryan C, Toomey RB, Diaz RM, Sanchez J. Lesbian, gay, bisexual, and transgender adolescent school victimization: implications for young adult health and adjustment. J Sch Health. 2011;81(5):223–30.
60. Kosciw JG, Palmer NA, Kull RM, Greytak EA. The effect of negative school climate on academic outcomes for LGBT youth and the role of in-school supports. J Sch Violence. 2013;12(1):45–63.
61. Heck NC, Flentje A, Cochran BN. Offsetting risks: high school gay-straight alliances and lesbian, gay, bisexual, and transgender (LGBT) youth. Sch Psychol Q. 2013;26(2):61–174.
62. Russell ST, Fish JN. Mental health in lesbian, gay, bisexual, and transgender (LGBT) youth. Annu Rev Clin Psychol. 2016;12:465–87.
63. Singh AA. Transgender youth of color and resilience: negotiating oppression and finding support. Sex Roles. 2013;68(11–12):690–702.
64. Craig SL, Tucker EW, Wagner EF. Empowering lesbian, gay, bisexual, and transgender youth: lessons learned from a safe schools summit. J Gay Lesbian Soc Serv. 2008;20(3):237–52.
65. PFLAG. Cultivating respect: safe schools for all [Internet]. 2017. Available from: https://www.pflag.org/publication/toptenwaystomakeschoolssafe.
66. Haas AP, Eliason M, Mays VM, Mathy RM, Cochran SD, D'Augelli AR, Silverman MM, Fisher PW, Hughes T, Rosario M, Russell ST. Suicide and suicide risk in lesbian, gay, bisexual, and transgender populations: review and recommendations. J Homosex. 2010;58(1):10–51.
67. Higa D, Hoppe MJ, Lindhorst T, Mincer S, Beadnell B, Morrison DM, Wells EA, Todd A, Mountz S. Negative and positive factors associated with the Well-being of lesbian, gay, bisexual, transgender, queer, and questioning (LGBTQ) youth. Youth Soc. 2014;46(5):663–87.
68. de Vries AL, Steensma TD, Cohen-Kettenis PT, VanderLaan DP, Zucker KJ. Poor peer relations predict parent-and self-reported Behavioral and emotional problems of adolescents with

gender dysphoria: a cross-national, cross-clinic comparative analysis. Eur Child Adolesc Psychiatry. 2016;25(6):579–88.

69. Testa RJ, Jimenez CL, Rankin S. Risk and resilience during transgender identity development: The effects of awareness and engagement with other transgender people on affect. J Gay Lesbian Ment Health. 2014;18(1):31–46.
70. Birkett M, Newcomb ME, Mustanski B. Does it get better? A longitudinal analysis of psychological distress and victimization in lesbian, gay, bisexual, transgender, and questioning youth. J Adolesc Health. 2015;56(3):280–5.
71. Gamarel KE, Reisner SL, Laurenceau JP, Nemoto T, Operario D. Gender minority stress, mental health, and relationship quality: a dyadic investigation of transgender women and their cisgender male partners. J Fam Psychol. 2014;28(4):437–47.
72. Bird JD, Kuhns L, Garofalo R. The impact of role models on health outcomes for lesbian, gay, bisexual, and transgender youth. J Adolesc Health. 2012;50(4):353–7.
73. Safer JD, Coleman E, Feldman J, Garofalo R, Hembree W, Radix A, Sevelius J. Barriers to health care for transgender individuals. Curr Opin Endocrinol Diabetes Obes. 2016;23(2):168–71.
74. Kosenko K, Rintamaki L, Raney S, Maness K. Transgender patient perceptions of stigma in health care contexts. Med Care. 2013;51(9):819–22.
75. Hagen DB, Galupo MP. Trans* individuals' experiences of gendered language with health care providers: recommendations for practitioners. Int J Transgend. 2014;15(1):16–34.
76. Hann M, Ivester R, Denton GD. Bioethics in practice: ethical issues in the care of transgender patients. Ochsner J. 2017;17(2):144–5.
77. Rafferty J, Committee On Psychosocial Aspects Of Child And Family Health. Ensuring comprehensive care and support for transgender and gender-diverse children and adolescents. Pediatrics. 2018;142(4):e20182162.
78. Hembree WC, Cohen-Kettenis PT, Gooren L, Hannema SE, Meyer WJ, Murad MH, Rosenthal SM, Safer JD, Tangpricha V, T'Sjoen GG. Endocrine treatment of gender-dysphoric/gender-incongruent persons: an Endocrine Society clinical practice guideline. J Clin Endocrinol Metabol. 2017;102(11):3869–903.
79. Coleman E, Bockting W, Botzer M, Cohen-Kettenis P, DeCuypere G, Feldman J, Fraser L, Green J, Knudson G, Meyer WJ, Monstrey S. Standards of care for the health of transsexual, transgender, and gender-nonconforming people, version 7. Int J Transgend. 2012;13(4):165–232.
80. Wylie K, Knudson G, Khan SI, Bonierbale M, Watanyusakul S, Baral S. Serving transgender people: clinical care considerations and service delivery models in transgender health. Lancet. 2016;388(10042):401–11.
81. American Psychological Association. Guidelines for psychological practice with transgender and gender nonconforming people. Am Psychol. 2015;70(9):832–64.
82. Turban J, Ferraiolo T, Martin A, Olezeski C. Ten things transgender and gender nonconforming youth want their doctors to know. J Am Acad Child Adolesc Psychiatry. 2017;56(4):275–7.
83. Hadland SE, Yehia BR, Makadon HJ. Caring for lesbian, gay, bisexual, transgender, and questioning youth in inclusive and affirmative environments. Pediatr Clin. 2016;63(6):955–69.
84. Austin A, Craig SL. Transgender affirmative cognitive behavioral therapy: clinical considerations and applications. Prof Psychol Res Pract. 2015;46(1):21–9.

Sex-Positive Approaches to Educating, Supporting, and Listening to TGD Youth in Clinical Encounters

6

Aida Manduley and Kira Manser

Introduction

Transgender and gender diverse (TGD) youth have a multitude of ways of relating to their bodies, relationships, and sexualities. Providers and clinicians working with this population (ranging from birth to 26 years of age) can take opportunities to invest in developing a sex-positive lens to address the unique and broad ways that sexual and romantic relationships can impact the mental health, sexual health, and overall wellness of their clients. Sex positivity has only recently begun to be articulated as an essential lens for clinicians to use when addressing sexuality and health issues [1]. This chapter articulates what a sex-positive approach entails, why it is essential when supporting TGD youth, as well as gives specific and relevant ways to incorporate it into clinical work supporting TGD youth who are navigating sexual and romantic relationships. While some suggestions apply across all ages, many have to be adapted, given how wide the developmental range is between birth and 26 years of age. For age-specific direction, please refer to the last section of the chapter.

A Sex-Positive Approach

Sex-positivity is a paradigm and social movement that embraces sexuality as a healthy and pleasurable aspect of humanity and recognizes that diversity of sexual expression is natural. It also emphasizes the important role of active consent within sexual relationships, the value and existence of pleasure, and the understanding that sexuality can also be a source of pain and harm, just not universally or exclusively so.

A. Manduley (✉)
Women of Color Sexual Health Network, Boston, MA, USA

K. Manser
Clinical Social Worker and Sex Educator in Private Practice, Pawtucket, RI, USA

M. Forcier et al. (eds.), *Pediatric Gender Identity*,
https://doi.org/10.1007/978-3-030-38909-3_6

The analysis of sex positivity articulated by Nuestifter, Underhill, and Manduley [2] will specifically help direct the recommendations in this chapter, particularly because it both integrates earlier works on the topic and is also tailored to clinical contexts. These authors advocate for sex positivity to include and recognize the ways sexuality intersects with every part of who we are. They describe sex positivity as requiring, in the broadest sense, only that people approach the reality of how diverse and different human sexual identities and expressions can be, with a sense of humility and curiosity, as opposed to judgment or superiority. Nuestifter, Underhill, and Manduley [2] also place great importance on practitioners committing to a constant process of building self-awareness of how they, and their clients, are socially located within oppressive systems, and how these social locations impact treatment, the clinical relationship, and the power within both.

An intentionally sex-positive approach, then, is essential to listening and opening a dialogue that may truly address patient needs and concerns around gender and sexuality [3]. This may have added value when clinicians talk about intimate aspects of health and identity with historically gender and sexual minoritized persons who have experienced bias, discrimination, and poorer care within the majority healthcare system. Historically, clinical interactions are more often sex-negative and evaluating for risk, disease, and treatment in ways that shame and alienate patients. Nuestifter, Underhill, and Manduley [2] describe sex-negative interactions as pathologizing and practiced in a context of imbalance of power. This can create interactions that are fear-based and add to sexual stigma. A sex-positive framework, instead, may help reduce shame, encourage patient honesty, and create an environment of openness and possibility that results in better care delivery. The following chapter offers tools for practitioners to intentionally expand their sex-positive approach so they are able to listen openly and provide sensitive, patient-centered care for TGD youth around romantic and sexual development.

Why Is Sex Positivity Essential While Working with TGD Youth?

An integrated sex-positive approach is important while working with TGD youth, and in fact, benefits all youth. While gender and sexuality are distinct parts of identity, they are deeply linked. For most people, the body is intimately connected to an internally felt sense of one's gender and is also the primary vehicle through which sexual experiences are gained. For TGD youth, the body can be a source of confusion and conflict, as well as pleasure and affirmation, as they navigate the somatic aspects of these complex parts of self. Unfortunately, while TGD youth are still often understood as having deviated from "normal" gender development, there is an increasing understanding and growing body of evidence that a patient-centered, affirming approach offers best practices for children and adolescents [4]. There is also evidence that sexual development in TGD youth is particularly important for clinicians to discuss, as they may have unique challenges to this developmental process [5]. Practitioners who work with TGD youth will very likely encounter and need to clinically respond to a broad and wide diversity of sexual expressions, desires, relationships, behaviors, lifestyles, and stories. This diversity could be related to TGD youth's ability to creatively cope, in both adaptive and potentially harmful ways, to a cultural context where people with diverse gender identities are routinely discriminated against and subjected to violence. The diversity of sexuality that is observed in TGD youth may also be related to how choices around sexuality can be utilized as an access point for self-determination, gender affirmation, unique self-expression, connection to others, and many other important social, emotional, and physical resources.

A sex-positive approach also helps providers to resist the tendency to universalize the narratives most visible from their social locations [6]. For example, the current dominant cultural narrative in the United States mainstream is that TGD people were born in the wrong body, and that there are specific and sequential medical treatments that people must access to relieve gender-related distress. The public and closely followed gender stories of celebrities like Caitlyn Jenner, Chaz Bono, and Janet Mock often seem to have become "the" trans narrative, instead of "a" trans narrative in a sea of many diverse gender stories. Within this narrative, medical treatment is generally aimed at making the TGD person more conforming to a cisgender ideal, and their physicality, sexual functioning, and desires (for others, for particular acts, etc.) are linked to that external arbitrary standard. While this narrative surely feels authentic and relevant for many gender diverse people, it is important that clinicians create opportunities for individual clients to share and develop their own unique gender and sexual narratives in treatment. This could be imagined as using a "salad bar" as opposed to "prix fixe" approach to facilitating conversations and treatment for TGD youth. Clinicians best support clients in accessing healthy and rewarding relationships with others—which can include but do not require romance and sex—by providing care that reflects and affirms that TGD people have an inherent right to a complex, dynamic, and self-determined relationships with their body, gender, and sexuality.

Working as a Sex-Positive Provider

Providers who work with TGD youth should have, as a primary lens, a self-awareness around how they are supporting their clients in making choices around their bodies, relationships, and sexual behaviors, and expressions. A sex-positive practitioner collaborates with clients to ensure that they have access to a robust menu of realistic options for their age group. This menu should be comprehensive, mindful of safety, and consensual—including considering and thinking creatively about the possibility that in the future they might want to make different choices [6]. Choices can be framed as correct in response to what the client needs now, while clinical conversation can also leave room to consider possible long-term impacts, and how their current actions will impact what choices will be available to them in the future. For example, if someone wants to undergo any medical intervention, clinicians should ensure that they discuss the impacts on sexual pleasure, reproductive capacity, possible chronic medical care needs, and how tissue changes may require a different type of safer sex regimen. While there are many areas of life where clients might not have a lot of control, it is essential that providers support patients in having an internal locus of control around the choices they make in regard to their sexuality, body, and relationships. This includes supporting them in developing resilience, change management skills, and psychological as well as somatic awareness of their desires and agency.

Tangible ways to support a patient in the process of making choices about their physical and sexual self, and specific sexual behaviors, might include supporting a client in moving toward measurable, relative, incremental goals versus achieving absolute, rigid, lofty goals. For example, if a client states "I want to stop floating away from my body when I'm having sex," a small redirection toward relative measures could look like suggesting the goal be "I want to float away from my body less frequently during sex." A clinician could also invite the patient to consider the steps they could take to be more aware of what situations or activities tend to send them into a dissociative state, suggest ways to be more present during sex, and how to communicate with partners about their needs. Also, it is important that alongside these interventions geared toward change, that providers are also actively teaching clients how to express self-compassion and the ability to tolerate distress related to feelings of shame and failure when change is not immediate, absolute, linear, or easy. It is most helpful for clinicians to prepare clients to be able to manage outcomes and their emotions, rather than unrealistically expecting stressors to be completely eradicated forever.

Unfortunately, most healthcare providers have not had much training or resources when it comes to providing sexuality-related counseling and care, and even less specifically while using a sex-positive framework and trauma-aware lens. Developing sex-positive skills and resources is a lifelong professional challenge, but is worth the investment, as it creates unique opportunities to engage with patients on a more real and intimate level. As providers, part of our role is to create safer spaces where the unique needs of each patient can be discussed and addressed. Developing a sex-positive framework for working with patients is a starting place for this type of safe, honest clinical relationship that can impact their well-being so deeply. This is especially true when patients who are gender diverse may be considering (or have already experienced) gender-affirming medical interventions that could impact how they experience and pursue intimacy. While in-depth engagement with every individual aspect of a client's sexuality will not be in the purview of every provider, seeing oneself as part of a care team where all have contributions to make in supporting this framing is integral to making it effective. As one hundred percent of our clinical populations experience gender and sexuality over their lifespan and in a variety of forms and trajectories, being sex and gender diversity positive is a generalizable package of knowledge and skills that benefit all our patients.

Given the breadth of human sexual and relational variance, as well as the ways they may influence a patient's risk profile and priorities, clinicians should strive to provide educational information across a broad spectrum of sexual practices and identities. Part of providing sex-positive care includes clinicians intentionally gathering resources and information as well as an awareness of their own values and assumptions about diverse sexual practices and relationships, including BDSM[1]

[1] BDSM is an overlapping acronym that refers to sensory and sometimes erotic practices involving any combination of bondage, discipline, dominance, submission, sadism, masochism, and often other practices that may be deemed non-mainstream [7].

(sometimes referred to as kink or kinky sex) and non-monogamous relationship arrangements (which include, but are not limited to, ones described as open, non-exclusive, or polyamorous). While these topics will not be relevant for all TGD youth, or may need to get addressed differently by age-group, not making assumptions and having medically accurate, affirming resources available for those who are engaging in (or curious about) these things communicates that their health and safety is a priority regardless of what type of sexual interests or identities they have. Practitioners do not have to become fluent in these topics, but a basic level of information and ease of asking relevant questions is helpful for providing culturally competent care and building trust with patients. Table 6.1 can serve as a guide for catalyzing these critical conversations from a sex-positive framework of choice and affirmative engagement. (Note: depending on the age and cognitive capacity of the youth, as well as other relevant factors, the language should be simplified or modified.)

Specific Approaches to Sex-Positive Counseling

Providers who take a comprehensive sexual history or are specifically asked to work with patients on sexuality concerns will go beyond the typical medical interview questions of: Are you sexually active? Do you use condoms and/or birth control? Providers taking a comprehensive sexual history may ask about current, previous, and potential future partners, types of activities patients enjoy, sexual concerns, types of activities that create anxiety or negative experiences, and histories of trauma. Additionally, appropriately assessing risk for sexually transmitted infections (STI) and potential unintended pregnancy requires specific understandings of what parts go where, and what are the transmission risks for STIs and creating a pregnancy.

By using a harm reduction approach—a framework that originally began as a way to address substance use through a social justice and human rights lens [8]—providers can empower their clients to make choices that work for them while minimizing their possible negative impacts. Harm reduction as a practice aims to minimize any possible negative health, social, and/or legal impacts of different behaviors, without limiting access to choices because they could have negative impacts. This approach is informed by the belief that self-determination, health, and wellness are human rights and that it is critical to meet clients "where they are at." This is especially notable in clinical settings, where the power dynamics usually privilege the practitioner as the source of all knowledge; harm reduction reframes the medical setting into one that is more collaborative and where the client's expertise is just as valuable to their care as that of the provider.

In the spirit of Don McVinney—a pioneer in harm reduction work in the United States—and his work on substance use, a way to conceptualize harm reduction as it relates to sex is to move away from locating problems as existing within a person and instead focus on the person's *relationship* to an act or substance (such as sex) instead. When patients bring up sexuality issues, successfully using this lens means

Table 6.1 Approaches to starting a conversation about sexual and romantic needs and choices

Different topics	Conversation starters	Affirmation and exploration
Choices around physical body	What sexual experiences or behaviors are meaningful for you now, or are you interested in being able to access in the future? What pleasurable bodily sensations or situations are meaningful for you now, or are you interested in being able to have in the future? What ways could your choices around medical interventions impact how you experience pleasure? Are there specific actions or situations that help you feel affirmed as your gender? Are there ones that make you feel invisible, misunderstood, or misgendered? Are there behaviors or ways of relating to people (or your own body) that you would want to explore if they had less of a gendered meaning for you?	Often, people are taught to think about sex, touch, and pleasure within a narrow script. I prefer to think about these in an expansive way that allows people to think about it in terms of what works for them, in their context. People experience pleasure in lots of different physical and psychological ways, and it is an important part of overall health and wellness. How people feel pleasure can also vary greatly over time. It is not just about genitals! Sometimes people attach a gendered meaning to specific actions, and they may make us more or less likely to do them. Being aware of what we move toward or away from (and how we feel about that movement) can help us figure out where we might want to see some change and where we are feeling good.
Choices around sexual identity	How do you identify your sexuality? What words do you feel are a good fit, or even a partial fit? What ways are you attracted to other people, if any? Do you find your attraction is specific to certain characteristics, genders, bodies, behaviors, something else?	People can use lots of words to refer to their sexuality- like straight, queer, kinky, demisexual, or dominant, among many others. Attraction can be felt as emotional, physical, intellectual, sexual, or romantic, among others. Who you are attracted to and how or how much you are attracted to them can change over time and be influenced by many different things, including stress and hormone levels.
Choices around relationships	Do you want to have sexual and/or romantic relationships now or in the future? What types of intimate relationships are you interested in having? Let's brainstorm all the components that could be part of a relationship with another person, such as non-sexual physical touch, living together, special words for each other, sharing finances, sexual activity, and more. Then, instead of putting them all in the "relationship bag," we go through each one and see how and if you want to put it in your relationship bag. We can do this process with various relevant persons in your life.	You get to decide what kinds of relationships you want to be in, and that can change over time. Intimate relationships can include numerous ways of connecting. For example, you can choose if you want to be: committed or casual, monogamous or non-monogamous, or sexually active or not. We are often taught that relationships are a specific package deal of behaviors, but what is in the package or "relationship bag" is not the same for everyone, or every relationship.

providers can listen with open and humble curiosity about the choices patients make, the specific behaviors they engage in, the dynamics between them and a target behavior/substance/person, and both the benefits and risks of their actions. A practitioner taking a harm reduction approach would want a client to have access to any relevant medically accurate information (including possible negative impacts), a non-judgmental space to consider options, and a wide range of resources relating to their options. This practitioner would also clearly validate the reasons a patient might want or not want to engage in sexual behaviors and relationships (e.g., trading sex for money, a place to live, to avoid violence) rather than putting the reasons on a hierarchy of "acceptable" and "unacceptable."

Furthermore, if a patient is engaging in "risky behavior" that's gender-affirming or doing something like using illegal substances to help them access sexual pleasure, it is valuable for a clinician to ask about the function of those behaviors or substances, and see what useful resources or experiences they are bringing to the client. Thus, if looking for ways to reduce harm, a clinician can help their client identify appropriate replacements that meet the same, or similar enough, needs while reducing a client's defensiveness and increasing the likelihood of them disclosing information more readily. In these moments, it is important that a clinician attune to the values of the client and what they frame as important, rather than imposing their values or definitions of safety and harm on the client. As a guide, Table 6.2 offers conversation scripts and starters that highlight some of the similarities and differences between conversations that focus on risk management versus harm reduction and beyond.

If and when a client is able to honestly voice their reasons for engaging in sex that may be deemed riskier and the needs they are attempting to meet, a practitioner may be able to provide referrals to other wraparound services, such as shelters, anti-violence programs, food assistance, rehabilitation facilities, and so on, based on what the clients' stated needs are. If the youth is a minor, special referrals and considerations may need to be taken into account due to state mandatory reporting requirements.

Working with TGD Youth Across a Psychosocial Developmental Framework

A psychosocial developmental framework can be used to organize sex-positive and gender-affirming interventions with families of young children, and children and youth from birth through early adulthood. A psychosocial framework supports a sex-positive approach because it frames physical and sexual development as occurring within a dynamic exchange with external social forces. It broadly assumes growth across the lifespan, that individuals contribute to their own development, and values cultural context. However, there are limits to this framework's alignment with sex positivity. One limit is that a psychosocial developmental framework primarily describes development as a linear process defined by replicating dominant ideals of what "successful" development includes. As a way of responding to this

Table 6.2 Sample scripts for starting harm reduction and sexual health conversations around some common sexual scenarios

Sexual behavior or situation	Risk focused conversation	Harm reduction conversation	Going further conversation
Client does not use condoms during receptive anal sex.	"You should use a condom each time you have receptive anal sex to prevent HIV infection."	"Can you tell me more about how you decide to use or not use a condom during receptive anal sex? What things might make it easier to use a condom during receptive anal sex?" "What are your concerns, if any, about having receptive anal sex without condoms? I can share more about things like STI risk, but I want to make sure we focus on addressing what feels important to you here."	"While receptive anal sex can be associated with greater risk for acquiring HIV, many people do not use condoms. Some people chose to accept that risk for getting HIV. More recently, some people take PreP daily to avoid acquiring HIV."
Client is into sex that involves kink and is nervous or afraid to disclose.	"Are you using condoms? Do you use other devices during sex? Do you have a process for consent?"	"There are a wide variety of sexual activities. Can you tell me more about what you do so we can talk about reducing possible harm?" "Depending on the kind of activities you're doing, and what your goals are, we can figure out which harms we might focus on reducing and which ones don't need to be addressed as much or at all."	"Many people enjoy kink, but do not bring it up with their provider. Thank you for sharing this with me so we can work together to help you have pleasurable interactions that minimize harm to you and your partner(s)." "If there's any behavior you're nervous to disclose, I understand, and want to assure you I'm not here to force you to do or stop doing anything. Whatever you say is meant to help me give you more relevant suggestions for how to care for yourself. Feel free to ask me any questions that would make you feel more comfortable sharing."

Client does not want to have sex, and reports having no sexual attraction to other people or much of a sex drive.	"Sometimes even people who do not want to have sex or feel attraction do end up having sex with others, or sometimes even experiencing assault. Have you had any sexual experiences lately that may have put you at risk for STIs, pregnancy, or anything like that?"	"Is this something that you identify as a problem? If yes, we can have a discussion about it, but I don't want to assume it's an issue. Furthermore, I know preferences and behaviors don't always align, so if you are engaging in sexual activity even infrequently we may want to discuss how to make that a safer experience for you."	"Sex drives and attractions can vary for many reasons, and no one should be forced into sexual activity they don't want. Whether or not you continue to feel this way, I am here to help you figure out what kinds of tools and resources fit your situation."
Client reports they enjoy pain during sexual activity.	"What kind of things are you doing during masturbation or sex? Is there risk of injury, bleeding, infection, etc.?"	"What types of behaviors have you been learning about? Do you have access to information about how to keep yourself and partners as safe as possible while exploring these types of sexual play?"	"Many people can find pleasure in intense sensations during sex. Being aware of the risks associated with different activities makes it easier to have the experiences you want while also taking care of you and your partner(s)."
Client reports they are submissive to their partner.	"Is this something you're choosing for yourself or is someone pressuring you into it? Do you feel you can say no to interactions?"	"Can you tell me more about how your submission relates to the ways you have sex and negotiate consent with your partner? That way we can figure out health strategies that make sense for your situation."	"Many people engage in power play with their partners. What agreements or boundaries have you and your partner made around this power dynamic?"

(continued)

Table 6.2 (continued)

Sexual behavior or situation	Risk focused conversation	Harm reduction conversation	Going further conversation
Client reports skepticism about dental dams, or does not want to use them because they do not fit their or their partners' genitals properly. (This is especially common for clients assigned female at birth who have had a metoidioplasty and/or been on testosterone for a long time.)	"There are many infections that can be spread through skin to skin contact, so having oral sex without a barrier is a risk though it is lower than unprotected genital sex, for example."	"Can you tell me more about what your concerns are about dental dams? What might make it easier or more pleasurable to use them?"	"Dental dams are sometimes challenging to find or wear. If the issue is sensation and fit, some people instead choose to cut up a latex or nitrile glove for protection instead. This would mean cutting the fingers (except the thumb) off the glove and creating a slit up the side where the pinky would be. This opens up the glove and leaves the thumb of the glove as a place to put the [clitoris or other appropriate word based on client preference] and provide greater sensation as well as coverage."
Client is having unprotected sex and is at risk for STI transmission.	"Having sex without protection puts you at risk for STI transmission and possibly unintended pregnancy if that is biologically relevant. It would be safer to use protection."	"What goes into your decisions to not use protection?" "Do you know other ways you could reduce some of the risks that are associated with unprotected sex? Do you know about PEP and PrEP? Would you like any more information or to have a conversation about whether that could be a good choice for you?"	"Some patients are not concerned about being exposed or being infected with STIs and HIV. If that is your situation, we can still talk about the benefits of regular screening or testing to offer early identification and treatment options for you if you become infected."

			"There are a few ways people can practice safer sex if they don't like using external condoms. Have you ever used an internal condom? Sometimes people like them more than external condoms because you can place them before beginning sexual activity. Do you have access to body safe lubricant? Using it on its own can reduce the chance that an STI will be transmitted if it is present, although using it with a barrier offers the most protection.
Client reports having sex while under the influence of controlled substances or chemicals that may alter their judgment.	"It can be really unsafe to have sex while using substances because they can alter judgment. In some cases it is not possible for someone to give consent to sex if they've been using substances."	"What is going into your decision to mix substances with sex? What do you think the impact is on you when you make that decision? What things do you do to take care of yourself while you are using substances?"	"What do you appreciate and what do you dislike about using substances or chemicals? Are there other ways to get the same effect that may be safer? Would you be interested in brainstorming ways to still have the benefits you enjoy, while minimizing side effects and other risks?"

limitation, providers might consider that there is huge variance and diversity in the goals and outcomes for individual human development. We offer specific sex-positive and gender-affirming suggestions for providers to consider using—with clinical judgment in their specific developmental and cultural contexts—to reflect the importance of nurturing sex-positive and gender-affirming clinical care for families, children, and youth.

Providing Sex-Positive Care Across All Ages for All Types of Providers

- Continuously work to be aware of implicit biases and regularly invest time to build self-awareness around internally held prejudices, assumptions, and beliefs about sexuality within a complex matrix of identities.
  - Resource for self-development: attend a Sexual Attitude Reassessment (SAR)—an intensive multimedia experience to help members evaluate their biases, values, attitudes, and feelings regarding a variety of sexuality topics. This can help people identify what areas they need further training in, discover new issues they feel strongly about, recognize triggering topics they may need support around, and more—all with the goal of self-knowledge and application into work contexts.
- Seek to understand clients' gender and sexual identities within their own cultural context using a strengths-based, wellness, and resilience-focused framework, while also understanding that it is normal and healthy for this to shift and change over time. For many, disclosure about gender or sexual diversity does not occur until well into adulthood, so it is important to ask patients of all ages.
- Support clients in connecting to others in ways that are functional for them, their values, and their social context. This includes not assuming that romantic or emotional interests must specifically precede, follow, or even be linked to sexual interests.
- Make valid what is present in the moment and affirm possibility of that shifting without leaning on or hoping for a later shift that makes the client more legibly fit dominant societal narratives.
- Develop a trauma-informed clinical approach. Given the high rates of trauma in the general population and especially TGD communities [9], it is essential to incorporate knowledge about the impact of different forms of violence (including emotional, financial, sexual, and so forth) on client behavior and clinical practice. A trauma-informed approach can look like actively offering all clients choices and self-determination in conducting conversations that include sexuality and gender content. For example, giving clients tools and options to open or shut down discussions that relate to their personal sexuality, gender, or body. This can also mean explaining procedures before they happen and as they are taking place, allowing for processing time for the client, reducing shaming language overall (e.g., "STIs are bad or dirty"), paying attention to nonverbal cues that dissociation may be taking place, offering information via various channels rather than just

one (e.g., verbally, in writing, etc.), and asking questions like "Is there anything in your history that might make this procedure or conversation challenging?" and "Is there anything I could do to make this a more comfortable experience for you?"
- Screen for domestic violence holistically (including between housemates, relatives, past and present partners, etc.) and do not make gendered assumptions about the existence or direction of possible violence. Center questions on a patient's feelings of safety, access to resources they need to live, their ability to make decisions, others' respect for their needs and boundaries, etc.
- Consider the overarching concept of diversity in gender and sexuality, which, while commonly discussed in pediatric settings, is actually a part of our youth's generational and cultural experience at this time in the United States. Consider that developing a clear and direct degree of honesty, transparency in communicating with youth about sexual diversity opens the door to improved patient-centered care in areas that youth may not have formal or professional guidance. When appropriate and developmentally relevant, allowing for frank conversations about diverse sexual identities and practices such as role-playing, BDSM and kink, polyamory, asexuality, pansexuality, and other practices can be useful to youth considering or already engaged in these practices. Opening the conversation to questions about consent, sexual boundaries, sexual violence, sexual pleasure, as well as risks, addresses a fuller context of our youth's experience and reality, and encourages patient-centered care with a shared decision-making, affirmation model. Providers need safe spaces to understand that sexual diversity is real and is an important health topic to address. Open communication and patient-centered care in these sometimes sensitive areas can work to build a stronger, more authentic provider–patient relationship and access to practically addressing more specific sexual needs and care.
- Resource Sharing:
  - The Center of Excellence for Transgender Health has developed a comprehensive set of protocols for primary care and gender affirmation for trans and gender diverse people – http://transhealth.ucsf.edu/protocols
  - "The Body Keeps the Score" by Bessel van der Kolk
  - "Healing Sex: A Mind Body Approach to Healing Sexual Trauma" by Staci Haines
  - "Adopting a Trauma-Informed Approach for LGBTQ Youth: A Two-Part Resource for Schools and Agencies" – a digital PDF resource developed by National Resource Center for Mental Health Promotion and Youth Violence Prevention – https://healthysafechildren.org/sites/default/files/Trauma_Informed_Approach_LGBTQ_Youth_1.pdf

Very Early Childhood (Birth–2 Years)

Most providers do not consider this an important developmental age to address sexuality or gender development. However, an enormous amount of growth occurs during this time, including the maturation of skills that parents bring to their parent–child relationship. Specifically, in the first couple years of life, children are gathering and interpreting information about gender and sexuality as important ways people are classified within their communities.

- Assess if clients' social context includes engagement with people of diverse gender and sexual expressions.
- Support caregivers in awareness of and intentionality with gendered language, as well as other options they may not have considered, such as gender-neutral terminology (possible even in heavily gendered languages such as Spanish).
- Introduce or reaffirm that while infants are often assigned a sex and gender at birth based on parts and hormones, gender is an evolving concept that will develop over time. For some children assigned gender at birth is consistent with their developing gender identity. For other children, gender identity may deviate from their assigned gender at birth, and that gender diversity can be a normal aspect of human development and important to support. It is also worth noting that some may also learn that they have an intersex condition or difference of sexual development that can impact both their felt sense of gender as well as their body.
- Normalize for caregivers that it is typical for children to masturbate and explore the pleasure potential in their bodies and genitals. Support caregivers in being able to direct children to engage in these behaviors in safe, private spaces.
- Resource Sharing:
  - "InterACT: Advocates for Intersex Youth" developed a guide for providers around how to provide affirming care for gender diverse youth – https://interactadvocates.org/wp-content/uploads/2018/09/interACT-Lambda-Legal-intersex-hospital-policies.pdf
  - "Gender Spectrum" is an advocacy group that provides resources for both parents and providers of TGD youth – https://www.genderspectrum.org/explore-topics/

Toddlerhood (2–3 Years)

Toddlers are often in the process of learning how to categorize people and themselves based on their culturally contextual understanding of gender. At this age, children begin to integrate language, concepts, and values as they experience a wide range of explicit and implicit messages.

- With cultural humility, encourage caregivers to allow children to express preferences in clothing, hair, toys, and play. Acknowledge that while there may be cultural expectations with a family or community setting to gender and/or sexuality, there is also a larger world beyond family that may serve as a resource to a child who explores diversity in their gender and sexuality.
- Offer parents, family members, childcare providers, schools, and coaches opportunities to encourage experimentation with broader concepts of gender expectations, with language and activities that open doors rather than narrow experiences.

- Provide psychoeducation to caregivers around how to model bodily autonomy in interactions with toddler (e.g., teaching caregivers to offer children choices around physical contact that is not required for care, encouraging caregivers to use and teach language so children can label their full body including their genitals).

Early School Age (4–6)

Generally, this is the time frame when many children develop a firm sense of themselves as gendered beings. During this time, many children engage in gender-based play and continue to expand their vocabulary and understanding of self in context.

- Provide information that uses medically accurate and culturally sensitive terminology in defining genitals as being distinct from gender and identity. Allow youth to use terminology that may make discussions more, rather than less comfortable, with the explicit understanding that these substitutes are there to help them be honest and accurate as well.
- Ensure caregivers know how to access and provide affirming messages about the diversity of bodies regarding race, color, ability, size, gender, and age.
- Minimize absolute "gendering" of specific roles, tasks, and identities allowing children to be exposed to a wide variety of activities and interactions. This may occur both in homes and families, and in larger education, faith, sports and activities centers. Identify key stakeholders in these groups and in your community who are willing to modify curriculum or agendas to support diversity.
- Suggest ways caregivers can intentionally model diverse relationships styles by providing access to inclusive and sex-positive books, social circles, and conversations.
- Resource Sharing:
  - "What Makes a Baby?" by Cory Silverberg is a fun, relevant to young children, accurate, and gender-inclusive book that helps adults and young children have conversations about reproductive health.
  - "Flamingo Rampant Press" is a small publisher of intentionally positive and affirming children's books for young people of all gender identities.

Middle Childhood (6–12)

During this stage, children are often interacting with peers outside of the family for the first time in a meaningful way. This is an important developmental period for children to develop an internal sense of pride in themselves versus inferiority.

- Advocate that children begin comprehensive and inclusive sex education before puberty.
- Provide resources and education that frames consent as a complex process that benefits when participants to have strong self-awareness and communication

skills. Continue from previous discussions of body autonomy in the preschool years to build verbal and physical strategies that youth may apply in situations where they need to set limits regarding consent and autonomy.

- Begin to engage young people who demonstrate critical thinking skills to consider what their sexual beliefs, values, and attitudes are and how they developed them. Allow for time and open-ended discussions when confronted with questions that might be difficult to answer yourself. Model honesty and critical thinking when confronted with difficult questions or concepts from a youth.
- Begin to provide education to caregivers and youth that frames sexuality as a complex and multidimensional axis of identity. Introduce the concepts of human and child development as ongoing, lifelong evolving understandings of self and others. Introduce gender and sexuality as a normative aspect of all persons growing into adulthood.
- Actively practice affirming, non-stigmatizing language to discuss a broad range of relational and sexual communities, concepts, and practices including, but not limited to, asexuality, consent, sexual boundaries, sexual pressure and violence, safer sex practices, pleasure (as opposed to solely focusing on risk, and especially important when discussing holistic care and topics like masturbation), and varied family structures and relational arrangements (e.g., monogamous and non-monogamous, nuclear and extended, blended, etc.). For some, youth will grow curious about sexual diversity at an early age and bring up topics like kink and explicit sexual material as well. Thus, providers who understand these issues, resources, and ways to explore discussions around them (including how to screen for possible abuse as needed) may offer youth developmentally appropriate and needed safe spaces for better understanding their own burgeoning sexuality and that of those around them.
- Assess if there is confusion or tension around either gender or sexual identity as a part of every clinical assessment as a child moves into puberty. This might include asking a youth to describe how they relate to or think about their body currently, as well as what information they have and how they feel about any expected or experienced sexual development.
- Ensure that TGD youth have access to and receive adequate support in decision-making around sexual health integrated into their overall healthcare plan. This includes providing information on local mental health resources that support gender exploration and affirmation, as well as medical providers who may offer hormone blockers and gender-affirming hormones that might have an impact on sexual functioning, desires, sexual self-esteem and gender-related concerns.
- When discussing bodies, make information available about the range of appearances of secondary sex characteristics and genitals, including the realities of intersex people and differences of sexual development.
- Resource Sharing:
  - The Circles of Sexuality considered for TGD people. (http://forge-forward.org/wp-content/docs/HANDOUT-circles-of-sexuality-eli-r-green.pdf)
  - “Sex is a Funny Word” by Cory Silverberg is an inclusive resource for children in this developmental stage about bodies, sexuality, and gender.

Adolescence (12–18)

This is the developmental stage in which many youths are actively exploring different social contexts, identities, and roles. It is important to not pathologize this exploration, and to support youth in accessing safe ways to explore a multitude of ways they could express and understand themselves. This is also a time when peer networks are vital, and some differentiation from the family will also likely occur.

- Treat youth as experts of their own journey with regard to social indicators of gender. These can include using a youth's preferred name as well as respecting clothing choices, engagement in activities, and pronouns. Create a clinical context to demonstrate that their choices will be affirmed and respected whether they are consistent and static, or evolving and dynamic. Identify yourself as a non-judgmental and supportive adult who is comfortable discussing and has information about diverse gender and sexuality issues. Present yourself as a safe and respectful clinician who may offer education, resources, and benefits for the many ways youth experience gender and sexuality.
- Assess if youth have regular access to accurate, sex-positive discussions at home and at school. What sort of sex health education has that youth experienced? Did it offer helpful information? Was it stigmatizing or traumatizing in the context of their individual experience?
- Assess if youth have regular access to safe contexts and relationships to explore gender and sexual expression.
- Support ability to assess safety and make self-valuing choices as youths' independence and mobility increase by providing clinical opportunities for TGD youth to assess safety. Discuss approaches to disclosure of a diverse gender or sexual identity, and develop resiliency around fear of both anticipated and actual range of outcomes.
- Help youth consider how, if, and what forms of physical and emotional intimacy can affirm their gender and sexuality (e.g., does a particular sexual act or language for their body parts make them feel seen as their gender, does a particular form of verbal affection make them feel more or less cared for, etc.). Alternatively, help youth identify what forms of intimacy may be at odds with their gender experience.
- Ensure sexually active youth, including youth who are sexual with self, have access to relevant and a broad variety of safer sex supplies and interventions including barriers, body safe lubricants, masturbation aids, and pleasure-inclusive sex education.
- Assess if youth experience any types of dissociation when they are engaging in sexual activity. Have an awareness that TGD youth are more likely to interact with their bodies and sexual encounters as being connected to fear, danger, or trauma while also exploring if there are ways their body or sexual practices bring them pleasure and increased possibility of connection and joy.
- Listen to possible concerns around if "they are normal" or "if other people feel like this" and help normalize the wide range of human sexual experience, espe-

cially for youth that may be clearly identifying as TGD or on the asexual spectrum. Connect these youth to relevant resources about these questions and peer support networks as appropriate so they can combat feelings of isolation and increase feelings of social connectivity.
- Incorporate the topics of pleasure and a sense of well-being into discussions of sexual functioning, gender identity or expression, and even topics such as stress management.
- Help youth develop discernment and analysis skills to evaluate the sometimes tangled feelings of unhappiness, discomfort, pubertal distress, emotional dysregulation, body or gender dysphoria, etc., as sometimes many varyingly rooted concerns may be lumped together into somatic complaints or short statements about discomfort with their bodies. This often means asking clarifying questions about what and how things feel "bad," what sorts of things have helped, and why they think that might be, as well as asking how they usually experience emotions such as fear, anger, and sadness.
- Ensure that youth have support in decision-making around medical care that includes information about how choices to access gender-affirming medical care could impact their body, relationships, and sexual functioning, in both positive and challenging ways in both present and future.
- Resource sharing:
  – "Coming Out as You!" A digitally available zine from Trevor Project: https://www.thetrevorproject.org/about/programs-services/coming-out-as-you/

Early Adulthood (18–26)

Youth in this stage generally have a similar level of basic information as adults, but often have not developed the psychosocial, experiential, or emotional maturity to use this basis of information to realistically consider the more nuanced or long-term impacts of their choices, especially if there are issues that have slowed or arrested their development. Again, this sex-positive inclusive care will also help providers not to forget to routinely offer anticipatory guidance for patients with cognitive delays, physical limitations, and other complex medical conditions.

- Deconstruct the narrative that bodies are either sexually functioning or sexually dysfunctional within your clinical interactions. Instead, focus on what types of sexual and sensate experiences and capacities a person is invested in having in their lives. Help patients understand that different sources of messaging may have informed those desires, and support people in thinking expansively about how to realistically access these interests.
- Continue providing support for building experience in assessing safety. This includes resilience around disclosure around gender or sexual identities, especially when navigating connections via technological means such as dating apps.
- Support TGD youth in communicating with their partners using emotional literacy and understanding of how trauma can present during sexual encounters so

neither partner incorrectly interprets a TGD person's shame, or reluctance to engage in certain sexual acts, as a rejection or relating to their worth as a sexual partner.

- Do not assume that people develop asexual or aromantic sexual identities in response to trauma. Instead, use curiosity to unpack if there are unconscious connections you might be assuming. Clinicians should always assess for, but never assume, a TGD young person has experienced trauma. Instead of always seeing asexuality as a static orientation, explore what the *function* of the identity might play in that person's life.
- Help clients think through what sexual terminology feels pleasurable, affirming, or fun and creative ways they can communicate that to any relevant partners. S. Bear Bergman and Tobi Hill-Meyer are good resources for this, and the poem "How To Make Love To A Trans Person" by Gabe Moses can be an artistic way to engage an older youth on this topic.
- Share narratives and other resources, including ones that provide TGD-specific sexuality education and how-tos, that can help a client see themselves reflected in media and understand the myriad ways TGD people can experience relationships and pleasure.
- Resource Sharing:
  - "Nerve Endings: The New Trans Erotic" edited by Tobi Hill-Meyer.
  - "Mira Bellwether's sex-positive zine focused on sex with trans women"
  - "Girl Sex 101" by Allison Moon
  - "Trans Bodies, Trans Selves" Edited by Laura Erickson-Schroth
  - The Kink Clinical Practice Guidelines Project (www.kinkguidelines.com) which is an ongoing endeavor spearheaded by a diverse team of health professionals to create and regularly update best practices and guidelines for working with people who are interested and/or involved in kink, BDSM, and/or fetish eroticism.
  - Guides to safer-sex for trans men or trans women - https://www.tht.org.uk/hiv-and-sexual-health/sexual-health/improving-your-sexual-health/sex-trans-man AND https://www.tht.org.uk/hiv-and-sexual-health/sexual-health/improving-your-sexual-health/sex-trans-woman
  - There are many ways to use sexual enhancement devices to support people in having gender-affirming sexual experiences, or being able to access a specific type of physical pleasure or orgasm. For more information, visit The Center for Sexual Pleasure and Health at www.thecsph.org.

Conclusion

The discussions and resources in this chapter are a helpful starting place for clinicians beginning to develop a comprehensive, sex-positive clinical approach for patients of all genders and sexualities across the lifespan. In order to effectively integrate sex positivity into their work with TGD youth, it is essential that providers engage in an ongoing and dynamic process of building awareness of self and values around sexuality. As with other aspects of clinically engaging with vulnerable and disadvantaged populations, understanding how our personal lens affects our professional care, as well as recognizing and valuing the patient's individual experience as most relevant to care, is helpful in building trust and offering patient-centered services. It would never be possible to have expert knowledge on every sexuality topic that will be relevant to clients' care, just as each client will come with an individual and unique experience of their sexuality. However, by doing the work to approach all conversations about sexuality from a place of curiosity and humility, and to offer options for care that respect diversity, providers can provide a clinical context that supports TGD youth in accessing the sexual health care that responds to their unique and individual needs. As sexuality is an important aspect of human development and can so greatly impact overall health and safety, it is important that all providers consider how to best listen to their patients and engage in sex-positive counseling across the lifespan.

References

1. Burnes T, Singh AA, Witherspoon RG. Sex positivity and counseling psychology: an introduction to the major contribution. Couns Psychol. 2017;45(4):470–86.
2. Neustifter R, Underhill A, Manduley A, Powell L, Sasso T, Pascoe L, Beaton J. Defining sex positivity in therapy. Manuscript Submitted for Publication. 2017.
3. Burnes T, Singh AA, Witherspoon RG. Graduate counseling psychology training in sex and sexuality: an exploratory analysis. Couns Psychol. 2017;45(4):504–27.
4. Rafferty J, Committee on Psychosocial Aspects of Child and Family Health, Committee on Adolescence, Section on Lesbian, Gay, Bisexual and Transgender Health and Wellness, American Academy of Pediatrics. Ensuring comprehensive care and support for transgender and gender-diverse Children and Adolescents. Pediatrics. 2018;142(4):e20182162. http://pediatrics.aappublicatio.org/content/142/4/e20182162.
5. Bungener S, Steensma T, Cohen-Kettenis P, De V. Sexual and romantic experiences of transgender youth before gender-affirmative treatment. Pediatrics. 2017;139(3):e20162283. https://doi.org/10.1542/peds.2016-2283.
6. Cruz C, Greenwald E, Sandil R. Let's talk about sex: integrating sex positivity in counseling psychology practice. Couns Psychol. 2017;45(4):547–69.
7. Dunkley C, Brotto L. Clinical considerations in treating bdsm practitioners: a review. J Sex Marital Ther. 2018;44(7):701–12. https://doi.org/10.1080/0092623X.2018.1451792.
8. Koyama E. Disloyal to feminism: abuse of survivors within the domestic violence shelter system. In: Color of violence: the incite! anthology. Cambridge, MA: South End Press; 2006.
9. James SE, Herman JL, Rankin S, Keisling M, Mottet L, Anafi M. Executive summary of the report of the 2015 U.S. transgender survey. Washington, DC: National Center for Transgender Equality; 2016.

Patient-Centered Care: Providing Safe Spaces in Behavioral Health Settings

7

Alison M. Jost and Agnieszka Janicka

> In my early professional years I was asking the question: How can I treat, or cure, or change this person? Now I would phrase the question in this way: How can I provide a relationship which this person may use for [their] own personal growth? – Carl Rogers

In the United States over the past couple of years, heated cultural debates have emerged over the existence of safe spaces in academic settings, particularly on college campuses [1–3]. LGBTQ students, students of color, and other historically oppressed groups have argued for the importance of metaphorical and physical spaces free from bias, marginalization, and acts of aggression. As the continued creation of such spaces in schools and elsewhere becomes threatened, it becomes all the more important to understand the need for and purpose of these spaces in clinical settings.

The power of a safe therapeutic space cannot be overstated. For many of our transgender and gender diverse patients, whose days are regularly marked by parental rejection [4–7], peer hostility [8–11], and minority stress [12–15] (to say nothing of the internalized transphobia many carry on their own [16]), the clinical space may be the *only* place where they are met with acceptance and validation. As physicians, therapists, and other care providers, we are in a unique position to create a refuge for patients who otherwise are met with chronic rejection.

Through our work with over 200 transgender and gender diverse patients, we have found that there are certain crucial elements to creating patient-centered spaces that are safe and affirming in a meaningful, sustained way. Through a developing case study, we will explore some of the components that are essential to creating such spaces. As the case unfolds, we will pause to discuss important considerations for the transhealth provider.

A. M. Jost (✉) · A. Janicka
Adult Gender and Sexuality Behavioral Health Program at Lifespan, Providence, RI, USA

M. Forcier et al. (eds.), *Pediatric Gender Identity*,
https://doi.org/10.1007/978-3-030-38909-3_7

"Tell Me Your Story" – The Importance of Taking Patients at their Word

A 13-year-old asserting female, natal male, Sophie, is brought into a psychiatric outpatient clinic by her parents, who are concerned about her recent pronouncement that she is a girl. A few months ago, at the start of 8th grade, she asked others to call her Sophie, began using female pronouns, and grew her hair long. Her parents explain that up until recently she had never shown any interest in "girly" things, and that it was only after she began watching YouTube videos posted by a transgender girl that she came out as trans herself: "We're worried," they say. "We think she's acting out. This has to be some kind of phase." At the start of the interview, Sophie is tearful as she says, "My parents don't believe me. My doctor doesn't believe me. I don't know how to explain it to them."

Regardless of our particular discipline, as practitioners we are trained to approach cases with a certain critical curiosity. What is happening beyond what we see on the surface? Are we missing something? Is the patient telling us everything? This sense of scrutiny can be further heightened when we are talking to a child or teenager. The patient is so young, we find ourselves thinking – how can they possibly know what they are feeling? What if they change their mind? While a critical mind is essential to being a good clinician, when expressed with an air of paternalism, it quickly becomes antithetical to creating a validating and safe space.

Think for a moment about how any of us feel when we are met with doubt or skepticism in a clinical encounter. Meeting a doctor or practitioner who fails to listen to us, or who seems unconvinced by our story, is unpleasant at best and traumatic at worst. It certainly does not lead one to want to go back to that clinician. And think, too, of the powerlessness one feels as a child when faced with an "all knowing" adult whose stance is that they know more and best – the invalidation of these moments can create wounds that last a lifetime. Add to this any number of other power differentials [17] – race, class, education level, able-bodiedness, cis-privilege – and we quickly begin to see how we, as care providers, hold a potentially enormous amount of power that demands great care and attention. In short, it takes time to create a safe, validating space for our patients, and only a moment for one raised eyebrow to take it all away.

Our first duty as transhealth providers, then, is to truly *listen* to the patient's story – and to take them at their word [18]. Our starting position is that the patient – not us, not their parents [19] – is the expert on their own thoughts and feelings. Certainly, we take the thoughts and observations of these other people into careful consideration, but we look *first* to the patient about what they are experiencing. But what does taking a patient at their word look like in actual practice?

Let us return for a moment to the case of Sophie, who, like many of our patients, feels doubted and misunderstood. We see it all the time – even loving and well-meaning people in a patient's life regularly ask "how do you know you're really trans?" or "are you sure you're not gay?" or will tell a child or teen that they are "just going through a phase" or are "confused" or suffering from other mental health issues. Because of this, by the time they come to our office, many patients, especially adolescents, feel pressure to *prove* their gender identity to us as providers.

In our practice, we aim to take away this pressure by first attending carefully to the therapeutic tone and language we use. Whether sitting with a young child or an older adolescent, our presence should be empathic and accepting. Statements meant to elicit information should be inviting rather than questioning. Instead of asking Sophie, as her parents and doctor have, "how do you know you're trans?" we might instead say any of the following: "Would you mind telling me about your story?" "What would you like for me to know about what you think and feel?" or "What don't people in your life understand about what you're going through?" In Sophie's case, once she knows that it is not her responsibility to prove anything to us, the hope is that her story will unfold on its own terms, authentically and without being unduly influenced by other people's needs or agendas.

Honoring Diversity of Gender Experiences and Ambivalence about the Gender Affirmation Process

> As the initial meeting with Sophie continues, she shares more: "My parents don't think I'm trans because I was never girly when I was younger. But when my body started changing last year, everything felt wrong to me. Not just uncomfortable, but wrong, like this isn't the body I'm supposed to have. But they say trans people know they're trans when they're super young. Maybe I should just tell them I always knew so that they'll finally believe me."

For too many of our patients, there is little if any room outside of the therapeutic space to voice questions or ambivalence about their experience of their gender or the gender affirmation process. Because their stories are regularly doubted or challenged by parents [19], other family members, peers, teachers, or the larger community, it is entirely understandable that they do not share the parts of their experience that might invite further scrutiny and skepticism. As a result, patients like Sophie, fearing they will not receive the gender-affirming treatment they need unless they can convince us of their experiences, often initially downplay or deny any understandable ambivalence they might have about what they are going through and where treatment might take them.

We believe that a safe therapeutic space allows for two things: first, it recognizes the wide variety of gender experiences among individuals, and appreciates that narratives of gender incongruence will be different from person to person. Second, it honors the fact that individuals can be certain about their gender identity while also experiencing ambivalence about various aspects of gender affirmation. Let us address each of these points in turn.

Some patients understand from a very early age that their sex assigned at birth does not match their internal sense of themselves, and they are insistent, consistent, and persistent about this gender mismatch from childhood onwards [20]. For other patients, though, their gender identity journey is much more gradual, and they do not identify as transgender until adolescence or adulthood. We have worked with many patients who, like Sophie, showed no signs of gender incongruence until puberty, when they developed secondary sex characteristics. And we have worked with adult patients who say they always struggled with the knowledge that something was "different" about them, but who, until recently, never had the concepts or language to express that this difference was rooted in gender incongruence. A safe therapeutic space makes clear to patients that their stories do not have to fit one particular mold, and that the process of transition is different for every individual.

Many of us know that life transitions, even good ones, can be a major source of stress for people. Starting a new job, getting married, moving to a new town – even while we welcome these events, we can simultaneously feel overwhelmed or unmoored by them. While the parallel between these events and the process of gender affirmation is not perfect, this latter series of events often comes with a natural mix of excitement, relief, hope, uncertainty, trepidation, and many other emotions. Patients regularly deal with uncertainty about all manner of aspects of their transition – when and how to come out as transgender to family, friends, and peers; how to cope if and when they face rejection; whether to begin puberty blockers or hormones. Oftentimes, especially for adolescents, these decisions come with excruciating trade-offs – the choice to live a life that is authentic to oneself can, for instance, spell the loss of everything from parental approval to more tangible things like financial support and even housing [21, 22]. We believe that a safe therapeutic space honors the ambivalence that is likely to arise in the face of such difficult choices. One of our roles as clinicians is to help patients navigate feelings of ambivalence so that their transition, should they choose to move forward, is authentic to themselves and reflective of their hopes, goals, and needs.

Taking One's Time: Embracing Complexity and Sitting with Diagnostic Uncertainty

> During the early stages of treatment, Sophie and her parents provide the following additional information: Aside from her recent pronouncement of being transgender, she has a history of anxiety that began in early childhood. From the time she was quite little, she would become highly distressed by changes in her routine and has always had intense interests. At age 10, after her younger sister died following a 2-year battle with leukemia, her anxiety worsened and she attended outpatient therapy for about a year. Although her anxiety has not been an issue lately, she and her parents both note that over the last year her mood has been down, she no longer socializes with the couple of friends she has, she sleeps a lot after school, and her grades have fallen. In addition, she is barely eating and has lost 15 pounds in the past 2 months.

In a behavioral health setting, it is the rare patient who comes through our doors with a "neat," straightforward presentation of gender dysphoria. More often, patients come to us in crisis and with multiple presenting issues – severe depression, anxiety, self-injurious behavior, a trauma history, few, if any, social supports – all in addition to gender-related distress. The urge to "figure out" what is going on can be quite strong, particularly for practitioners trying to select the most appropriate and effective psychiatric medications. This urge is often heightened by the fact that many parents are desperate for answers about what is happening with their child, and they are looking to the clinician to provide them.

In a case like Sophie's, the various differential diagnoses can feel almost dizzying. Based on what is known so far, a clinician open to all possibilities would consider everything from a major depressive episode, to a complicated grief reaction, to an autism spectrum disorder, to an eating disorder like anorexia, all in addition to gender dysphoria. Her lack of eating and weight loss alone raise various possibilities: Is this a classic neurovegetative symptom of depression? Or perhaps this is anorexia, and she is purposely restricting her food intake to avoid weight gain. Or perhaps what looks like anorexia is not driven by a fear of becoming fat in and of itself, but rather by a fear of entering further into puberty. By restricting her food intake, she can stave off developing further secondary sex characteristics, thereby lessening the intensity of her gender dysphoria. All of these would be reasonable suppositions, and nothing but time and more information will bring greater diagnostic clarity.

To those ends – taking time and obtaining more information – we rely on the strength of the therapeutic rapport to ensure that patients return to us beyond the first clinical encounter, and allow us to obtain collateral information from other relevant sources. Indeed, because so many of the cases we see are highly complex, the information obtained from a patient's parents, primary care physicians, past therapists, and even teachers and other relatives can be invaluable in trying to determine the diagnoses and best course of treatment. Where Sophie's parents state that she has never expressed ambivalence about her gender before, for example, a past therapist or teacher might have observed otherwise.

Learning to sit with and even appreciate diagnostic uncertainty is not always easy, but there are several reasons to build tolerance for this. First, so many of these cases, especially in a psychiatric setting, are highly complex. Even cases that initially seem rather straightforward often end up being more nuanced over time. The more we come to expect this, the less daunting the work will be. Second, given that our patients are dealing with uncertainty all the time – what is happening to them? Will their parents and peers accept them? Will they "pass?" Are they safe to move about in the world? – it can be highly therapeutic for us to model what it looks like to accept that we do not always have all of the answers, and that uncertainty, while uncomfortable, is not something we must avoid.

Importantly, taking time to conceptualize a case does not necessarily mean taking the same amount of time to provide various indicated treatments, including puberty blockers and hormones. Full control of depression, anxiety, and other symptoms may not be possible in the context of significant gender dysphoria. Careful consideration of each condition and the interconnections among them is necessary in determining treatment, and often cotreatment of multiple conditions is necessary (for example, puberty blockers, antidepressants, and psychotherapy).

Fostering Future Orientation

As Sophie progresses in weekly outpatient psychotherapy, the extent of her depression becomes increasingly apparent. Although she makes clear that she would never commit suicide – "I'd never do that to my parents" – she endorses feeling chronically passively suicidal – "I wish I could go to sleep and never wake up. It'd be easier. I don't really care what happens to me."

Suicide is a major mental health concern among transgender children and adolescents [23].The rates of prior suicide attempts in transgender adolescents and young adults have ranged from 9% up to 30% [24–30]. It is critical that clinicians regularly monitor the nature and intensity of any suicidal ideation they observe in their patients. This should be done through the ongoing use of standardized assessment tools [31, 32] and through discussions in sessions with patients and their parents. But once a clinician has determined to the best of their ability that a patient like Sophie is not at risk of imminent harm, the task of getting treatment "off the ground" can feel equally challenging. How does one move treatment forward when a patient is mired in hopelessness and apathy? There are no easy answers to this question, but in our experience, one function of a safe therapeutic space is to enable a patient to identify the various factors that cause them to feel stuck in the first place. To an adolescent like Sophie, for instance, we might ask, "What seems easier about going to sleep forever? What wouldn't you have to face?" The point here is not to overemphasize the sources of a patient's hopelessness – in fact, the temptation as providers is often to rush past these topics because they make us feel so powerless – but to understand the causes of pain and despair in order to work through them.

For many of our patients, feelings of hopelessness emerge with particular intensity during puberty. If puberty is an uncomfortable time even for cisgender adolescents, then for transgender and gender diverse teens, this is a time when dysphoria often reaches unbearable levels. For some, like Sophie, it is not until the relative androgyny of their prepubescent body begins to disappear that they first express to others how "wrong" their developing bodies feel [33]. Understandably, many teens feel that the loss of control, confusion, and helplessness they feel during puberty is how they will *always* feel. We believe that another crucial function of a safe space is to make it easier for patients to access an imagined future where some of the issues they are dealing with now are resolved, and where they inevitably have more control over their lives [34].

To these ends, the therapeutic space becomes one in which a patient can explore what a future living their authentic self might look like. The clinician encourages this process by asking such questions as, " If you could totally be yourself, what would you look like? What kinds of things would you be doing? Who would you be with? Where would you live?" For patients whose parents do not provide permission for puberty blockers or hormonal treatment, it can be empowering to identify the possibilities that will be available to them when they are of legal age to make medical decisions. When this is many years off for a patient, the clinician can help extend the safety and hope of the therapeutic space by connecting the patient to local LGBTQ youth support groups, which can serve as a lifesaving reminder that a patient is not alone in their experience. If resources in the community are lacking, clinicians themselves may bring patients together for group therapy sessions that are adjunctive to individual psychotherapy.

Ideally, imagining a better life with the patient focuses on the near- *and* long-term future, addressing the real challenges of the present, while enabling the patient to see that these challenges are not permanent or insurmountable.

After four months in therapy, and with the addition of an SSRI, Sophie's depressive symptoms are gradually lessening. She no longer reports feeling passively suicidal, her appetite has improved, and she is engaging in schoolwork once again. She has begun attending afterschool activities at an LGBTQ community center, and she and her parents have attended several family therapy sessions. She has also met with an endocrinologist to discuss starting hormonal treatment. When asked about her progress in treatment, Sophie puts it this way: "I still have good days and bad days. It's not like everything is suddenly great or perfect. But at least now I care if I live, and I want to live, because there are things I want to do in the future. That's a good feeling. It keeps me going."

Conclusion

The approaches that we have outlined above are not new or revolutionary. They have been the mainstays of good psychotherapy for many decades now. But too often, because these cases can be confusing, complicated, uncomfortable, and full of urgency, we forget to ground ourselves in what we know. We know, because we have had the privilege of seeing it time and time again, that creating safe therapeutic spaces can make all the difference for a struggling transgender or gender diverse child or adolescent. When a patient knows that they will be taken at their word, when they hear that it is okay to feel ambivalent about certain aspects of transitioning, and that their story doesn't have to fit one particular mold, when the complexity of their struggles is honored and given room, and when they can imagine and take steps toward a better future, then at least they have one space in the world that is safe enough to be authentically themselves. From there, many things are possible.

References

1. Perez-Pena R, Smith M, Saul S. University of Chicago strikes back against campus political correctness. New York Times [Internet]. 2016 [cited 2019Mar5]. Available from: https://www.nytimes.com/2016/08/27/us/university-of-chicago-strikes-back-against-campus-political-correctness.html.
2. Jaschik S. Chicago professors fire back. Inside Higher Ed [Internet]. 2016 [cited 5 Mar 2019]. Available from: https://www.insidehighered.com/news/2016/09/14/u-chicago-professors-issue-letter-safe-spaces-and-trigger-warnings.
3. Ho K. Tackling the term: what is a safe space? [Internet]. Harvard Political Review. 2017 [cited 5 Mar 2019]. Available from: http://harvardpolitics.com/harvard/what-is-a-safe-space/.
4. Klein A, Golub SA. Family rejection as a predictor of suicide attempts and substance misuse among transgender and gender nonconforming adults. LGBT Health. 2016;3(3):193–9.
5. Ryan C, Huebner D, Diaz RM, Sanchez J. Family rejection as a predictor of negative health outcomes in white and latino lesbian, gay, and bisexual young adults. Pediatrics. 2009;123(1):346–52.
6. Olson KR, Durwood L, McLaughlin KA. Mental health of transgender children who are supported in their identities. Pediatrics. 2016;137(3):e20153223.
7. Ryan C, Russell ST, Huebner D, Diaz R, Sanchez J. Family acceptance in adolescence and the health of LGBT young adults. J Child Adolesc Psychiatr Nurs. 2010;23(4):205–13.
8. Russell ST, Ryan C, Toomey RB, Diaz RM, Sanchez J. Lesbian, gay, bisexual, and transgender adolescent school victimization: implications for young adult health and adjustment. J Sch Health. 2011;81(5):223–30.

9. Sterzing PR, Ratliff GA, Gartner RE, Mcgeough BL, Johnson KC. Social ecological correlates of polyvictimization among a national sample of transgender, genderqueer, and cisgender sexual minority adolescents. Child Abuse Negl. 2017;67:1–12.
10. Kosciw JG, Greytak EA, Giga NM, Villenas C, Danischewski DJ. The 2015 National school climate survey: the experiences of lesbian, gay, bisexual, transgender, and queer youth in our nation's schools [Internet]. GLSEN. 2016 [cited 5 Mar 2019]. Available from: https://files.eric.ed.gov/fulltext/ED574780.pdf.
11. Out in the Open. Education sector responses to violence based on sexual orientation and gender identity/expression. Paris: United Nations Educational, Scientific and Cultural Organization; 2016.
12. Hatzenbuehler ML, Pachankis JE. Stigma and minority stress as social determinants of health among lesbian, gay, bisexual, and transgender youth. Pediatr Clin N Am. 2016;63(6):985–97.
13. Pearlin LI, Schieman S, Fazio EM, Meersman SC. Stress, health, and the life course: some conceptual perspectives. J Health Soc Behav. 2005;46(2):205–19.
14. Hendricks ML, Testa RJ. A conceptual framework for clinical work with transgender and gender nonconforming clients: an adaptation of the minority stress model. Prof Psychol Res Pract. 2012;43(5):460–7.
15. Human Rights Campaign. Violence against the transgender community in 2017 [Internet]. Human Rights Campaign. 2019 [cited 5 Mar 2019]. Available from: https://www.hrc.org/resources/violence-against-the-transgender-community-in-2017.
16. Rood BA, Reisner SL, Puckett JA, Surace FI, Berman AK, Pantalone DW. Internalized transphobia: exploring perceptions of social messages in transgender and gender-nonconforming adults. Int J Transgend. 2017;18(4):411–26.
17. Nimmon L, Stenfors-Hayes T. The "handling" of power in the physician-patient encounter: perceptions from experienced physicians. BMC Med Educ. 2016;16(1):114.
18. Parens E. Taking people at their word [Internet]. Bioethics Forum. The Hastings Center. 2006 [cited 5 Mar 2019]. Available from: https://www.thehastingscenter.org/taking-people-at-their-word/.
19. Littman L. Rapid-onset gender dysphoria in adolescents and young adults: a study of parental reports. PLoS One. 2018;13(8):e0202330.
20. Meier C, Harris J, American Psychological Association. Fact sheet: gender diversity and transgender identity in children. Washington, DC: American Psychological Association; 2013.
21. Cochran BN, Stewart AJ, Ginzler JA, Cauce AM. Challenges faced by homeless sexual minorities: comparison of gay, lesbian, bisexual, and transgender homeless adolescents with their heterosexual counterparts. Am J Public Health. 2002;92(5):773–7.
22. Keuroghlian AS, Shtasel D, Bassuk EL. Out on the street: a public health and policy agenda for lesbian, gay, bisexual, and transgender youth who are homeless. Am J Orthopsychiatry. 2014;84(1):66–72.
23. Grossman AH, Daugelli AR. Transgender youth and life-threatening Behaviors. Suicide Life Threat Behav. 2007;37(5):527–37.
24. Spack NP, Edwards-Leeper L, Feldman HA, Leibowitz S, Mandel F, Diamond DA, et al. Children and adolescents with gender identity disorder referred to a pediatric medical center. Pediatrics. 2012;129(3):418–25.
25. Olson J, Schrager SM, Belzer M, Simons LK, Clark LF. Baseline physiologic and psychosocial characteristics of transgender youth seeking care for gender dysphoria. J Adolesc Health. 2015;57(4):374–80.
26. Reisner SL, Vetters R, Leclerc M, Zaslow S, Wolfrum S, Shumer D, et al. Mental health of transgender youth in care at an adolescent urban community health center: a matched retrospective cohort study. J Adolesc Health. 2015;56(3):274–9.
27. Kaltiala-Heino R, Sumia M, Työläjärvi M, Lindberg N. Two years of gender identity service for minors: overrepresentation of natal girls with severe problems in adolescent development. Child Adolesc Psychiatry Ment Health. 2015;9(1):9.
28. Holt V, Skagerberg E, Dunsford M. Young people with features of gender dysphoria: demographics and associated difficulties. Clin Child Psychol Psychiatry. 2014;21(1):108–18.

29. Peterson CM, Matthews A, Copps-Smith E, Conard LA. Suicidality, self-harm, and body dissatisfaction in transgender adolescents and emerging adults with gender dysphoria. Suicide Life Threat Behav. 2016;47(4):475–82.
30. Eisenberg ME, Gower AL, Mcmorris BJ, Rider GN, Shea G, Coleman E. Risk and protective factors in the lives of transgender/gender nonconforming adolescents. J Adolesc Health. 2017;61(4):521–6.
31. The Lighthouse Project [Internet]. The Columbia lighthouse project. 2019 [cited 5 Mar 2019]. Available from: http://cssrs.columbia.edu/.
32. Suicide Prevention Resource Center. Suicide assessment five-step evaluation and triage for mental health professionals [Internet]. Available from: https://www.integration.samhsa.gov/images/res/SAFE_T.pdf.
33. Pattillo M. Gender dysphoria study faces criticism. Brown Daily Herald [Internet]. 2018 [cited 5 Mar 2019]. Available from: http://www.browndailyherald.com/2018/09/04/gender-dysphoria-study-meets-criticism/.
34. It Gets Better. Available from: https://itgetsbetter.org/about/.

Primary Care

8

Jaye Watts and Chelsea Graham

Objectives

1. To illustrate primary care as a key model for the delivery of health care for gender diverse individuals. This includes an interdisciplinary, patient-centered medical home, practice management, care coordination, and electronic health records.
2. To describe the elements of primary care for transgender youth, including preventive health and screening: substance use, depression and anxiety, vaccines, contraception, sexual health, education, and home safety.

Primary Care: An Important Healthcare Delivery Model

Gender-affirming care is primary care. The World Professional Association for Transgender Health (WPATH) supports primary care providers (PCPs) as a cornerstone in healthcare delivery [1]. PCPs are charged with providing a holistic, comprehensive assessment and longitudinal approach to care plans. Becoming familiar over many years, with both a youth and their family, allows for patients and providers to create a therapeutic, trusting relationship. Establishing a strong, respectful relationship between patient and provider is critical to improving long-term transgender health outcomes. The US Transgender Survey (USTS) reports that 33% of people who saw a doctor in the last year had at least one negative experience and 23% did not seek health care for fear of being mistreated [2].

PCPs are the pillars of community-centered, patient-responsive care, in that they promote and ensure physical and emotional health as well as social well-being. PCPs should model acceptance, affirming language and destigmatize transgender/gender diverse (TGD) identities for both patients and parents. It is essential for the PCP to

J. Watts · C. Graham (✉)
Thundermist Health Center and Brown Family Medicine Residency, Pawtucket, RI, USA
e-mail: chelseagr@thundermisthealth.org

M. Forcier et al. (eds.), *Pediatric Gender Identity*,
https://doi.org/10.1007/978-3-030-38909-3_8

develop a nonjudgmental partnership that equally affirms the experiences of both the patient and their parents [3], given the important role of parent support in improving TGD youth health outcomes. High-quality, knowledgeable, respectful medical care is essential to building a strong partnership with all patients, including gender and/or sexual minority patients.

PCPs offer anticipatory guidance in addition to providing gender-affirming care, but both are clearly complementary and build upon each other in promoting long-term reduction of morbidity and promoting healthier outcomes. Transgender individuals face additional barriers to long-term positive health outcomes and are less likely than their cisgender peers to have their preventive care needs met [4]. A trans-competent PCP can thus promote general preventive health care and quality of life, as they support their patient's gender identity and offer broad-based gender-affirming options for care.

PCPs who provide anticipatory guidance to children, adolescents, and young adults offer a paradigm of screening and early intervention in regard to a wide variety of pediatric health issues, including family connectedness, peer and school engagement, safety, nutrition, substance use, sexual development, and mental health concerns. This model, the HEADSSS (Table 8.1) wellness and risk screening exam, forms the basis for youth wellness visits and can provide young people who are questioning their gender identity an opportunity to confide in their providers from an earlier age. This format creates a safe space because patients are given permission to talk about a wide variety of sensitive subjects. Thus far it appears that earlier identification and support may reduce internalized stigma and psychological distress [5].

When youth disclose a TGD identity to their families, a family's first inclination may be to reach out to their primary care provider for information and support. Providers who have a well-established relationship with a family already have some degree of familiarity and trust and can offer a wonderful opportunity to model careful listening and acceptance for families. Parents most often want to help their children and have fears about their safety, health, and well-being in general that can be escalated when a child discloses that they are TGD. PCPs can reassure caregivers that listening carefully to their child, accepting and loving the authentic child, and following a child's lead as they explore and learn more about their unique gender identity is critical to all children's healthy development. PCPs who incorporate a gender history in their patient interview and care for all of their patients, cis or trans, promote honest discussions about healthy human development that can move both children and families toward acknowledgment, acceptance, and even celebration of a youth moving toward an increasing independent and healthy development.

Gender-Affirming Preventive Health, Development, and Risk Assessment

Primary care providers play an integral role in preventive health, and health maintenance for all youth, including our gender diverse patients. WPATH supports primary care providers as a cornerstone for accessible, comprehensive healthcare

Table 8.1 HEADSSS screening tool for adolescent and young adult anticipatory guidance for gender diverse youth

Home	Who do you live with? Tell me about your family.
	Who have you disclosed to in the home, family setting?
	Do you have family support?
	If not biologic family support, who is your family of choice?
Education/ employment	Are you in school, which school? Are you disclosed at school to: friends, all students, faculty/staff?
	What grade are you in? How is school/work going? What grades do you get?
	How do you get along with your peers? What types of supports are offered for TGD students? Who is a good point of contact for support?
	Any bullying?
	Future goals?
Activities	Tell me about your friends. Who are you disclosed to? How did you disclose and how are your friends supporting or not supporting you?
	What are your interests? What do you do for fun? Are you engaged in any LGBTQ+ support or activity groups at school or in your community?
	How much screen time are you using? Do you have an online presence and online TGD friends and contacts that you go to for support and information?
Drugs/ substance use	Many young people experiment with drugs. Have you or your friends tried anything (tobacco/alcohol or illicit substances)? This also includes drugs not prescribed to you or hormones not prescribed to you. It is helpful for me to know, not to judge you, but to have an idea of what your exposures and risks might be (i.e., framing why for sensitive questions)
Safety	Do you have any history of trauma? This may include bullying, child abuse, domestic or dating violence.
	Are you currently experiencing trauma? This can be emotional, physical, or sexual.
	Have you ever felt pressured or pushed to have sex? Have you been in situations where you feel physically unsafe? Where/what are these situations?
Suicide/ mental health	Have you ever struggled with depression and/or anxiety?
	Have you ever tried to harm yourself? How have you tried to hurt yourself?
	Have you ever thought about dying or not being alive? Have you ever fantasized about hurting or killing yourself?
	Have you ever tried to commit suicide?
	Have you ever been hospitalized for your mental health?
Sexuality	What kinds of people are you attracted to (sexual orientation)?
	Are you in a relationship, romantic, sexual, or other?
	Do you have any sexual partners? Tell me about them (their sex and gender). How many partners have you had? In the past six months? In the past year?
	If sexually active, what parts of your body do you use for sex? This helps us to better screen for sexually transmitted infections (i.e., framing)
	Have you ever been treated for an infection from sex?
	Have you ever been pregnant or involved with a pregnancy?
	Do you want to be pregnant now or in the future?
	If not, what do you do to protect yourself from infection and/or pregnancy?
	Have you ever exchanged sex for money, drugs, a place to stay, or anything?

delivery [1]. There are a variety of online resources for primary care providers to deliver trans-sensitive and relevant primary care for their gender diverse youth and adult patients [6, 7]. As with their cisgender peers, TGD children and adolescents should be comprehensively screened and offered information about healthy decision-making and behaviors. Primary care services for all youth include vaccinations, contraception, family planning, sexually transmitted infection (STI) screening as well as promoting and ensuring physical, emotional, and social well-being.

When taking a complete medical and psychosocial history for youth, it should include a gender history. Not all youth who have questions about their gender will present with that chief complaint. Instead, they might show signs of depression or poor school performance or engage in risky behaviors because they are struggling with their identity [8, 9]. It is important to ensure confidentiality and ask these questions separately from the caregiver, as is done with the HEADSSS exam (Table 8.1). We recommend taking a gender history from an early age. You may present the question like this, 'For many youth, their gender and sexuality is an important part of their identity. Have you ever had questions about your gender identity?' In well child checks, the clinician can start asking patients and their families about gender as early as age 3. Initial questions for the patients and their parents may be about child play, friends, hairstyles, and dress preferences. The earlier providers ask, the less likely they are to miss key developmental stages. Taking a gender history on all children and adolescents not only helps to recognize gender diverse youth, but it normalizes conversations about gender and plants seeds for future allies.

Another crucial piece of anticipatory guidance for adolescent development that primary care clinicians can address is puberty. When discussing puberty with youth, ask people how they feel in their bodies. Ask questions such as, "What do you like about your adolescent developing body and self; what do you not like?" This allows the clinician to capture youth who may be experiencing gender dysphoria as secondary gender characteristics begin to declare themselves physically. Timing is important because the risk of suicide, depression, and self-destructive behaviors for TGD and all youth increases with puberty [9]. Identifying gender dysphoria at this stage can be lifesaving.

PCPs have the option to offer appropriate referrals to mental health and medical persons who specialize in gender. These gender experts can recommend a variety of puberty suppressing endocrine therapies if the person is in early puberty (i.e., tanner stage 2). PCPs are increasingly able to start hormone therapy themselves in many primary care settings, given an increase in education and training opportunities in medical school, residency, and continuing medical education settings [1, 10]. For prepubertal youth who are considering social transition, no medications or interventions are required other than the primary care provider supporting their parents in creating a gender affirmative space to explore their gender identity with completely reversible efforts via dress, hairstyles, name, and pronouns [11].

Primary Prevention

Primary prevention and anticipatory guidance for TGD youth follow guidelines for cisgender peers with the caveat that screening should take into consideration current hormone therapy and anatomy. As with their cisgender peers, TGD youth should be offered early childhood vaccines as well as vaccines during the adolescent years including the following: tetanus, diphtheria, and pertussis (Tdap), human papillomavirus (HPV), hepatitis A, and meningitis. For all adolescents, the HPV vaccine is recommended, as early as age 9, and at least by ages 11 or 12, prior to sexual debut. The HPV vaccine may prevent some oncogenic strains of HPV from oral, rectal, penile, and cervical cancers. It is currently offered as a two-dose series before age 15, and a three-dose series now extended into later adulthood. Adolescents may be tested for immunity or offered the hepatitis A and hepatitis B vaccine series to prevent transmission of these food- and fluid-borne diseases. MenACWY, one of the meningococcal vaccines, is recommended for all youth. MenB, the other meningococcal vaccine, can be offered based on an individual basis with the target ages between 16 and 23 years. All patients should receive the annual influenza vaccine [12].

Home

All adolescents should be asked about their living situation to assess safety in their home environment. In one survey, 32% of youth in homeless shelters left home because of emotional, physical, or sexual abuse. In this cohort, approximately 45% ran away or were rejected from home because of their sexual orientation or gender identity. Parental rejection has been shown to lead to homelessness and increased risk of suicidality [13, 14]. The evidence seems to consistently demonstrate that even small decreases in parental rejection offer youth protective long-term health outcomes against depression, suicide, and substance use [15, 16].

Transgender and gender diverse individuals are especially vulnerable in the areas of housing insecurity, with subsequent implications for health and well-being. The USTS 2015 survey reports that TGD individuals are overrepresented in homeless populations. Thirty percent of respondents report experiencing homelessness at some point in their lifetime and 25% of respondents who reported being homeless in the past year report avoiding shelters due to safety concerns [2]. Because of these housing and financial disadvantages, TGD individuals are more at risk for needing to rely on sex work for economic security, trading sex for shelter, food, or substances of abuse [17]. TGD persons may experience higher incarceration rates related to these deficits in home support, economic and educational engagement, as well as traditional system safety nets. Providers should be aware that social safety net resources to which you refer cisgender patients may not be safe or appropriate for transgender individuals.

Education

School and social settings are an important part of socialization and identity formation for all youth. A nationwide internet survey conducted by the University of Connecticut and the Human Rights Campaign showed that 73% of lesbian, gay, bisexual, transgender, and queer (LGBTQ+) students received verbal threats because of their identity [18]. Bullying is even more prevalent for TGD youth of color because of racism, where four out of five youth report being a victim of racism. In this study, half of the transgender girls reported being physically threatened [18]. Additionally, teachers and administrators in school settings may tolerate these bullying activities, ignore, or participate in harassment. Bullying can then lead to minority stress [see Chap. 5. Minority Stress & The Impact of Acceptance] and put youth at increased risk for engaging in substance use and other risk behaviors that can lead to poor health outcomes [19]. In particular, bathrooms and locker rooms may become a point of contention and provide obstacles to a smooth transition in some school settings. National and state laws may offer or exclude protections for TGD individuals [18].

Resiliency is supported and promoted in schools that have Gay Straight Alliances and other school-based networks to support gender and sexual minority youth create protective factors that decrease stress, risky behaviors, and mitigate negative experiences [17]. Although PCPs may not participate intensively in creating specific educational plans, they may guide the families toward requesting appropriate interventions including an individualized education plan (IEP). In instances where bullying is undermining academic progress, they can request an IEP. PCPs can also involve their behavioral health and social work colleagues to help create this safe learning environment.

Activities

TGD youth are more likely to suffer from disordered eating which is often related to body dissatisfaction prior to the gender affirmation process [20]. Sports teams and other clubs based on gender may also present obstacles for TGD youth from integrating seamlessly into larger social networks. Lack of shared experiences or bullying may mean some TGD youth are less connected, supported, and more socially isolated than cisgender peers. Peer relationships are important developmental tasks and help youth meet developmental milestones that move a youth toward their adult identity.

Drugs/Substance Use

Annual adolescent anticipatory guidance visits should include questions about substance use, including tobacco, alcohol, marijuana, and illicit drugs. The Teen Health and Technology Study showed that gender minority youth have earlier and increased use of tobacco, alcohol, marijuana, and other illicit substances in the last 12 months when compared to cisgender peers [19]. Substance use was also correlated with increased rates of bullying [19]. As with all adolescents, screening for substance use should be regularly updated.

Sexual Health and Family Planning

As part of the psychosocial adolescent history, it is important to take an inclusive sexual history. This should include an organ inventory of current anatomy, partners, practices, as well as a history of prior activities and STIs [21]. Discussions should promote a nonjudgmental inquiry that attempts to look at specific behaviors that can lead to both increased risk as well as increased opportunities for preventive interventions. Safer sex practices with regular screening, consistent use of barrier methods, as well as pre- and postexposure (PrEP and PEP) practices to prevent human immunodeficiency virus (HIV) offer youth opportunities to improve self-efficacy and self-care in an important area of adolescent and young adult development.

The Center for Disease Control (CDC) suggests that all adolescents begin screening for HIV at age 13. Screening intervals then depend on sexual practices. Transgender women are estimated to have a high prevalence of HIV in the United States (14.1%) and an even higher prevalence in Black transgender women (44.2%) [22, 23]. Recommendations for STI screening in transgender adolescents and young adults can be extrapolated from current CDC guidelines, as there is limited data in the literature specific to this population. Screening for gonorrhea and chlamydia in sexually active transgender youth should be annual, based on general guidelines for assigned cisgender anticipatory guidance, specific sexual practices and at least annually done until age 24 [21]. Transgender females who have receptive anal sex with assigned males are also at higher risk and should be offered chlamydia and gonorrhea screening at least annually at points of contact (oral, urethra, and rectum). Hepatitis C and syphilis screening should be offered to young transgender women who have sex with assigned males [22]. TGD youth who engage in sex work should also be STI screened on a routine basis and considered eligible for PrEP.

Family planning is an important aspect of sexual anticipatory guidance for all youth. Patients with a uterus and ovaries can become pregnant even on testosterone and without experiencing periods. Patients with sperm and testes can create a pregnancy even on estrogen. If transgender males want to prevent pregnancy and are having sperm–egg sex, clinicians can offer effective long-acting reversible contraceptives such as intrauterine devices, the etonogestrel implant, progestin injections, or combined estrogen–progesterone birth control medications. It is important to note that testosterone is a teratogen and is contraindicated in pregnancy. Some of these methods also help with cessation of menses for patients suffering from dysphoria during menses, in addition to providing contraception.

The Reproductive Health Access Project and Bedsider.org have patient-friendly information that includes birth control options for patients across the gender spectrum [24, 25]. It is important to have these conversations in an inclusive and affirming manner to avoid unintended pregnancies and allow patients to have autonomy over their body and reproductive system. Additionally, full scope family planning recognizes that some transgender persons may at some point want to explore genetic parenting. Transgender males and females who want to have genetic children should be referred to reproductive endocrinology to discuss oocyte cryopreservation and urology for sperm banking.

Safety, Suicide, and Mental Health

All adolescents should be screened for depression, anxiety, self-injurious behaviors, and suicide risk. Depression and anxiety are common mental health concerns in TGD populations [26–28]. Even more concerning is the high rate of suicidality and suicide attempts [29, 30]. Minority stress, lack of support, stigma, and discrimination are directly linked to the increased rates of mental health concerns listed above [31]. We also recommend screening for intimate partner violence and any history of childhood trauma or abuse, as modeled in Table 8.1.

Understanding the increase in prevalence of mental health and safety concerns can lead to more in-depth screening and appropriate referrals to gender-affirming mental health providers. It is helpful for the PCP to learn more about local and regional mental health experts who are comfortable and knowledgeable about the intersectionality of gender and mental health care. Youth and families should not be expected to educate their mental health providers on the basics of gender care and sequelae of TGD identity in contemporary cultures.

Practice Management

Patient engagement in primary care involves more than provider knowledge and skills, it includes a whole clinic experience. A patient's experience begins with the first point of contact, from when a patient calls to make an appointment. It continues through patient registration and the forms patients are asked to complete and then on to questions during medical assistant intakes that may include taking medication and surgical histories. The visit may conclude with orders for labs and studies after discharge. Nurses need access to information about medications, prior authorizations, and how to manage telephone encounters that might come up in the course of providing care. Having gender knowledgeable staff offers additional supports and models for an affirmative medical experience [32, 33].

Particular care should be taken to train all support staff including call center and reception employees [34]. Asking every patient what their asserted name and pronouns are is respectful and not only indicates a certain cultural sensitivity to the trans experience, but also reflects overall patient-centered care. When providers or staff misgender or make mistakes, clear and honest acknowledgment and apologies offer clinic personnel a means to connect and improve future care. One should also take care not to *over*apologize and create a scenario where the personnel's guilt becomes the focus of the interaction.

Billing personnel must be aware of common issues related to insurance including claim denials due to incongruent gender markers between the practice and insurance provider, and insurance policies that continue to place exclusions on the use of certain codes for gender-affirming care. For efficiency, all forms, workflows, and operating procedures should be reviewed to make sure they address the unique needs of transgender individuals. Small adjustments can eliminate the need for either special processes for transgender individuals and more importantly reduce barriers or problematic situations (see Table 8.2).

Table 8.2 Potential pitfalls and patient-centered alternatives for practice management

Instead of this	Try this
When a new patient calls to register, guessing the gender based on their name and voice	Ask each patient what gender marker they want on their record
Only collecting information about a patient's legal name	Ask each patient if there is a different name that they would like you to use for them and create a system for everyone who uses the record to be notified of a patient's affirmed name
Forms that say ☐ Male ☐ Female (check one)	Gender: ______________ or Use 2-step method asking assigned sex at birth and current gender identity [35]
Guessing at a person's pronouns based on their appearance	Create a space on your intake form that asks: What pronouns do you use? (ex. he, she, they, etc…) Have documentation Ask all patients' names and pronouns for office use
Calling patients from the waiting area by the name on their record	Ask patients how they would like to be addressed when called from the waiting area or Use an anonymous pager system that will alert a patient when it is their turn
Sending out patient letters addressing the patient by the name on their record	Use a system that will populate affirmed names, when present, on letters addressed to the patient (with the patient's permission)
Gendering restrooms that are single occupancy	Clearly indicate that single occupancy restrooms are gender neutral
Requiring someone to use the gender marker on health record that is filed with their health insurance company	Make a billing note to submit bills with the gender marker on their health insurance and use their affirmed gender marker on their record; Be prepared to change the gender marker (on the bill) and resubmit bills that are denied due to mismatched gender markers

Electronic Health Records

A key component of trans-affirmative practice management involves the ease with which the Electronic Health Record (EHR) captures and operationalizes information about the TGD individuals it proposes to serve. An optimal system would include multiple gender identities and affirmed names in functional places and on identifying materials. However, many systems require 'workarounds' to make sure that the system captures a person's affirmed name, pronouns, and identity. Trouble spots include systems that 'helpfully' exclude a certain diagnosis or lab orders based on the gender on a patient's record and structured data fields that do not inform or connect to other parts of the EHR in any sort of meaningful or useful manner. For example, in one system that has an option to identify a patient as transgender, the information interacts with the clinical decision support system by suppressing all preventive screening alerts, rendering that system useless for monitoring preventive health screening for transgender individuals. A possible solution could include an organ inventory option that connects to the preventive screening alerts.

There have been some recent improvements, including federal requirements for EHRs certified under Stage 3 of Meaningful Use to include structured data on sexual orientation and gender identity [36, 37]. Providers or practices which are considering switching or upgrading their EHR should be asking questions about how the system functions regarding TGD individuals. Systems will not change, unless administrators demand better options. Instead of asking the patient to adapt to the limitations of the system, we must be asking why the system is not adapting to the needs of the patient.

Patient-Centered Medical Homes

An interdisciplinary, patient-centered medical home is a great model for TGD-sensitive and savvy health services. TGD individuals who can receive care for preventive health and chronic conditions in the same place as their gender-affirming hormone treatment may be more likely to adhere to treatment plans and stay engaged with those providers [38]. The services offered within a patient-centered medical home also offer tangible resources and supports for individuals who struggle with health literacy, anxiety, and organization recognizing that intersectionality of disparities will additionally affect care.

Community health centers that focus on caring for marginalized and vulnerable populations may offer same-day urgent appointments, sliding scales, or free care for people who are uninsured or underinsured. A study looking at underserved transgender adults in Massachusetts found that common barriers to care included a younger age, low income, and low educational attainment [39]. Marginalized populations and individuals are more likely to also experience lower levels of health literacy making it especially difficult to navigate the healthcare system without additional supports. Community health centers utilizing an integrated care approach, including behavioral health clinicians, case managers, nurse care managers, or peer navigators, may help to reduce these barriers and keep high-risk patients engaged. Addressing known social determinants of health including risks especially prevalent in TGD populations that include suboptimal housing, food insecurity, transportation issues, and financial barriers is a part of primary care.

Care Coordination

It is likely at some point a transgender patient will need to be referred for some sort of specialty care. The PCPs should take extra care in ensuring that the provider to which they refer is also prepared to care for gender diverse individuals. This may include contacting the specialist in advance and ensuring the referral includes patient's gender identity, affirmed name, and pronouns if these are different from the legal name in the EHR. In the event a patient has a negative experience, PCPs should follow up with the specialist about the patient's concerns. PCPs should also be prepared to work together with behavioral health providers, surgeons, and others involved in the patient's gender-affirming care, particularly around referrals for surgery and possibly preoperative or postoperative health concerns. PCPs can help to ensure required documentation is sent to the surgeon with the referral to streamline the process of prior authorization and obtaining a surgical consultation. [See Chap. 20.].

Conclusion: Creating a Longitudinal Partnership with Youth

The PCP's role is to partner with patients and their families from a young age to create a healthy, longitudinal relationship. They are often the first providers that patients will meet and can incorporate routine gender histories, nonjudgmental interviewing techniques, application of appropriate names and pronouns, demonstrating that they will provide excellent full scope health services. If patients have had a prior negative experience with health care, it may take them even longer to build trust with their current providers. In addition to building trust and creating inclusive environments, PCPs are well placed to build alliances with their patients and communities. PCPs can open new doors to healthcare services, previously not explored by many TGD patients, by working to understand their experiences, fears, and barriers, and being knowledgeable about area resources. PCPs have an opportunity to provide TGD-sensitive care, as they offer general medical anticipatory guidance or specific affirming health services for TGD individuals seeking primary care. PCPs have opportunities to connect, to promote well-being, and to support TGD patients at all stages of identity development and across the life span.

References

1. Coleman E, Bockting W, Botzer M, Cohen-Kettenis P, DeCuypere G, Feldman J, et al. Standards of care for the health of transsexual, transgender, and gender-nonconforming people, version 7. Int J Transgend. 2012;13(4):165–232. https://doi.org/10.1080/15532739.2011.700873.
2. James SE, Herman JL, Rankin S, Keisling M, Mottet L, Anafi M. The report of the 2015 US transgender survey, 2018.
3. Rafferty J, Committee on Psychosocial Aspects of Child and Family Health. Ensuring comprehensive care and support for transgender and gender-diverse children and adolescents. Pediatrics. 2018;142(4):e20182162.
4. Erickson-Schroth L, editor. Trans bodies, trans selves: a resource for the transgender community. Oxford: Oxford University Press; 2014. p. 215–22.
5. Olson KR, Durwood L, DeMeules M, McLaughlin KA. Mental health of transgender children who are supported in their identities. Pediatrics. 2016;137(3):1.
6. Deutsch MB, editor. Guidelines for the primary and gender-affirming care of transgender and gender nonbinary people. San Francisco: University of California; 2016.
7. Cavanaugh T, Hopwood R, Lambert C. Informed consent in the medical care of transgender and gender-nonconforming patients. AMA J Ethics. 2016;18(11):1147–55.
8. Brill S, Kenney L. The transgender teen: a handbook for parents and professionals supporting transgender and non-binary teens. San Francisco: Cleis Press; 2016.
9. Lopez X, Stewart S, Jacobson-Dickman E. Approach to children and adolescents with gender dysphoria. Pediatr Rev. 2016;37(3):89–96; quiz 97–8. https://doi.org/10.1542/pir.2015-0032.
10. Hembree WC, Cohen-Kettenis PT, Gooren L, Hannema SE, Meyer WJ, Murad MH, Rosenthal SM, Safer JD, Tangpricha V, T'Sjoen GG. Endocrine treatment of gender-dysphoric/gender-incongruent persons: an endocrine society clinical practice guideline. J Clin Endocrinol Metabol. 2017;102(11):3869–903. https://doi.org/10.4158/1934-2403-23.12.1437.
11. De Vries AL, Klink D, Cohen-Kettenis PT. What the primary care pediatrician needs to know about gender incongruence and gender dysphoria in children and adolescents. Pediatr Clin. 2016;63(6):1121–35. https://doi.org/10.1016/j.pcl.2016.07.011.
12. Recommended immunization schedule for children and adolescents aged 18 years or younger. United States: Centers for Disease Control and Prevention; 2018. https://www.cdc.gov/vaccines/schedules/downloads/child/0-18yrs-child-combined-schedule.pdf. Accessed 8 Dec 2018.
13. Durso LE, Gates GJ. Serving our youth: findings from a national survey of services providers working with lesbian, gay, bisexual and transgender youth who are homeless or at risk of becoming homeless. New York: The Williams Institute with True Colors Fund and The Palette Fund; 2012.
14. Klein A, Golub SA. Family rejection as a predictor of suicide attempts and substance misuse among transgender and gender nonconforming adults. LGBT Health. 2016;3(3):193–9.
15. Katz-Wise SL, Rosario M, Tsappis M. LGBT youth and family acceptance. Pediatr Clin N Am. 2016;63(6):1011–25.
16. Ryan C, Russell ST, Huebner D, Diaz R, Sanchez J. Family acceptance in adolescence and the health of LGBT young adults. J Child Adolesc Psychiatr Nurs. 2010;23(4):205–13.
17. Heck NC, Flentje A, Cochran BN. Offsetting risks: high school gay-straight alliances and lesbian, gay, bisexual, and transgender (LGBT) youth. Sch Psychol Q. 2011;26(2):161–74.
18. Kahn E, Johnson A, Lee M, Miranda L. LGBTQ Youth Report. Human rights campaign and University of Connecticut. 2018. https://assets2.hrc.org/files/assets/resources/2018-Youth-Report-NoVid.pdf?_ga=2.11537844.1062138234.1538506864-1830849074.1538506864. Accessed 1 Dec 2018.
19. Reisner SL, Greytak EA, Parsons JT, Ybarra ML. Gender minority social stress in adolescence: disparities in adolescent bullying and substance use by gender identity. J Sex Res. 2015;52(3):243–56.

20. Jones BA, Haycraft E, Murjan S, Arcelus J. Body dissatisfaction and disordered eating in trans people: a systematic review of the literature. Int Rev Psychiatry. 2016;28(1):81–94.
21. Schmidt E, Rizzolo D. Disease screening and prevention for transgender and gender-diverse adults. JAAPA. 2017;30(10):11–6. https://doi.org/10.1097/01.JAA.0000524709.87224.57.
22. Workowski KA. Centers for disease control and prevention Sexually Transmitted Diseases Treatment Guidelines. Clin Infect Dis. 2015;61(Suppl 8):S759–62.
23. Becasen JS, Denard CL, Mullins MM, Higa DH, Sipe TA. Estimating the prevalence of HIV and sexual behaviors among the US transgender population: a systematic review and meta-analysis, 2006–2017. Am J Public Health. 2019;109(1):e1–8.
24. Birth control across the gender spectrum. https://www.reproductiveaccess.org/wp-content/uploads/2018/06/bc-across-gender-spectrum.pdf. Aug 2018.
25. Shah M. Birth control across the gender spectrum. https://www.bedsider.org/features/1070-birth-control-across-the-gender-spectrum. July 2017.
26. Witcomb GL, Bouman WP, Claes L, Brewin N, Crawford JR, Arcelus J. Levels of depression in transgender people and its predictors: results of a large matched control study with transgender people accessing clinical services. J Affect Disord. 2018;235:308–15.
27. Millet N, Longworth J, Arcelus J. Prevalence of anxiety symptoms and disorders in the transgender population: a systematic review of the literature. Int J Transgend. 2017;18(1):27–38. https://doi.org/10.1080/15532739.2016.1258353.
28. Marshall E, Claes L, Bouman WP, Witcomb GL, Arcelus J. Non-suicidal self-injury and suicidality in trans people: a systematic review of the literature. Int Rev Psychiatry. 2016;28(1): 58–69.
29. Taliaferro LA, McMorris BJ, Rider GN, Eisenberg ME. Risk and protective factors for self-harm in a population-based sample of transgender youth. Arch Suicide Res. 2018;23(2):203–21. https://doi.org/10.1080/13811118.2018.1430639. [Epub ahead of print] PubMed PMID: 29461934.
30. Toomey RB, Syvertsen AK, Shramko M. Transgender adolescent suicide behavior. Pediatrics. 2018;142(4):e20174218.
31. Valentine SE, Shipherd JC. A systematic review of social stress and mental health among transgender and gender non-conforming people in the United States. Clin Psychol Rev. 2018; 66:24.
32. Wichinski KA. Providing culturally proficient care for transgender patients. Nursing. 2015;45(2):58–63. https://doi.org/10.1097/01.NURSE.0000456370.79660.f8.
33. Felsenstein DR. Enhancing lesbian, gay, bisexual, and transgender cultural competence in a Midwestern primary care clinic setting. J Nurses Prof Dev. 2018;34(3):142–50. https://doi.org/10.1097/NND.0000000000000450.
34. National LGBT Health Education Center. Affirmative care for transgender and gender non-conforming people: best practices for front-line health care staff, 2016.
35. Cahill S, Singal R, Grasso C, King D, Mayer K, Baker K, et al. Do ask, do tell: high levels of acceptability by patients of routine collection of sexual orientation and gender identity data in four diverse American community health centers. PLoS One. 2014;9(9):1–8.
36. Fenway Health. Landmark decision by Dept. of Health and Human Services will reduce health disparities experienced by LGBT people. Fenway Health Newsroom. 2015 Oct 7. http://fenwayfocus.org/2015/10/landmark-decision-by-dept-of-health-and-human-services-will-reduce-health-disparities-experienced-by-lgbt-people/. Accessed 11 Nov 2018.
37. Radis E. Preparing for and understanding your 2018 uniform data system (UDS) submission webinar. HRSA. 2018 Oct 11. https://bphc.hrsa.gov/sites/default/files/bphc/datareporting/reporting/preparing-and-fenunderstanding-your-uds-2018.pdf
38. Sevelius JM, Carrico A, Johnson MO. Antiretroviral therapy adherence among transgender women living with HIV. J Assoc Nurses AIDS Care. 2010;21(3):256–64.
39. White Hughto JM, Rose AJ, Pachankis JE, Reisner SL. Barriers to gender transition-related healthcare: identifying underserved transgender adults in Massachusetts. Transgend Health. 2017;2(1):107–18.

Mood, Anxiety, and Other Mental Health Concerns

9

Marijn Arnoldussen and Annelou L. C. de Vries

Introduction

When considering the mental health of transgender and gender diverse (TGD) children and adolescents, it is easy to imagine how the significant challenges of navigating this experience may be a source of stress, with resultant consequences for mental health. Although this chapter shows that indeed TGD youth may be a vulnerable population in this respect, there are clearly subgroups that function well and show few mental health difficulties. For example, pubertal adolescents who are supported by their parents, accepted by their peers, and receive medical gender affirming treatment at specialized gender clinics may function well. Prepubertal gender diverse children who grow up with a supporting environment may not show any co-occurring psychiatric condition. Nonetheless, in this chapter, we discuss the mental health difficulties that TGD children and adolescents may present with. Chapter 10 focuses on neurodevelopmental concerns. Many studies reveal concerning clinical range scores on depression scales and suicidality and parent and self-reported measures of emotional and behavioral problems that are often comparable to mental health clinic-referred populations. Though, differences exist between clinics and samples. For clinical practice, it is important to not only be aware of the mental health vulnerabilities that exist in gender diverse youth, but also understand factors related to the psychological difficulties to help build resilience. This chapter discusses the factors that have been studied, as well as clinical implications.

M. Arnoldussen · A. L. C. de Vries (✉)
Department of Child and Adolescent Psychiatry, Center of Expertise on Gender Dysphoria, Amsterdam UMC, VU University Medical Center, Amsterdam, The Netherlands
e-mail: alc.devries@amsterdamumc.nl

M. Forcier et al. (eds.), *Pediatric Gender Identity*,
https://doi.org/10.1007/978-3-030-38909-3_9

Prevalence of Mental Health Difficulties in Various Samples of TGD Youth

Historically, most studies on psychopathology and psychological functioning of TGD youth have been performed in specialized gender identity clinics and came from just a limited number of such clinics. Most of the prepubertal children coming to these clinics met the diagnostic criteria for the diagnostic category used in the DSM-III-R and DSM-IV: gender identity disorder, and most pubertal adolescents had a request for medical affirmative treatment (gender reassignment at the time). The recent increase in visibility and recognition of gender diversity in youth has been paralleled by an increase in publications on other populations: high school samples, community samples, and Internet-recruited self-identified samples. In addition, several recent publications come from newer clinics presenting their chart data of a rapidly growing number of referrals, sometimes compared with matched controls. It is clear that the variability of the samples and used methods to measure mental health limit the comparability of the results. Still, most of these studies reveal high rates of mental health problems, although some exceptions exist.

Participants in early studies on this subject were mainly gender diverse prepubertal children [1–5]. More recent studies, however, also focused on the psychological functioning of gender diverse adolescents. The results of these studies were that the prevalence rates of co-occurring mental health difficulties in gender diverse children and adolescents were higher when compared to children and adolescents from the general population. Two chart review studies that were conducted in the United Kingdom and the United States found that a significant proportion of the adolescents who were assessed at a gender clinic experienced depressive symptoms [6, 7]. Other, more recent clinical-sample-based studies reported that depression and anxiety disorders were two of the most common coexisting diagnoses in transgender and gender diverse adolescents [8–14]. A chart review study that was published in 2016 on 218 gender diverse youngsters (mean age 14 years) reported that 45.7% of the assigned males at birth (AMABs) and 39.4% of the assigned females at birth (AFABs) experienced low mood/depression and that more than 20% of these youngsters (21.0% of AMABs and 23.4% of the AFABs) showed symptoms of anxiety [9]. A more recent chart review study on 1082 referred adolescents who identified as transgender or gender diverse matched with 21,317 cisgender enrollees (mean age unknown, age range 10–17 years) revealed that depressive disorders were found in 48.5% of the AMABs and 61.5% of the AFABs and that anxiety disorders were found in 37.2% of the AMABs and 38.9% of the AFABs. Both disorders occurred about five times more often among TGD adolescents compared with their matched cisgender peers [11]. Finally, a chart review study of 180 adolescents who identified as transgender and 180 matched cisgender-referred controls (mean age 19.6 years) reported that transgender youth had a twofold to threefold increased risk of depression and anxiety disorders [14]. Besides clinical sample-based studies that retrieved data regarding mental health directly from the subject's file, there are also studies that measured the psychological functioning and occurring related difficulties of gender diverse adolescents through respondent-based psychiatric interviews or psychological questionnaires [15–17]. De Vries et al. examined coexisting related difficulties in 105 TGD adolescents (mean age 14.6 years) who were referred to a gender identity clinic through the Diagnostic Interview Schedule for Children (DISC), a respondent-based psychiatric interview assessing all common DSM-IV Axis I mental disorders in children and adolescents [15, 18]. It was found that the majority (67.6%) of the 105 referred adolescents had no concurrent psychiatric disorder, while 32.4% had at least one and 15.2% had two or more comorbid diagnoses. Disorders that were the most common were social anxiety disorder (9.5%), major depression (8.6%), oppositional defiant disorder (8.6%), and specific phobia (7.6%). Anxiety disorders were the most common in the referred adolescents (21%), followed by mood disorders (12.4%) and disruptive disorders (11.4%). These relatively low percentages of psychiatric conditions compared to some other clinic samples were explained by the authors by the fact that the studied sample may be a selected sample supported by parents and growing up in an accepting (Dutch) environment [15].

The above studies used different measurements to examine coexisting related difficulties. However, since some of the studies used similar measures, cross-clinic comparisons can be made. For example, three studies that were performed in gender identity clinics in Los Angeles, Toronto, and Amsterdam used the Beck Depression Inventory II to measure whether there were depressive symptoms in the participating adolescents [16, 17, 19, 20]. A study that aimed to describe the baseline characteristics of gender diverse adolescents (mean age 19.2 years) seeking care at a transgender youth clinic in Los Angeles found that 24% of the sample had Beck depression scores in the mild-to-moderate depression range and 11% had scores in the severe-extreme depression range [16]. Another study on 203 gender diverse adolescents (mean age 16.3 years) who were assessed in a transgender youth clinic in Toronto found that 41.6% of the AFABs and 34.4% of the AMABs had Beck depression scores in the severe-extreme depression range [17]. On the other hand, a Dutch follow-up study of 70 adolescents (mean age 16.6 years) who received puberty suppression reported that the mean baseline Beck depression score of the adolescents was below the clinical range [19]. These lower rates of depression might reflect that these adolescents trust that they are helped and supported by receiving puberty suppression to prevent suffering from puberty development. However, it is unclear what the reasons are for the different results between clinics; it might be due to different cultural, social, and clinical environments.

In addition to aforementioned occurring emotional difficulties among TGD adolescents, there are also studies that found that adolescents who identify as gender diverse or transgender have a higher risk of developing an eating disorder [7–9]. Three chart review studies reported prevalence rates of eating disorders in referred gender diverse adolescents ranging from 4.8% to 13.3% [7–9]. However, these results concern young people who were referred to specialized gender identity clinics, and it is unclear whether these percentages also apply to gender diverse young people in the rest of population.

Finally, up until now, only one case report of a gender diverse adolescent with psychosis has been published [21]. In this case report, Meijer et al. described a

17-year-old adolescent AFAB who was diagnosed with bipolar schizoaffective disorder and who started with hormonal treatment at age 19 after his counselors from the gender clinic and his treating psychiatrist concluded that his gender dysphoria was a possible factor in the onset of his psychotic symptoms. Although when this person was 25 years old, after a mastectomy, hysterectomy, and metoidioplasty were performed, he experienced his second and last full-blown psychotic episode, his transgender identity never changed, and it was concluded that satisfaction with the gender-affirmative therapy was high and that gender-affirmative treatment could be possible and safe in this vulnerable population.

The above results are all based on gender diverse adolescents who presented for care at gender identity clinics which means that these may be different for gender diverse adolescents in the general population who may not have similar rates of mental health difficulties. However, two large community sample-based studies on mental health of TGD youth report similar results as the aforementioned studies [22, 23]. Clark et al. found that gender diverse adolescents (mean age unknown, age range 12–18 years), compared to their cisgender peers, reported a significantly higher rate of depressive symptoms (41.3% vs. 11.8%) [22], and Veale et al. described that these youngsters (mean age unknown, age range 14–18 years) experienced significantly more emotional distress than their peers who do not experience gender incongruence [23].

The results discussed so far demonstrate that mental health difficulties occur more often in gender diverse children and adolescents compared to their cisgender peers. Nonetheless, there are two studies that showed that socially transitioned prepubertal transgender children and young transgender adolescents who are supported in their gender identity have developmentally normative levels of depression and only minimal elevations in anxiety [24, 25]. Like studies of selected clinical adolescent gender diverse samples that feel supported and trust that they will receive medical gender-affirming treatment [e.g., 15, 19], this suggests that social support and affirming transgender youth in their experienced gender identity instead of their sex assigned at birth may lead to better, or even normative, mental health outcomes.

A specific mental health concern in adult transgender individuals is the alarming reported high rates of suicide attempts [26]. There are also various studies that have focused on self-harm and suicidality in transgender and gender diverse children and adolescents. There is one clinical sample-based study in which exclusively prepubertal children (mean age unknown, age range 3–12 years) participated [27]. This study found that, by parent report, TGD children show an increased rate of self-harm/suicidality as they get older. Most of the studies in which adolescents participated are clinical sample based, and despite the fact that their methods differ greatly, their results are quite similar indicating that self-harm and suicidality are more common among TGD youth in comparison with their cisgender peers [7–11, 13, 14, 16, 17, 28–31]. An American study that was published in 2007 revealed that nearly half of the 55 participants (mean age 17.5 years), who were recruited at two community centers providing services to LGBTQ+ youth in New York City, reported serious thoughts about attempting suicide and one quarter reported a history of suicide attempts [28]. A chart study on 125 adolescents who were seeking medical care at a gender identity clinic in London (mean age 13.6 years) that was published a few years later reported that 14% of the participants had thoughts of inflicting self-injury, 24% of the participants inflicted self-injury, and 10% of the participants made a suicide attempt before they were referred to the gender identity clinic [29]. When comparing AMABs with AFABs, it was found that the number of suicide attempts did not differ but that thoughts of inflicting self-injury were more common in AMABs and that inflicting self-injury was more common in AFABs. In one of the most recent retrospective chart review studies (mean age 17.1 years), in which a psychosocial assessment administered by medicine physicians was used to measure the prevalence of self-harm and suicidality among the participants, findings were that 41.8% of the adolescents who identified as transgender self-harmed and that 30.3% of these adolescents made at least one suicide attempt [30]. It was also found that compared to AMABs, AFABs more frequently reported a history of suicide attempts and self-harming.

The results of the aforementioned studies on suicidality and self-harm are all based on gender identity clinic-referred adolescents and, therefore, may not be representative of the young gender diverse population as a whole. However, there are only a few population-based studies on self-harm and suicidality among TGD adolescents [22, 23, 32]. One of these studies, utilizing data collected through a survey that was held among New Zealand secondary school students in 2012 (mean age unknown, age range 12–18 years), reported that 45.5% of the students who identified as transgender self-harmed in the past 12 months and that 19.8% of the these students attempted suicide in the past [22]. In another study that was based on data derived from American high school students (mean age 15.4 years) who participated in a survey between 2013 and 2015, findings were that the prevalence of past 12-month self-reported suicidal ideation was nearly twice as high for gender diverse youth compared with nontransgender youth [32]. The study also reported that depressive symptoms and school-based victimization were both significantly associated with a higher risk of developing suicidal ideation among gender diverse adolescents. From the above, it can be concluded that self-harm and suicidality are of significant concern also for young transgender and gender diverse people and require the clinicians' full attention during the counseling of young gender diverse people.

Factors Related to Mental Health of Gender diverse and Transgender Youth

Different factors may be related to the mental health difficulties of TGD youth. Apart from the distress of their gender dysphoria, one important hypothesis is that these problems are related to minority stress. That is, the increased distress stemming from prejudice and rejection first observed in lesbian, gay, and bisexual minorities compared to heterosexual individuals [33]. Community sample studies show that youth who are gender diverse and have a gender different from their sex assigned at birth may experience *gender minority* stress; compared to cisgender youth, the higher rates of bullying (up to 80%), harassment, and peer victimization mediate the higher odds of substance use, psychological distress, low life satisfaction, depression, suicidal ideation, and self-harm [14, 34–39]. In a longitudinal study following a sample of middle-school age children over time, children who appraised themselves as gender nonconforming and also felt pressure to conform to gender norms were most likely to have internalizing problems [40]. Programs that increase acceptance and tolerance and help gender diverse youth to come out in schools improve the well-being of transgender youth [41].

In clinic-referred TGD youth, poor peer relation is one of the strongest investigated predictors for behavioral and emotional problems. Although not a direct measure of victimization, these studies define poor peer relations by positive answers to parent-rated [42], teacher-rated [43], or self-rated [44] items like "Doesn't get along with other kids," "Gets teased a lot," and "Not liked by other kids." In three such studies, a direct comparison was made between youth referred to a Canadian and a Dutch gender identity clinic. Parents, teachers, and youth reported significantly more behavioral and emotional problems in the Canadian compared to the Dutch youth [2, 45, 46]. In all three studies, poor peer relations fully explained the differences in emotional and behavior problems across the two clinics [45, 46]. A more recent study on psychological functioning and peer relationship problems in adolescents across four European specialist gender services (The Netherlands, Belgium, the United Kingdom, and Switzerland) found differences across Europe. Overall, emotional and behavioral problems and peer relationship problems occurred most in adolescents from the United Kingdom, followed by Switzerland and Belgium. Adolescents from the Netherlands showed the least behavioral and emotional problems, and their peer relations were best [47]. Cross-clinic differences may, thus, reflect that in some societies there is more peer acceptance and tolerance to gender diverse youth than in others, and that accepting environments may foster superior mental health outcomes. This knowledge is important when developing programs that help to improve the worrisome psychological functioning of transgender youth.

Of course the most important support one can get should come from the direct family. Young children, in particular, are fully dependent on their parents for receiving help and acceptance regarding their gender diverse behavior. But adolescents as well are seldom able to seek affirming care without their parents' support. Despite increased tolerance in Western societies, coming out as transgender is for many youth still difficult out of fear for their parents' reaction, whether it is justified or not. Adolescents who feel that their families accept and tolerate their sexual and/or gender minority identities have better self-esteem, social support, and general health, as well as less depression and suicidal ideation [48]. In contrast, LGBT adolescents who have parents who try to change their gender-diversity or sexual orientation, either by themselves or by sending them to a religious leader, have more depression, suicidality, and less educational attainment in young adulthood [49]. Interventions that help to increase parents' acceptance are needed.

Clinical Approach

The young TGD population is a vulnerable group in which mental health difficulties occur more often than in their cisgender peers. Since these difficulties are related to gender minority stress, creating a society that accepts and understands gender diversity in youth and decreasing stigmatization around gender-diversity are of pivotal importance. Positive media attention, accepting school climates, and activities that empower LGBT youth may all be helpful in reaching that goal. For the individual gender diverse child or adolescent, however, it is crucial to identify occurring mental health difficulties in time, and when treatment is needed, refer the adolescent to a mental health clinician. When a specialized gender clinic is far from home, mental health support should preferably occur in the surroundings of where the adolescent lives. The referring clinician should keep in mind that these local health-care providers might need support in working with gender diverse adolescents from transgender specialists [50].

When medical affirming treatment is considered, it is important to recognize and observe emerging mental health difficulties, but mental health difficulties in themselves are not an absolute contraindication to starting medical interventions [51]. It has to be estimated, however, whether a decision regarding medical treatment with lifelong consequences can be deliberately considered and complied within the adolescent's particular situation. If mental health difficulties interfere with a proper assessment of the feelings of gender dysphoria or if they impede a gender-affirmative treatment, specialized mental health care might be needed prior to the start of medical interventions.

In addition to mental health problems, other factors also play a part in deciding whether or not to start with gender-affirmative treatment. These factors include the capability to conform to a medical trajectory and the decision-making capacity of the adolescent. The decision-making capacity refers to one's ability to utilize information about treatment options and to make a choice that is in line with one's own values and preferences [52]. The decision-making capacity can vary per adolescent and per situation, and it is therefore essential to be estimated on a case-by-case basis.

Another factor that influences the decision regarding medical treatment is whether the adolescent is supported by their social environment. Some families experience a lot of stress because of the gender diversity and the desire for gender-affirmative treatment of the adolescent. One of the problems that might arise, for example, is when parents have different views on the diagnosis or treatment of their child [50]. When this is the case, it is necessary to reach out to both parents and to emphasize the importance of support from parents and the recognition of the gender identity of their child. In the most favorable situation, both parents support the decision to start with medical interventions before the treatment actually begins. Unfortunately, however, this is not always the case. If it is in the best interest of the adolescent, sometimes, this decision should be made without the approval of one or more caregivers, while taking into account certain relevant legal and ethical guidelines [50, 53].

During the process of clinical assessment and transition, it is important to pay attention to issues such as support and social environment. Supportive therapy or counseling could help adolescents if they experience unpleasant or disappointing events during their transition [50]. Joining support groups or service-users groups could also offer empowerment to transitioning adolescents. Finally, clinicians should keep in mind that there are adolescents who have unrealistic expectations regarding their medical treatment and their transition. It is important to place these expectations in perspective so that disappointments can be avoided as much as possible [50].

Clinical Vignette

Ian is a 15-year-old, who was assigned female at birth. From a young age, Ian has known that he does not feel like a girl but like a boy. Ian socially transitioned at age 14 and has lived since then in the boy's role, but he is upset about his changing body. Ian often feels worthless and gloomy, and he is very anxious about what his peers think of him. At certain times, his mood is so bleak and he is so anxious that he does not manage to attend school. Ian does not receive treatment for his mental health difficulties.

Ian's father acknowledges the fact that his child is suffering from gender dysphoria, but he does not support Ian's identity. For example, Ian's father still refers to Ian using a female name and pronouns. Ian's father's greatest concern is the fact that Ian does not attend school. Ian and his father often argue about Ian's school absenteeism. Ian's father indicates that Ian should try harder to attend school, and Ian states that it is not that simple. Ian's mother is not involved in his care.

What could the clinician do?

It is important that the clinician establish a good relationship with Ian so that mutual trust arises.

Ian should be referred to psychiatric care for his mood and anxiety complaints. A point of attention in this treatment should be the self-image and self-acceptance of Ian. It is also important to involve Ian's teachers at school and his school psychologist in his treatment, so they become aware of Ian's situation. They can provide insight into the quality of his peer relations, and they can offer him extra support when needed. Furthermore, family counseling should be provided in which father can learn to understand the importance of parental support and the recognition of Ian's gender identity. Ian and his father can also work on developing a better relationship during this therapy. In addition, referring Ian to a support group may be considered. A support group could offer Ian recognition for his feelings and could provide empowerment. Finally, since Ian is suffering from his changing body, starting medical treatment once Ian and his father have adequate care should be considered, as discussed in Chap. 14.

Financial Support This chapter received no specific grant from any funding agency or commercial or not-for-profit sectors.

Conflict of Interest The authors declare that they have no conflict of interest.

References

1. Zucker KJ, Bradley SJ. Gender identity disorder and psychosexual problems in children and adolescents. New York: Guildford Press; 1995.
2. Cohen-Kettenis PT, Owen A, Kaijser VG, Bradley SJ, Zucker KJ. Demographic characteristics, social competence, and behavior problems in children with gender identity disorder: a cross-national, cross-clinic comparative analysis. J Abnorm Child Psychol. 2003;31:41–53.
3. Wallien MS, Swaab H, Cohen-Kettenis PT. Psychiatric comorbidity among children with gender identity disorder. J Am Acad Child Adolesc Psychiatry. 2007;46:1307–14.
4. Pleak RR, Meyer-Bahlburg HF, O'Brien JD, Bowen HA, Morganstein A. Cross-gender behavior and psychopathology in boy psychiatric outpatients. J Am Acad Child Adolesc Psychiatry. 1989;28:385–93.
5. Zucker KJ, Bradley SJ, Lowry Sullivan CB. Traits of separation anxiety in boys with gender identity disorder. J Am Acad Child Adolesc Psychiatry. 1996;35:791–8.
6. Di Ceglie D, Freedman D, McPherson S, Richardson P. Children and adolescents referred to a specialist gender identity development service: clinical features and demographic characteristics. Int J Transgend. 2002;6(1):97–103. http://www.symposion.com/ijt/ijtvo06no01_01.htm.
7. Spack NP, Edwards-Leeper L, Feldman HA, Leibowitz S, Mandel F, Diamond DA, et al. Children and adolescents with gender identity disorder referred to a pediatric medical center. Pediatrics. 2012;129:418–25.
8. Khatchadourian K, Amed S, Metzger DL. Clinical management of youth with gender dysphoria in Vancouver. J Pediatr. 2014;164:906–11.
9. Holt V, Skagerberg E, Dunsford M. Young people with features of gender dysphoria: demographics and associated difficulties. Clin Child Psychol Psychiatry. 2016;21:108–18.
10. Chen M, Fuqua J, Eugster EA. Characteristics of referrals for gender dysphoria over a 13-year period. J Adolesc Health. 2016;58:369–71.
11. Becerra-Culqui TA, Liu Y, Nash R, Cromwell L, Flanders WD, Getahun D, et al. Mental health of transgender and gender nonconforming youth compared with their peers. Pediatrics. 2018;141:e20173845. https://doi.org/10.1542/peds.2017-3845.
12. Kaltiala-Heino R, Sumia M, Työläjärvi M, Lindberg N. Two years of gender identity service for minors: overrepresentation of natal girls with severe problems in adolescent development. Child Adolesc Psychiatry Ment Health. 2015;9:9.
13. Nahata L, Quinn GP, Caltabellotta NM, Tishelman AC. Mental health concerns and insurance denials among transgender adolescents. LGBT Health. 2017;4:188–93.
14. Reisner SL, Vetters R, Leclerc M, Zaslow S, Wolfrum S, Shumer D, et al. Mental health of transgender youth in care at an adolescent urban community health center: a matched retrospective cohort study. J Adolesc Health. 2015;56:274–9.
15. de Vries AL, Doreleijers TA, Steensma TD, Cohen-Kettenis PT. Psychiatric comorbidity in gender dysphoric adolescents. J Child Psychol Psychiatry. 2011;52:1195–202.
16. Olson J, Schrager SM, Belzer M, Simons LK, Clark LF. Baseline physiologic and psychosocial characteristics of transgender youth seeking care for gender dysphoria. J Adolesc Health. 2015;57:374–80.
17. Chiniara LN, Bonifacio HJ, Palmert MR. Characteristics of adolescents referred to a gender clinic: are youth seen now different from those in initial reports? Horm Res Paediatr. 2018;89:434–41.
18. Ferdinand RF, van der Ende J. NIMH-DISC-IV: diagnostic interview schedule for children. Geautoriseerde Nederlandse vertaling; 2000.
19. de Vries AL, Steensma TD, Doreleijers TA, Cohen-Kettenis PT. Puberty suppression in adolescents with gender identity disorder: a prospective follow-up study. J Sex Med. 2011;8:2276–83.
20. Beck AT, Steer RA, Ball R, Ranieri W. Comparison of beck depression inventories -IA and -II in psychiatric outpatients. J Pers Assess. 1996;67:588–97.

21. Meijer JH, Eeckhout GM, van Vlerken RH, de Vries AL. Gender dysphoria and co-existing psychosis: review and four case examples of successful gender affirmative treatment. LGBT Health. 2017;4:106–14.
22. Clark TC, Lucassen MF, Bullen P, Denny SJ, Fleming TM, Robinson EM, et al. The health and well-being of transgender high school students: results from the New Zealand adolescent health survey. J Adolesc Health. 2014;55:93–9.
23. Veale JF, Watson RJ, Peter T, Saewyc EM. Mental health disparities among Canadian transgender youth. J Adolesc Health. 2017;60:44–9.
24. Olson KR, Durwood L, DeMeules M, McLaughlin KA. Mental health of transgender children who are supported in their identities. Pediatrics. 2016;137:e20153223.
25. Durwood L, McLaughlin KA, Olson KR. Mental health and self-worth in socially transitioned transgender youth. J Am Acad Child Adolesc Psychiatry. 2017;56:116–23.
26. Marshall E, Claes L, Bouman WP, Witcomb GL, Arcelus J. Non-suicidal self-injury and suicidality in trans people: a systematic review of the literature. Int Rev Psychiatry. 2016;28:58–69.
27. Aitken M, VanderLaan DP, Wasserman L, Stjoanovski S, Zucker KJ. Self-harm and suicidality in children referred for gender dysphoria. J Am Acad Child Adolesc Psychiatry. 2016;55:513–20.
28. Grossman AH, D'Augelli AR. Transgender youth and life-threatening behaviors. Suicide Life Threat Behav. 2007;37:527–37.
29. Skagerberg E, Parkinson R, Carmichael P. Self-harming thoughts and behaviors in a group of children and adolescents with gender dysphoria. Int J Transgend. 2013;14:86–92.
30. Peterson CM, Matthews A, Copps-Smith E, Conard LA. Suicidality, self-harm, and body dissatisfaction in transgender adolescents and emerging adults with gender dysphoria. Suicide Life Threat Behav. 2017;47:475–82.
31. Fisher AD, Ristori J, Castellini G, Sensi C, Cassioli E, Prunas A, et al. Psychological characteristics of Italian gender dysphoric adolescents: a case-control study. J Endocrinol Invest. 2017;40:953–65.
32. Perez-Brumer A, Day JK, Russell JK, Hatzenbuehler ML. Prevalence and correlates of suicidal ideation among transgender youth in California: findings from a representative, population-based sample of high school students. J Am Acad Child Adolesc Psychiatry. 2017;56:739–46.
33. Meyer IH. Prejudice, social stress, and mental health in lesbian, gay, and bisexual populations: conceptual issues and research evidence. Psychol Bull. 2003;129:674–97.
34. Grossman AH, D'Augelli AR. Transgender youth: invisible and vulnerable. J Homosex. 2006;51:111–28.
35. McGuire JK, Anderson CR, Toomey RB, Russell ST. School climate for transgender youth: a mixed method investigation of student experiences and school responses. J Youth Adolesc. 2010;39:1175–88.
36. Toomey RB, Ryan C, Diaz RM, Card NA, Russell ST. Gender-nonconforming lesbian, gay, bisexual, and transgender youth: school victimization and young adult psychosocial adjustment. Dev Psychol. 2010;46:1580–9.
37. Liu RT, Mustanski B. Suicidal ideation and self-harm in lesbian, gay, bisexual, and transgender youth. Am J Prev Med. 2012;42:221–8.
38. Birkett M, Newcomb ME, Mustanski B. Does it get better? A longitudinal analysis of psychological distress and victimization in lesbian, gay, bisexual, transgender, and questioning youth. J Adolesc Health. 2015;56:280–5.
39. Timmins L, Rimes KA, Rahman Q. Minority stressors and psychological distress in transgender individuals. Psychol Sex Orientat Gend Divers. 2017;4:328–40.
40. Yunger JL, Carver PR, Perry DG. Does gender identity influence children's psychological well-being? Dev Psychol. 2004;40:572–82.
41. Russell ST, Toomey RB, Ryan C, Diaz RM. Being out at school: the implications for school victimization and young adult adjustment. Am J Orthopsychiatry. 2014;84:635–43.
42. Achenbach TM, Edelbrock CS. Manual for the child behavior checklist and revised child behavior profile. Burlington: University of Vermont, Department of Psychiatry; 1983.

43. Achenbach TM, Edelbrock CS. Manual for the teacher's report form and teacher version of the child behavior profile. Burlington: University of Vermont, Department of Psychiatry; 1986.
44. Achenbach TM. Manual for the youth self-report. Burlington: University of Vermont, Department of Psychiatry; 1991.
45. Steensma TD, Zucker KJ, Kreukels BP, VanderLaan DP, Wood H, Fuentes A, et al. Behavioral and emotional problems on the teacher's report form: a cross-national, cross-clinic comparative analysis of gender dysphoric children and adolescents. J Abnorm Child Psychol. 2014;42:635–47.
46. de Vries AL, Steensma TD, Cohen-Kettenis PT, VanderLaan DP, Zucker KJ. Poor peer relations predict parent- and self-reported behavioral and emotional problems of adolescents with gender dysphoria: a cross-national, cross-clinic comparative analysis. Eur Child Adolesc Psychiatry. 2016;25:579–88.
47. de Graaf NM, Cohen-Kettenis PT, Carmichael P, de Vries AL, Dhondt K, Laridaen J, et al. Psychological functioning in adolescents referred to specialist gender identity clinics across Europe: a clinical comparison study between four clinics. Eur Child Adolesc Psychiatry. 2018;27:909–19.
48. Ryan C, Russell ST, Huebner D, Diaz R, Sanchez J. Family acceptance in adolescence and the health of LGBT young adults. J Child Adolesc Psychiatr Nurs. 2010;23:205–13.
49. Turban JL, Beckwith N, Reisner S, Keuroghlian AS. 4.10 exposure to conversion therapy for gender identity is associated with poor adult mental health outcomes among transgender people in the US. J Am Acad Child Adolesc Psychiatry. 2018;57:S208.
50. De Vries AL, Klink D, Cohen-Kettenis PT. What the primary care pediatrician needs to know about gender incongruence and gender dysphoria in children and adolescents. Pediatr Clin North Am. 2016;63:1121–35.
51. Coleman E, Bockting W, Botzer M, Cohen-Kettenis PT, DeCuypere G, Feldman J, et al. Standards of care for the health of transsexual, transgender and gender non-conforming people, version 7. Int J Transgend. 2011;13:165–232.
52. Karlawish J. Assessment of decision-making capacity in adults 2017. https://www.uptodate.com/contents/assessment-of-decision-making-capacity-in-adults. Accessed 1 Dec 2018.
53. Olson KA, Middleman AB. Consent in adolescent health care 2018. https://www.uptodate.com/contents/consent-in-adolescent-health-care. Accessed 1 Dec 2018.

Caring for Transgender and Gender Diverse Youth with Co-occurring Neurodiversity

10

Roy H. T. van Vlerken, Coralie E. Fuchs, and Anna I. R. van der Miesen

Introduction

Gender is thought to be a developmental process, and for some youth, gender identity may continue to shift and develop throughout childhood and into adolescence or adulthood. Diverse aspects of social, emotional, and identity development may be influenced by the presence of autism spectrum disorder (ASD), and increasingly, the co-occurrence of gender diversity and ASD is a focus of study. While most clinicians are aware of the potential co-occurrence of several psychological symptoms in transgender and gender diverse (TGD) children and adolescents [1, 2], less is known about the seemingly higher prevalence of ASD and/or social developmental impairments in TGD children and adolescents seen in specialized gender services. A growing body of literature has attempted to characterize and quantify the presence of ASD characteristics in TGD youth. This work started in the nineties with descriptions in case reports [e.g., 3]. In 2010, the first systematic study was performed investigating diagnoses of ASD in children and adolescents referred for gender dysphoria (GD) assessment [4]. Since then, the number of publications on the co-occurrence of GD/TGD and ASD has increased every year [5]. So, what do we know now about this potential co-occurrence? For example, can GD be diagnosed in youth with ASD? Likewise, can ASD be diagnosed in TGD youth? Also, what should every clinician working with TGD youth with (characteristics of) ASD know? This chapter describes the

R. H. T. van Vlerken (✉) · A. I. R. van der Miesen
Amsterdam UMC, VU University Medical Center, Department of Child and Adolescent Psychiatry, Center of Expertise on Gender Dysphoria, Amsterdam, The Netherlands
e-mail: r.vanvlerken@amsterdamumc.nl

C. E. Fuchs
Amsterdam UMC, VU University Medical Center, Department of Medical Psychology, Center of Expertise on Gender Dysphoria, Amsterdam, The Netherlands

M. Forcier et al. (eds.), *Pediatric Gender Identity*,
https://doi.org/10.1007/978-3-030-38909-3_10

current state of the literature regarding this co-occurrence and addresses important clinical aspects with regard to assessment and gender affirmative treatment.

What Is Autism Spectrum Disorder?

The two main characteristics of ASD are (i) persistent impairments in social communication and interaction (criterion A) and (ii) restricted, repetitive patterns of behavior, interests, or activities (criterion B) [6]. The umbrella term ASD encompasses conditions that were previous referred to in the DSM-IV-TR as autistic disorder, Asperger's syndrome, pervasive developmental disorder not otherwise specified (PDD-NOS), and childhood disintegrative disorder [7]. This creates some challenges in comparing literature over time and similarly reflects a changing and growing lexicon as well as growing body of evidence across the ASD frameworks, also visible in TGD data and frameworks.

Characteristics of ASD usually manifest from early infancy onward [6]. ASD is heterogeneous with respect to clinical presentation and severity [8]. The extent to which characteristics manifest depends on the severity of the ASD characteristics as well as on the developmental level and chronologic age [6]. Difficulties in establishing, maintaining, and understanding social relations in youth with ASD vary from a lack of social interaction and play to difficulty adjusting one's social behavior to different social settings (criterion A). Individuals with ASD might also struggle to share thoughts and feelings with others, to use nonverbal communication, such as eye contact or gesturing, and might find it difficult to respond to social situations or find these situations overwhelming. An example of the B criterion of repetitive behaviors typical for ASD could be a tendency to order toys instead of playing with them, or simple motor stereotyped behaviors such as hand flapping, rocking, or spinning [6]. Children and adolescents with ASD might also show a tendency to sameness, as can be apparent from a resistance to change and rigid patterns of thinking (e.g., getting upset by a small change in routines). The limited and fixed interests seen in ASD are often unusual in focus and intensity [6], for example, an intense interest in trains. Sometimes, these interests might be correlated with being oversensitive or under-sensitive to sensory input or with an unusual interest in the sensory aspect of the environment (e.g., the urge to touch certain fabrics, dislike of specific food textures, or fascinations with shiny objects) [6].

The prevalence of ASD in the general population has recently been estimated around 1%, with a prevalence rate that is two to three times higher in males assigned at birth [8]. The exact cause of ASD is unknown. It has been suggested that ASD has a multifactorial origin, resulting from genetic and nongenetic risk factors (and their interaction) that might interfere with typical neurodevelopment [9]. ASD is often described as a neurodevelopmental condition. A more non-pathologizing approach is to view ASD as a neurodiverse condition resulting from developmental variation or as neurodiversity [10], instead of a disorder per se.

Co-occurrence

A growing body of literature suggests that neurodiversity and GD/TGD intersect more frequently than might be anticipated by chance. Existing literature has for the most part framed this as a categorical question, attempting to quantify rates of co-occurrence of GD and ASD. Studies have differed in the methods used (both qualitative and quantitative), the samples investigated (TGD individuals and individuals with ASD, respectively), and the use of control groups. The literature with regard to the co-occurrence of GD and ASD in children and adolescents was first described in several case reports [e.g., 3, 11]. The first quantitative study was a Dutch study that examined ASD in children and adolescents consecutively referred to a gender clinic by formally assessing an ASD diagnosis, using the Diagnostic Interview for Social and Communication Disorder [12]. An ASD incidence of 7.8% was found ($n = 16$ meeting the full criteria of ASD out of a total of $N = 204$) [4]. Other quantitative studies investigated the characteristics of ASD instead of ASD diagnoses in TGD children and adolescents [13–19]. These studies included sample sizes ranging from 25 to 490 TGD children and adolescents. Using different measures, such as the Social Responsiveness Scale [15, 17] or the Asperger Syndrome Diagnostic Scale [18], while using neurotypical [e.g., 13] or ASD reference groups [19], all studies that investigated clinical range ASD percentages found increased percentages of individuals that met the cut-off for a potential ASD diagnosis ranging from 14.5% to 68%. It should be noted, however, that none of these studies used a clinical control group, and therefore, general conclusions about these studies should be made carefully [20].

Conversely, one study investigated GD diagnoses in children with ASD [21]. This study found that children with ASD were over four times as likely to be diagnosed with GD, compared to children from the general population. In addition, four studies investigated gender variance (GV), defined as the wish to be of the other gender, in samples of children and adolescents diagnosed with ASD [22–25]. They found elevated levels of GV compared to the general population, with percentages ranging from 4% to 6.5%. One study also found increased levels of GV in individuals with attention-deficit/hyperactivity disorder [24], and therefore, any conclusions about the specificity of these findings should be made with caution. One recent study investigated TGD and ASD in a community-based general population sample of children and found that increased ASD characteristics were associated with increased TGD characteristics [26].

Although the literature strongly points out a more frequent intersection of TGD and neurodiversity, some additional conceptualizations are relevant. Diagnosing ASD properly can be challenging, even more so in clinic-referred youth. In general, more research with validated measures is necessary to investigate the co-occurring prevalence rates. Also, the social cognitive challenges that have been found in TGD youth might represent a distinct phenomenon from ASD; TGD individuals might score higher on social cognitive measures due to a high prevalence of minority stress and poor peer relations, instead of reflecting an ASD diagnosis [20].

How Could the Possible Co-occurrence of GD/TGD and ASD Be Explained?

In the literature, several ideas have been forwarded to make sense of the possible co-occurrence of GD/TGD and ASD. These can be subdivided into biological, psychological, and social mechanisms or a combination of those, as suggested by van der Miesen et al. [27] and will be discussed below.

Biological Factors

It may be hypothesized that the intersection between GD/TGD and ASD is related to shared, brain-based factors. In ASD research [28], as well as research related to the potential GD/TGD–ASD co-occurrence, one hypothesis is based on the extreme male brain (EMB) theory [29]. This theory posits that, on average, neurotypical males have a stronger drive to systemize than empathize, while neurotypical females have a stronger drive to empathize than systemize. Empathizing is the drive to understand and respond properly to another person's thoughts and emotions, while systemizing is the drive to analyze, understand, or construct systems [29]. According to the EMB theory, the brain type – with regard to these cognitive profiles – of individuals with ASD has shifted toward an extreme male type, with on average more systemizing than empathizing [29]. Increased prenatal testosterone exposure has been suggested as one of the contributing factors underlying this shift and might influence the development of the brain in the male or female direction [30]. Furthermore, the EMB theory has been suggested to be involved in the GD–ASD co-occurrence [31], as increased intrauterine testosterone exposure could lead to both increase in autistic characteristics or ASD, and also GD, especially in assigned females at birth. While some studies indeed partly support the EMB theory by indirect evidence, most other studies do not support the EMB theory as an explanation [e.g., 19]. In addition, the EMB theory would only explain why assigned females at birth with ASD might have more co-occurring TGD/GD, and therefore, more research is needed to see if and how the EMB theory might be an underlying factor.

Psychological Factors

For clinicians assessing children or adolescents with ASD who exhibit gender diverse behavior (e.g., cross-dressing), it is important to consider whether this behavior might reflect the sometimes limited, fixed, and intense or focused interests, which are one of the B criteria for ASD [6]. Correspondingly, authors of several case reports have suggested that TGD in persons with ASD might originate from ASD-related preoccupations or fixations [3, 11, 32]. The first author who suggested this hypothesis described two boys with gender diverse behavior that was thought to be the result of a tendency to unusual objects [33]. In line with this hypothesis, one study investigated obsessions and compulsions in children referred for GD and found that both obsessions and compulsions were elevated compared to nonreferred individuals [16]. In the children assigned male at birth referred for GD, themes in obsessions and compulsions were significantly more gender-related compared to their male siblings. In contrast, no differences were found among those assigned female at birth. Another study investigating different subdomains of the ASD spectrum (e.g., social problems, orientation problems, stereotyped behavior, and resistance to change) in children and adolescents referred for GD found elevations on all subdomains of the ASD spectrum in both assigned boys and girls at birth, respectively [19]. These findings imply that factors contributing to the potential co-occurrence of GD–ASD might not be specific to obsessional interests in individuals with ASD as previously suggested, but rather be related to more than one subdomain of ASD. Thus, it remains unclear whether obsessional interests in cross-gender themes occur in the context of ASD or are in fact related to gender identity development [16, 20]. These interests might be a way of communicating their gender identity, especially when confronted with resistance from, for example, the family, or stem from minority stress or stigma, instead of ASD-related characteristics [15, 16]. TGD youth might, therefore, also score higher on ASD measures in general [20]. Further, other subdomains of ASD, such as hyper- or hyporesponsiveness and developmental rigidity, have been suggested [4] to contribute to TGD in individuals with ASD, but more research is needed to see whether this can be supported by empirical evidence [27].

Social Factors

Children and adolescents with ASD might be less aware of stereotypical societal gender norms and, therefore, be less hampered to express TGD, allowing them to follow their own creative gender path [24, 34]. Differences in social learning and this lack of awareness may lead to a less concrete, socially determined concept of being a binary "gendered" individual. The experiences of individuals with ASD, with regard to gender, might be very insightful in deconstructing society's binary view of gender [34]. One study in adults has investigated different ASD characteristics and found support for the hypothesis that individuals with ASD might be more resistant to social gender conditioning [35].

Children with ASD might find it difficult to form relationships with peers and to establish and maintain friendships [6]. Some reasons for these social difficulties include having a lack of shared interests and being less aware of the feelings and needs of others. Being ostracized or bullied might make it extra difficult to fit in with their own peer group. As a result, it has been hypothesized that children might develop a dislike of their own gender and develop feelings of belonging to the other gender [4, 11]. This phenomenon might even be reinforced if children feel that they are more tolerated or accepted by members of the other gender. For example, an assigned boy at birth who is not good at soccer, and therefore is bullied by other assigned boys at birth but is readily accepted by a group of assigned girls at birth, might develop a dislike toward being a boy and a greater sense of belonging to the group of girls. Likewise, an assigned girl at birth who does not understand the unwritten social rules that apply to a group of assigned girls at birth and shares certain interests or skills with assigned boys at birth (e.g., playing with dinosaurs) might identify more with a group of boys. One study in adults with ASD investigated social identification and found lower social identification with gender groups and less positive feelings (self-esteem) about gender groups compared to neurotypical individuals. In addition, TGD adults with ASD reported lower gender identification and self-esteem than non-TGD individuals with ASD [36]. However, this hypothesis has not been directly investigated with regard to gender identity development and remains, therefore, speculative.

Assessment and Treatment

Children and adolescents with ASD or ASD characteristics might present gender-related concerns to health professionals in different settings, for example, to their general practitioner, pediatrician, or mental health specialist. Questions might arise regarding the implications that co-occurring ASD might have on assessment and treatment of TGD children and adolescents. The following section addresses clinical aspects regarding assessment and treatment of TGD youth and co-occurring ASD together with a vignette example. To date, only initial clinical guidelines based on expert consensus for the care of TGD adolescents with ASD were published [37].

Assessment

While co-occurring ASD might come with challenges in assessment, there is clinical consensus that TGD and ASD can co-occur independently and that an ASD diagnosis should not be an exclusion criterion for a GD diagnosis in children and adolescents nor for gender-affirming treatment in adolescents [37]. It is recommended to screen TGD children and adolescents for ASD and to refer for ASD diagnostics if indicated. Likewise, it is also advisable to screen youth with ASD for gender-related questions [37]. Individuals with (characteristics of) ASD who seek help for feelings of TGD could best be assessed by professionals with both expertise in TGD and ASD or by those with TGD expertise in close collaboration with ASD experts [37].

The role of the mental health provider in general may include assessment for GD/TGD, including affirmative and open exploration of the gender identity, assessment for/treatment of coexisting mental health conditions, to educate and advocate, to provide information on peer support, and to inform about/refer for gender affirmative medical interventions [38].

What ASD-specific characteristics should clinicians take into consideration during the diagnostic process? Youth with ASD who seek help for gender-related concerns might not always present as their experienced gender or find it difficult to socially transition due to social anxiety and impaired executive functioning (e.g., planning, organizing, and abstract thinking). Also, it might be more difficult to present socially in the experienced gender role before any gender affirmative treatment has taken place

[37]. For clinicians and parents, such a presentation could give rise to second thoughts about the credibility of their experience. Nonetheless, many of these youth might have persistent feelings of GD and should not be denied access to the assessment of GD. Instead, these individuals should be referred to professionals who might help them explore their gender identity and goals in a safe and supportive setting that incorporates appropriate integration of any ASD impact on executing an affirmation plan.

Assessment could additionally be complicated due to difficulties in communication and expressing/exploring gender-related feelings [37]. Individuals with ASD might be less aware of how they feel about their body, and identity in general, which could make it difficult to discuss feelings with regard to gender identity. Also, because of a tendency to use "black-and-white" thinking rather than "gray," individuals with ASD might find it difficult during assessment to explore gender from a continuous perspective, instead of a binary concept [37]. Additionally, understanding of the long-term impacts of treatment might be difficult for youth with ASD if they have limited ability to envision the future.

When assessing youth with ASD for GD, it is therefore advisable to have information on their strengths and challenges (e.g., cognitive functioning, communication abilities, executive functioning) and to take ASD-related features into account by, for example, adjusting language to their cognitive level or making use of visual supports. Treatment for specific ASD-related challenges or needs, such as problems with emotion recognition or social communication problems, can be advised, both prior (during the diagnostic phase) and parallel to gender affirmative treatment [37].

Vignette: Sam

Sam, a 14-year-old assigned male at birth, was diagnosed with ASD at age 8. In early childhood, Sam's development differed from peers in several areas. While growing up, Sam had several fixations, among others for dinosaurs, later for aliens and elves. Sam had a different way of interacting with peers, misunderstanding the intentions of others, and feeling left out and bullied. Sam also had a friendship with Ellen, a same aged assigned girl at birth living next door. They liked to play together with dolls and dress up as princesses. Sam never talked about gender identity questions till age 12. At that age, Sam mentioned the strong wish to be like Ellen. When presenting at the gender clinic, Sam could at first only describe what Ellen had that Sam also wished for, like having clothes with glitters and having more friendships with girls. Sam also told the clinician that Sam likes her name because it could both be a boy and girl name. During the assessment of GD, it took Sam several months to disentangle their own feelings and thoughts from the picture Sam had made of Ellen. Sam went to a therapist experienced in ASD to enable her to give words to her feelings. During these sessions, the despair became apparent that Sam felt because of the bodily changes caused by puberty. Sam's parents were supportive, adding examples of gender diverse behavior from early infanthood on, and giving room to Sam in discovering her own identity.

It can sometimes be challenging to disentangle GD/TGD from ASD-related characteristics. Clinicians and/or caregivers might be worried that TGD feelings might stem from ASD-related characteristics such as fixations/obsessions, special interests, or a need for certain sensory input. It is to be advised to take an individual approach, with sometimes an extended assessment period [27, 37].

Youth with ASD might report experiences of TGD since elementary school [39]. However, sometimes children with ASD might be devoid of any self-reference to gender when they are younger and might be less aware of social gender norms. They might not think about gender at all when they are little, becoming aware of gender only in late childhood or adolescence, for example, when secondary sex characteristics develop [34, 35]. Involvement of family or caregivers is important because a history from parents or caregivers can provide valuable information of gender identity development in (early) childhood. Moreover, family support can play a very important role in psychological health and well-being [38].

Also, in some studies, an elevation of emotional and behavior problems, especially affective, anxiety, and somatic problems, has been found in individuals with ASD and co-occurring TGD, compared to individuals with ASD alone [25]. Clinicians should, thus, be alert of these and other co-occurring conditions during assessment and incorporate these in the treatment plan or refer individuals to specific services.

Nonmedical Interventions: A Stepwise Approach, Psychoeducation, and Gender Exploration

There is often no clear distinction between assessment and treatment of GD in youth with ASD, and assessment and treatment might partly overlap [37]. ASD-related problems in future thinking might lead to difficulties in envisaging how something in the future will be or feel. Steps in social transition should be evaluated in a stepwise approach, with regard to GD-related distress and general well-being [37]. This careful evaluation of the stepwise approach often continues during gender affirmative treatment, such as hormone treatment.

Vignette: Sam (continued)

The assessment of GD was helped by the parallel treatment with the ASD therapist. Sam was able to express her feelings by, for example, describing difficult situations in a diary, making a painting of herself and formulating steps necessary to become more happy with herself. Sam discovered a more expansive way of understanding her gender diverse thoughts, feelings, and experiences, by separating her gender identity, gender expression, gender assigned at birth, and physical or emotional attraction toward others. One of the more difficult subjects was Sam's wish to be more socially accepted in the group of girls at school. Although she became more at ease with herself, she still experienced challenges in social interactions. It took Sam much effort to understand and accept that not everything would improve after transitioning.

Extended psychoeducation for neurodiverse youth, as well as for parents/caregivers, is an important part of supporting youth and their parents to help develop a broad range of possible gender outcomes and increase flexibility in thinking about gender, self-awareness, and social insight [37, 39]. During consultations with youth, it is often helpful to explore gender as a continuum instead of a binary, to provide alternative gender outcomes (such as gender fluid, a-gender), and to inform them about the options of embodying various aspects of another gender without having a full medical transition.

Youth with ASD should be encouraged to explore their gender identity, various options within the gender spectrum, and gender role/expression in their own pace, before possible irreversible medical treatment interventions. As youth with ASD might be inclined to "all or nothing" thinking, it can be challenging to take a gradual approach in exploring gender-affirming steps [37].

Incorporating aspects of the experienced gender, before medical interventions have started or completed, can be confusing or provoke anxiety. Also, exploration beyond what is familiar or what feels safe can provoke anxiety. When youth with ASD find it complex to initiate or complete a social transition due to, for example, executive functioning problems, rigid thinking, or anxiety, caregivers should be involved to facilitate gender exploration and to support or give guidance regarding any difficulties. Such difficulties can vary from problems with coming out to using makeup or finding an own and satisfactory clothing style. Also, it can be helpful to offer a certain structure in themes to be explored, for example, clothing, hairstyle, and hobbies, and each step should be evaluated carefully.

During this stepwise approach, it is important to monitor the process, and therefore, appointment compliance is important. As youth with ASD find it sometimes difficult to come to sessions, involvement of caregivers and support with planning can be helpful [37].

Medical Treatment

Vignette: Sam (continued)

After a period of assessment, the distress caused by the potential virilization of her body became very apparent (e.g., panic attacks because of the feeling of having facial hair, avoiding the confrontation with her body by refusing to take a shower). A treatment with puberty blockers was started as a first step to release this distress and to help Sam take the time to further discover her own unique identity. A big step was coming-out at school. Sam had first planned to transition over the summer holiday, even wanting to change school in order to avoid the confrontation with the in-between phase. Finally, with the help of her teacher, she accepted to change her plans and be open about her feelings in her own class. Much to her surprise, her peers were accepting Sam's transition. At age 16, Sam started gender-affirming hormones, already feeling a lot more at ease with herself.

TGD adolescents with ASD have undergone gender affirmative medical treatment [4]. It has been suggested that gonadotropin-releasing hormone (GNRH) analogues (puberty blockers) to suppress puberty development and gender-affirming cross-sex hormone (CSH) therapy in adolescents with GD are associated with alleviation of GD and improvement of mental health [40, 41]. Long-term follow-up studies in TGD adolescents with ASD on either the use of GNRH analogues and CSH are lacking, and it is, therefore, until now unsure what the outcomes of gender affirmative treatment are in individuals with ASD. Because of possible difficulties with future thinking, when it comes to medical treatment to relieve GD, prudence should be taken regarding irreversible effects of medical treatment and regarding having realistic expectations for treatment. To be able to consent for treatment, benefits and risks of treatment should be discussed in a way taking the adolescents' thinking style into account [37].

The literature on gender-affirming surgery in adolescents is scarce and mainly comprises gender-affirming bilateral mastectomy [42]. Several studies have shown benefits of mastectomy in adolescents [42], yet no research has been done in adolescents with co-occurring ASD. Long-term follow-up studies are needed to see whether individuals with ASD will equally benefit from gender-affirming surgery as neurotypical individuals.

Conclusion

A growing body of literature suggests that neurodiversity and GD/TGD intersect more frequently than might be anticipated by chance. Underlying biological, psychological, and social hypotheses for this potential co-occurrence have been proposed, but empirical evidence for any of these hypotheses is lacking. It has also been suggested that due to minority stress in TGD individuals, they might show characteristics that resemble ASD but are a result of GD/TGD. Further research is needed to investigate if and why GD/TGD and ASD co-occur more frequently.

The experience and expression of gender may be different depending on whether someone is neurodiverse or not. With regard to assessment and treatment, there is clinical consensus that GD and ASD can co-occur independently. Individuals with ASD who seek help for their feelings of GD might come with specific challenges during assessment and treatment. However, ASD should not be an exclusion criterion, and therefore, these individuals should have access to gender affirmative treatment. Future research is needed on the sometimes clinically challenging co-occurrence of GD/TGD and ASD, for example, on the development of specific assessment tools and on long-term follow-up of treatment.

Acknowledgment The authors thank A. Natisha Nabbijohn for the helpful contribution during the draft of the manuscript.

Financial Support This chapter received no specific grant from any funding agency or commercial or not-for-profit sectors.

Conflict of Interest The authors declare that they have no conflict of interest.

References

1. Ristori J, Steensma TD. Gender dysphoria in childhood. Int Rev Psychiatry. 2016;28:13–20.
2. Leibowitz SF, de Vries ALC. Gender dysphoria in adolescence. Int Rev Psychiatry. 2016;28:21–35.
3. Mukaddes NM. Gender identity problems in autistic children. Child Care Health Dev. 2002;28:529–32.
4. de Vries ALC, Noens ILJ, Cohen-Kettenis PT, van Berckelaer-Onnes IA, Doreleijers TAH. Autism spectrum disorders in gender dysphoric children and adolescents. J Autism Dev Disord. 2010;40:930–6.
5. Øien RA, Cicchetti DV, Nordahl-Hansen A. Gender dysphoria, sexuality and autism spectrum disorders: a systematic review. J Autism Dev Disord. 2018;48:4028–37.
6. American Psychiatric Association. Diagnostic and statistical manual of mental disorders. 5th ed. Washington, DC: American Psychiatric Publishing; 2013.
7. American Psychiatric Association. Diagnostic and statistical manual of mental disorders. 4th ed., Text Revision ed. Washington, DC: American Psychiatric Publishing; 2000.
8. Lai M-C, Lombardo MV, Baron-Cohen S. Autism. Lancet. 2014;383:896–910.
9. Park HR, Lee JM, Moon HE, Lee DS, Kim BN, Kim J, et al. A short review on the current understanding of autism spectrum disorders. Exp Neurobiol. 2016;25:1–13.
10. Baron-Cohen S. Editorial perspective: neurodiversity – a revolutionary concept for autism and psychiatry. J Child Psychol Psychiatry. 2017;58:744–7.
11. Tateno M, Tateno Y, Saito Y. Comorbid childhood gender identity disorder in a boy with Asperger syndrome. Psychiatry Clin Neurosci. 2008;62:238.
12. Wing L. Diagnostic interview for social and communication disorders. Manual. Bromley: Centre for social and communication disorders; 1999.
13. Akgül GY, Ayaz AB, Yildirim G, Fis NP. Autistic traits and executive functions in children and adolescents with gender dysphoria. J Sex Marital Ther. 2018;44:619–26.
14. Di Ceglie D, Skagerberg E, Baron-Cohen S, Auyeung B. Empathising and systemising in adolescents with gender dysphoria. Opticion 1826. 2014;16:1–8.
15. Skagerberg E, Di Ceglie D, Carmichael P. Brief report: autistic features in children and adolescents with gender dysphoria. J Autism Dev Disord. 2015;45:2628–32.
16. VanderLaan DP, Postema L, Wood H, Singh D, Fantus S, Hyun J, et al. Do children with gender dysphoria have intense/obsessional interests? J Sex Res. 2014;52:213–9.
17. VanderLaan DP, Leef JH, Wood H, Hughes SK, Zucker KJ. Autism spectrum disorder risk factors and autistic traits in gender dysphoric children. J Autism Dev Disord. 2015;46:1742–50.
18. Shumer DE, Reisner SL, Edwards-Leeper L, Tishelman A. Evaluation of Asperger syndrome in youth presenting to a gender dysphoria clinic. LGBT Health. 2016;3:387–90.
19. van der Miesen AIR, de Vries ALC, Steensma TD, Hartman CA. Autistic symptoms in children and adolescents with gender dysphoria. J Autism Dev Disord. 2018;48:1537–48.
20. Turban JL, van Schalkwyk GI. "Gender dysphoria" and autism spectrum disorder: is the link real? J Am Acad Child Adolesc Psychiatry. 2018;57:8–9.e2.
21. Hisle-Gorman E, Landis CA, Susi A, Schvey NA, Gorman GH, Nylund CM, et al. Gender dysphoria in children with autism spectrum disorder. LGBT Health. 2019;6:95–100.
22. Janssen A, Huang H, Duncan C. Gender variance among youth with autism spectrum disorders: a retrospective chart review. Transgend Health. 2016;1:63–8.
23. May T, Pang K, Williams KJ. Gender variance in children and adolescents with autism spectrum disorders from the National Database for Autism Research. Int J Transgend. 2017;1 8:1–9.
24. Strang JF, Kenworthy L, Dominska A, Sokoloff J, Kenealy LE, Berl M, et al. Increased gender variance in autism spectrum disorders and attention deficit hyperactivity disorder. Arch Sex Behav. 2014;43:1525–33.
25. van der Miesen AIR, Hurley H, Bal AM, de Vries ALC. Prevalence of the wish to be of the opposite gender in adolescents and adults with autism spectrum disorder. Arch Sex Behav. 2018;47:2307–17.

26. Nabbijohn AN, van der Miesen AIR, Santarossa A, Peragine D, de Vries ALC, Popma A, et al. Gender variance and the autism spectrum: an examination of children ages 6–12 years. J Autism Dev Disord. 2019;49:1570–85.
27. van der Miesen AIR, Hurley H, de Vries ALC. Gender dysphoria and autism spectrum disorder: a narrative review. Int Rev Psychiatry. 2016;28:70–80.
28. Greenberg DM, Warrier V, Allison C, Baron-Cohen S. Testing the empathizing-systemizing theory of sex differences and the extreme male brain theory of autism in half a million people. PNAS. 2018;115:12152–7.
29. Baron-Cohen S. The extreme male brain theory of autism. Trends Cogn Sci. 2002;6:248–54.
30. Hines M, Constantinescu M, Spencer D. Early androgen exposure and human gender development. Biol Sex Differ. 2015;6:3.
31. Jones RM, Weelwright S, Farrel K, Martin E, Green R, Di Ceglie D. Brief report: female-to-male transsexual people and autistic traits. J Autism Dev Disord. 2012;42:301–6.
32. Parkinson J. Gender dysphoria in Asperger's syndrome: a caution. Australas Psychiatry. 2014;22:84–5.
33. Williams P, Allard AM, Sears L. Case study: cross-gender preoccupations in two male children with autism. J Autism Dev Disord. 1996;26:635–42.
34. Ehrensaft D. Double helix rainbow kids. J Autism Dev Disord. 2018;48:4079–81.
35. Walsh RJ, Krabbendam L, Dewinter J, Begeer S. Brief report: gender identity differences in autistic adults: associations with perceptual and socio-cognitive profiles. J Autism Dev Disord. 2018;48:4070–80.
36. Cooper K, Smith LGE, Russel AJ. Gender identity in autism: sex differences in social affiliation with gender groups. J Autism Dev Disord. 2018;48:3995–4006.
37. Strang JF, Meagher H, Kenworthy L, de Vries ALC, Menvielle E, Leibowitz SF, et al. Initial guidelines for co-occurring autism spectrum disorder and gender dysphoria or incongruence in adolescents. J Clin Child Adolesc Psychol. 2018;47:105–15.
38. Coleman E, Bockting W, Botzer M, Cohen-Kettenis PT, DeCuypere G, Feldman J, et al. Standards of care for the health of transsexual, transgender and gender non-conforming people, version 7. Int J Transgend. 2011;13:165–232.
39. Strang JF, Powers MD, Knauss M, Sibarium E, Leibowitz SF, Kenworthy L, et al. "They thought it was an obsession": trajectories and perspectives of autistic transgender and gender-diverse adolescents. J Autism Dev Disord. 2018;48:4039–55.
40. de Vries ALC, Cohen-Kettenis PT. Clinical management of gender dysphoria in children and adolescents: the Dutch approach. J Homosex. 2012;59:301–20.
41. Schagen SEE, Cohen-Kettenis PT, Delemarre-van de Waal HA, Hannema SE. Efficacy and safety of gonadotropin-releasing hormone agonist treatment to suppress puberty in gender dysphoric adolescents. J Sex Med. 2016;17:1125–32.
42. Mahfouda S, Moore JK, Siafarikas A, Hewit T, Ganti U, Lin A, et al. Gender-affirming hormones and surgery in transgender children and adolescents. Lancet Diabetes Endocrinol. 2019;7:484–98.

Considerations for Acute Care of TGD Youth

11

Zheala Qayyum, Erin Ursillo, Kristen Sayles, and Gerrit Van Schalkwyk

Introduction

Given the high rates of mental health concerns among transgender and gender diverse (TGD) youth (see Chap. 9), these young people may require acute psychiatric care, including treatment in inpatient, partial hospital (PHP), and intensive outpatient (IOP) settings.

Growing up within a body that is developing in an incongruent manner to one's gender identity can create significant stress for transgender and gender diverse (TGD) youth. Adolescents who experience dysphoria related to this incongruence suffer high rates of internalizing psychopathology that may lead to inpatient psychiatric hospitalization [1]. It is reported that 40% of transgender adults have attempted suicide, of whom 92% report attempting it before the age of 25. Historically, growing up in a culture where minoritized populations experience direct and indirect stigma and discrimination is demonstrated to create significant stress and is linked to poorer health outcomes for TGD persons. Rejection from family and peers, discrimination, bullying, and threats of violence all can contribute to worsening suicidal ideation and serious psychological distress [1].

Acute care in the psychiatric setting can either offer support or invalidate this already vulnerable population. TGD people are at higher risk of coming across challenges in accessing health care, as well as encountering health-care systems that are not geared toward recognizing, validating, and supporting their gender identities.

Z. Qayyum
Yale University School of Medicine (Department of Psychiatry), New Haven, CT, USA

E. Ursillo · K. Sayles
Butler Hospital, Providence, RI, USA

G. Van Schalkwyk (✉)
Warren Alpert School of Medicine, Brown University, Providence, RI, USA
e-mail: GVanschalkwyk@Butler.org

M. Forcier et al. (eds.), *Pediatric Gender Identity*,
https://doi.org/10.1007/978-3-030-38909-3_11

While the immediate priority of the inpatient psychiatric hospitalization is, therefore, first and foremost to ensure safety, providing a gender-affirming environment is paramount in laying the foundation for these youth to continue being engaged in care, rather than invalidating their identity, which could discourage them from seeking care after discharge. Invalidating experiences can be traumatizing for these youth who may enter acute treatment already at higher risk for suicide with comorbid mental health concerns.

This chapter discusses

- Key ways in which psychiatric systems may create an affirming environment at the policy and organizational level.
- How inpatient units and hospitals environments can be affirming, including a perspective on how staff can be trained to be effective in this context.
- Clinical considerations that may inform the individual care of TGD individuals in crisis.

An Affirming Environment in the Broader Treatment Environment

Embarking on the mission to create a safe and affirming PHP, IOP, or inpatient treatment environment for patients in the LGBTQ+ communities can have its challenges, but the reward of working around these challenges is great. In a perfect world, an agency would have full control over all factors of patient care; however, more often, the reality is that agencies begin this mission with suboptimal circumstances that are not easily influenced due to internal agency problems and/or broader healthcare system-related issues. This does not mean that the charge is futile. Success is attainable if the organization is committed to the mission of providing safe and affirming care, and if the agency problem solves creatively and plans ahead for potential road blocks. Of those organizations who do make a verbal commitment to improvement, unfortunately many do not succeed in the actual mission of providing LGBTQ+ informed care.

In order to stand out as a leading organization that does succeed in providing affirming healthcare, an agency should focus on three major areas: physical environment, staff education and engagement, and continued accountability [2].

Physical Environment

The overall goal when it comes to revamping the hospital's physical environment – whether it be an inpatient unit, PHP, or IOP – would be to modify the space in a way that promotes a welcoming, affirming, and safe setting for patients and visitors. Although the infrastructure of the building itself is not something that can often be altered, there are cost-effective modifications that can be made that do not include pricey renovations. If an agency has funds to spend on physical modifications, there are more expensive alterations that provide ideal benefit.

Modifying physical settings to provide accessible and safe bathroom options is an initial and critical start to greeting TGD youth and families. When single-occupant bathrooms exist on the premises, changing all single-occupant gender-based bathroom signs from male/female images to "all-gender" or "gender-neutral" images is an example of a low-cost modification. Doing so will create a welcoming atmosphere when patients enter new settings in crisis. A more costly approach would be to add single-occupant bathrooms if none exist on site.

Many organizations have multiple-occupant gender-segregated bathrooms which can pose both safety and privacy concerns for transgender individuals. Organizations can consider changing these bathroom types to all-gender restrooms even when there are single gender-neutral bathroom options on site. In keeping safety and privacy at the forefront of decision-making, there are several safety/privacy enhancements that the Human Rights Campaign recommends to aid in this goal (all of which vary in price); install flaps on the outer edge of stall doors to cover the gap between the door and the stall wall, extend stall doors and walls from floor to ceiling, and extend privacy dividers between urinals further out from the wall and to a higher level [2].

Establishing LGBTQ+ friendly resource centers in public areas with materials supportive to gender affirmation will not only provide useful education but will also demonstrate the hospital's support and competence in this area (little to no cost). Expanding upon the décor of the hospital to include artwork that embraces gender fluidity or diversity can be appealing and within a reasonable price point. Integrating safe zone images throughout the space (printed images at little to no cost that represent a safe and confidential space or person that welcomes people as their authentic selves) will send a visual message that people can discuss a variety of topics without fear of discrimination or retaliation [3]. There is no one set standard when it comes to safe zone signs. An agency can print images that already exist online or create a safe zone sign that relates to their own organization. Another way to display the standard within an organization that gender identity should not be assumed is to provide staff and patients with the option to display the pronouns they use on them with either a pin or a sticker.

Staff Engagement and Education

Agencies can create a culture that supports affirming care by starting with clear and consistent messaging and expectations about what it means to offer affirmative care. An agency may be successful in implementing that care and reaching goals by providing education and resources for staff to carry out this mission. Leadership can create institutional cultural improvements by offering: fundamental training for all staff, training on the latest medical record documentation, advanced clinical training for all clinicians, and consistent evaluation of the patient experience and staff success.

What to say....	Instead of...
What pronouns do you use?	**Assuming pronouns**
What is your gender? **How do you identify your gender?**	**Assuming gender**
What is your name?	**What name do you prefer*?**
How can I help you?	**How can I help you sir?**
Do you have a significant other?	**Do you have a husband, wife, boyfriend, girlfriend?**
Is the name on your insurance card different than your name?	**Did you legally change your name or what is your preferred* name?**
Hello everyone...	**Hello guys, ladies, etc.**

*Prefer indicates choice. Avoid in regards to name and pronoun usage

Fig. 11.1 Key points on language

Fundamental training includes everyone employed at the agency – from the first telephone encounter to discharge planning. Training begins with a review of appropriate terminology and concepts and with a discussion of affirming care. Training should offer opportunities for staff at all levels to be aware of their part in creating an affirming environment.

As this is a rapidly changing field, where concepts and terminology change regularly, initial education begins with updating staff on what we currently understand about gender identity and gender expression. While it is human and understandable for employees to come to work with their own biases and opinions, staff members have professional treatment responsibilities as it pertains to patient care and will need to monitor and manage their own biases at work. To assist with this, staff can be led through trainings that explore how personal biases could potentially interfere with their success in providing affirming care. Training may address assumptions we make about gender in our everyday language, ways people can adjust language to avoid assumptions (Fig. 11.1), and ways people can respectfully apologize if they make a mistake.

All staff will need to commit to asking every patient the name and pronoun they use rather than making assumptions. Although this practice may feel controversial for some, making this routine is crucial if an agency is committed to providing affirming care. There is no way to know someone's gender without asking. Incorrect assumptions make for a traumatic patient experience and are contradictory to the overall mission.

A common concern is that one could offend a cisgender patient by asking their gender. If the true goal is to provide affirming care, is it not far better to explain to a cisgender person why you asked them their gender than to make an incorrect assumption and offend a transgender person? An example of a response that would be appropriate is as follows: "I apologize. I did not ask you that to offend you. We as an organization will not assume anyone's gender based on our own assumptions. We ask every single patient to tell us who they are rather than us assuming."

Teaching staff how to ask questions about gender identity as well as role-playing potential scenarios with staff can help them feel confident and prepared for all potential interactions. Having staff introduce themselves to all patients using their own name and pronoun will act as a model for any patients who do not understand gender identity and will lead to opportunities for staff to spread the appropriate message about gender. It will be helpful to provide staff with a variety of practice scenarios to prepare them for potential interactions about gender so that they feel confident in these circumstances; apologizing for their mistake or redirecting an individual who is being disrespectful, clarifying gender identity for someone who does not understand, etc.

Reputable resources should be provided at the conclusion of these trainings, which will allow employees to do further research from reliable sources if they so choose. National organizations such as Pride, Youth Pride, The Health Equality Index, The National LGBT Health Education Center, Fenway Health, LAMBDA Legal, TGI Network, PFLAG, and the Human Rights Campaign are reliable options.

Creating a TGD responsive electronic medical record (EMR) is a large and system-wide task. In an ideal setting, documentation would be streamlined with clear standards that incorporate the diversity of gender identities, names, and pronouns. Many EMRs do not allow for flexibility in documenting on gender as gender is considered an identifier for insurance companies. In many settings, it may not be feasible to upgrade programming; therefore, creating affirmative work-arounds in the original EMR may be created and implemented systemically by staff. Attention to paper documents given to patients that ask them to select gender may be adapted to include more than the binary male/female options. Establishing responsible persons in EMR administration who will serve as a change leader can ensure that organizations stay up to date with best documentation practices since standards are ever evolving.

Advanced clinical trainings should be delivered to staff that have more of a clinical role with patients (physicians, clinicians, nurse practitioners, etc.). Discussion points on gender diversity, the different ways people affirm their gender, minority stress, biopsychosocial risk factors, and the most up-to-date clinical interventions will be vital. World Professional Association for Transgender Health (WPATH) is a reliable source that provides clinically relevant trainings on these topics.

Unfortunately, even with the installation of the above-mentioned levels of in-house training, it is unrealistic to expect that an agency full of experts on this topic will result. It will be pertinent to seek out in-house leaders; staff members who show a special interest in affirming care. Offering these leaders additional external continuing education training so that they can keep up with the ever-changing and evolving information on gender will be a great benefit to the organization as a whole. These agency point persons will be able to share the most up-to-date information with other employees, and they will serve as a motivating presence in the workspace as it pertains to affirming care.

Continued Accountability

While it is important to focus attention on the physical environment and staff education and engagement, in order to ensure success and stand out as a leader in affirming care for TGD individuals, close monitoring of the patient experience and staff conduct will be paramount. Feedback on patient experience is essential in determining areas of strength and weakness within an organization. Offering a posttreatment survey focused on the affirming experience is a considerate way of eliciting feedback from patients in an anonymous and voluntary manner. It would be helpful to consider establishing an in-house committee to monitor survey feedback and collaborate on solutions for areas of concern. Instituting conduct objectives within an employee's traditional job evaluation that highlights their own personal role in providing affirming care will allow management to hold staff members accountable and to assess for strengths and areas of potential improvement for each staff person. This will also reinforce the message to all employees that affirming care is the standard within the organization.

Inpatient Settings: A Case Study in Achieving Culture Change

An inpatient environment should seek to affirm the gender narrative described by the patient to allow them to receive the best possible psychiatric care. In order to facilitate an affirming inpatient environment, it is necessary that clinical staff are not only educated, but that there is a collective commitment to the mission. It is critical that unit leadership seeks to assertively develop and support an environment in which gender diverse youth may thrive; at the same time, this will not be successful if clinical staff is left behind by the process. On our inpatient adolescent unit at Butler Hospital, this was achieved through a multistep process that was both gradual and assertive. Core principles were as follows:

- *Exposure and Education*: Experts in the area of pediatric gender were invited to speak to clinical staff on multiple occasions. This was combined with implementing lessons learned as relevant clinical situations occurred.
- *Crucial Conversations*: Clinical staff were engaged around their own preconceived notions and potential areas of bias, and these were anticipated and addressed prior to patients arriving on the unit in order to ensure that barriers to affirming care were resolved without impacting the experience of individual patients. This approach drew on the concept of "crucial conversations" – a set of techniques for having productive discussions around emotionally charged topics [4].
- *Staff Engagement at All Levels*: Responsibility for an affirming environment was shared between physicians, nurses, mental health workers, occupational therapy, social services, and administrative staff. This approach reflected the principles of "shared governance," a well-articulated approach to manage complex challenges in professional environments [5].

- *Implementing Agreed-Upon Changes in Steps*: New approaches (e.g., bathroom or room assignment based on identified gender) to address TGD-specific needs were implemented in response as clinical situations arose, allowing staff to process barriers and participate in a collective effort to support gender diverse youth.

With these guiding principles, change was achieved through the following staff development procedures:

- *Case Studies*: These included an existing space for weekly, multidisciplinary case discussions and to identify areas for improvement in affirming care. These case studies provided an opportunity to identify preconceptions and bias and provided a safe platform in which these barriers could be explored and processed.
- *Informal Educational Interventions*: These include ad hoc conversations regarding appropriate pronoun usage and open-ended conversations to understand the current beliefs, level of understanding, and skill of individual staff in supporting gender diverse youth.
- *Formal Educational Interventions*:
  - Nursing grand rounds – A four-hour training was provided by a local physician expert on best practices for supporting gender diverse youth, for which continuing education credit was available.
  - Staff meetings – Additional trainings were provided by unit leadership, which utilized the Joint Commission LGBT Field Guide [6].
  - Optional trainings – Staff were encouraged to take the training offered by the Human Rights Campaign 2018 [2], which was made available for free through an institutional license.
- *Continued Education*: Existing platforms for clinical discussion such as weekly rounds, staff meetings, and weekly case discussions were thoughtfully enhanced to provide ongoing reinforcement of principles expounded during more formal education approaches

Practical Approaches

Achieving an affirming environment required both institutional change and circumventing complex challenges with practical solutions. It is possible to facilitate an affirming patient experience, even if longer-term challenges remain in addressing structural sources of bias within medical systems. The following steps were taken on our inpatient unit:

- *Name and Identifiers*: As noted previously, institutions vary in their ability to consistently display preferred names in electronic medical records, and regulations require that legal names appear on certain forms to facilitate inpatient admission, consent to care, and insurance. In order to balance this limitation with an effort to create an affirming environment, asserted names can be displayed on areas visible to the patient, which do not constitute legal documents – such as the unit name board, and whenever names are listed for unit activities. Staff can reference these sources where reminders are required regarding patients asserted name. Individual clinics and providers may be creative in work arounds that include patients asserted names being listed on wristbands, as this may be a low-risk opportunity to provide affirmation.

- *Bathrooms*: In order to maximize the positive experience of all patients while providing an affirming environment, communal bathrooms were used and gender diverse youth were allowed to use the bathroom that they were most comfortable with – an approach which has been implemented without incident over the last several years.
- *Room Assignment*: Preferences of the patient, the desire to be affirming, and the needs of other patients were considered and weighed. Although it may seem optimal to always room patients with other patients of their affirmed gender, this does not consistently reflect the desires of patients or may be challenging for other reasons. A single room is frequently a stated preference for gender diverse youth who are undergoing hormonal or surgical changes, and this is made available in these instances. Youth who have not begun any hormonal or surgical intervention may be most comfortable with roommates of their assigned at birth gender. When gender diverse youth express a desire to have a roommate of their affirmed gender, this should be facilitated as long as it does not expose the patient to undue risk; patients may experience trauma if they are roomed with a peer who articulates stigmatized views toward the patient. Available guidelines for Lambda Legal suggest that where patients object to having a gender diverse roommate, this should be problem solved through a discussion with the patient, or moving the patient who expresses the concern [6, 7]. In practice, we have found it is almost always possible to provide an environment, which is affirming, safe, and therapeutic for all patients.
- *TDG-Affirmative Resources and Materials*: The physical space included resources and materials for youth to see examples of gender diversity and to explore their own gender. Developmentally appropriate and affirming materials are made available, which provide concrete explanation and facilitate exploration of a patient's individual gender narrative.

Ongoing Challenges

Much work remains to be done to ensure that gender diverse youth have more consistent access to affirming inpatient care. Even within an environment, which seeks to prioritize this mission, challenges remain:

- *Barriers*: Privacy laws may be violated if potential roommates are made aware of a youth's gender diversity; not involving the roommate in such a discussion creates a real risk for inappropriate comments or behavior toward the roommate should they come to this realization in other ways. Parents of both patients and

roommates may not hold affirming views around gender diversity, and it may not be in the youth's best interest for this to derail psychiatric treatment.
- *Personal Bias*: Despite intense efforts at education, there may be areas of ignorance and a lack of commitment to an overall "culture change" among staff.
- *Issues of Intersectionality*: Youth in mental health settings may experience an intersection between their gender-related concerns, mental health concerns, and other socioeconomic factors that impact long-term health outcomes. More clinical study is indicated to best inform how to balance attention to the gender narrative during periods of crisis in order to optimize mental health treatment and ensure that youth receive the best care. Taking the lead from the patient seems to be a promising approach to this challenge – this is discussed in further detail below.

Clinical Approach

As there may be different reasons why a young transgender youth would find themselves in an acute treatment setting, there may also be a variety of unique gender issues specific to each patient.

TGD youth may disclose gender dysphoria or their transgender identity for the first time during the course of hospitalization or intensive outpatient care. This is more likely to occur if they have formed a trusting relationship with their clinician. These youth may be engaged in the process of exploring their gender identity and what it means to them. There may not be a commitment or crystallization of their gender as of yet. For these youth, it is important to not impose an artificial burden of having to make a decision about their gender. A clinician's best work is done supporting this process of emerging identity and allowing them a safe space to explore their gender identity. Relevant information regarding important and emerging aspects of gender may be communicated to staff and their outpatient team. Some youth may request more information and resources and referrals to gender-specific services as they approach discharge. Knowing your community providers and allies may help facilitate these next steps.

There are also youth who experience fluctuations in their gender identity or consider themselves outside the gender spectrum (i.e., nonbinary). These nonbinary identities may be encountered during acute treatment. Some fluctuations may arise when patients experience unsupportive attitudes and bias [8]. Nonbinary youth also tend to experience less support from their family and friends, putting them at greater risk for suffering [9]. Some youth experience understandable ambivalence about the cost and hardships encountered during the process of undertaking gender-affirming steps and long issues that may arise. Some youth do not continue to identify as transgender into their adulthood [10]. Regardless, having a safe environment and trusted relationships in which to discover who they are is the key component of any psychiatric treatment. In case of multiple psychiatric hospitalizations or periods of PHP/IOP treatment, where the patient has demonstrated variance in their gender identity or gender expression, clinicians and staff should maintain a nonjudgmental and validating approach toward the patient. Educate staff members that this variance may be a normal part of exploring gender identity for some youth. It is not necessary that one particular gender will be adhered to as part of the process of discovering one's most authentic self [10, 11].

There are other transgender youth admitted to acute care settings who are clear about their transgender identity and have not yet disclosed it to their family. In such cases, it is important that the clinician openly discusses what the young patient is comfortable disclosing to their family and when. Here, the role of the clinician is to support the patient while facilitating a discussion to enhance the family's understanding of the youth's gender identity. Often parent support and guidance are needed after the disclosure. The family should be supported in processing the information as they come to a place where they can mourn the loss of the idealized child and be more welcoming and accepting of the real person in front of them [8]. Understanding the family dynamics and environment in which the youth will be discharged is key in safe discharge planning.

Helpful Tips for Disclosure

1. Create a therapeutic alliance with the parents.
2. Inquire about the parental experience of their youth's journey. Often parents are already aware of the TGD youth atypical journey of gender development.
3. Explore parental beliefs about gender diversity and human development based on their social, cultural, and religious background.
4. Support the TGD youth when they are ready to disclose to their family, based on the individual youth's expressed needs.
5. Create a safe space both for the TGD youth and family to process together and individually. Set a supportive and nonjudgmental tone that does not stigmatize the TGD youth.
6. Provide psychoeducation to the family. Clarify that gender diversity is a normal human expression. It is also helpful to discuss that various trajectories such as persistence, nonconformity, phasing out, or adoption of atypical gender expression cannot be predicted.
7. Highlight the important role of parental support and involvement with the TGD youth. Although they do not influence their child's gender expression, they have a much greater influence on their physical, emotional, and psychological well-being, and social adjustment
8. Provide support in case of parental crisis. Explore parental fears.
9. Make a plan with the family to provide safety and support for the TGD youth.
10. Make referrals for family therapy and marital therapy if indicated.

There are instances when transgender youth are not ready to disclose their transgender identity to their family just yet. They may have previously experienced an invalidating environment or other forms or trauma or abuse that makes it difficult for them. Here the clinician must take the patient's lead. The focus should be respecting the patient's autonomy while helping them to build resilience to cope with the outside world and gain a greater sense of empowerment. Referrals and resources that are gender affirming outside the family setting can be helpful. Gendercool Project, the GSA network, Campus Pride, and Youth Policy Institute (YPI) are some examples where TGD youth can connect with peers and access support for themselves. It is also essential that the patient preference is seamlessly communicated to all members of the team involved in taking care of the patient, to ensure inadvertent disclosure does not occur.

As with their cisgender peers, TGD youth may require acute psychiatric treatment for a variety of mental health needs. Thorough psychiatric assessments for anxiety, mood, and substance-use disorders along with trauma are necessary and should not be overlooked [12]. Transgender identity can at times serve as a focus for other displaced conflicts, whether with their family, peers, or themselves. In some cases, there may be additional stressors that can compound the experienced minority stress, while in other cases, preexisting mental health issues can surface as result of the difficulties the TGD youth is experiencing. It is important to explore these both independently, and as they relate to the TGD identity [13]. Focusing on appropriate treatment modalities for comorbid disorders should be integrated into gender-affirming care and prioritized based on severity and impact on the individuals psychological and social functioning.

Psychopharmacological intervention may be indicated as part of the comprehensive treatment plan to alleviate symptoms of anxiety and depression that can result from minority stress and internalized bias, particularly when they impair functioning. It is also ideal to access appropriate consultation when indicated for psychoeducation about gender affirmation, hormonal therapy, and surgical interventions. The acute care setting is well suited for a multidisciplinary meeting to address these issues with the family while drawing in expertise from clinicians who will continue to follow-up with the patient after discharge. Questions may arise as to the timing of hormonal therapy for which input from a physician who specializes in these treatments can be extremely helpful. The treatment team should facilitate discussions as the next steps toward gender affirmation are discussed in a way that is most appropriate and supportive.

TGD youth in acute treatment settings deserve a full risk assessment upon admission and discharge, as well as developing a conceptual framework of their social and familial supports. A thorough discussion of a safety plan as well as follow-up treatment should be undertaken with the patient and the family. There is indeed an opportunity to take the time and holistically view the needs of the TGD youth and to make referrals that will best support the patient. There is now greater initiative in establishing specialized programs for LGBTQ youth in order to better address their mental health needs in a gender-affirming environment. Coordination with the school may also be necessary for those youth requiring academic support or interventions in the school environment.

Additionally steps should be taken to set up social and community supports for the transgender youth. As mentioned earlier, PFLAG, Campus Pride, Camp Aranu'tiq, the Trevor Project, and others serve as great resources to make these connections. Online resources can be accessed through www.genderspectrum.org.

Conclusion

Transgender and gender diverse youth face an unfair problem; although they may have greater needs for acute mental health treatment, they are less able to receive this treatment in environments that are appropriately supportive. Although practical challenges exist, there are many opportunities to create both small and larger institutional changes that would benefit these youth and families, educating and developing staff and clinicians who have the necessary skills to treat mental health concerns, while supporting and affirming the dynamic process of gender exploration.

References

1. James S, Herman J, Rankin S, Keisling M, Mottet L, Anafi MA. The report of the 2015 U.S. transgender survey. Washington, DC: National Center for Transgender Equality; 2016.
2. The Human Rights Campaign [Internet]. Healthcare equity index. 2018. [cited 11.29.2018]. https://www.hrc.org/hei.
3. The Safe Zone Project [Internet]. 2018 [cited 11.29.2018]. https://thesafezoneproject.com/.
4. Patterson KJ, Major K, Abderrahman EA, Sweeney JI. Crucial conversations – tools for talking when the stakes are high. Am J Nurs. 2013;113(4):66–70.
5. Barden AM, Griffin MTQ, Donahue M, Fitzpatrick JJ. Shared governance and empowerment in registered nurses working in a hospital setting. Nurs Adm Q. 2011;35(3):212–8.
6. Commission TJ. Advancing effective communication, cultural competence, and patient- and family-centered care for the lesbian, gay, bisexual, and transgender (LGBT) community. 2014. https://www.jointcommission.org/lgbt/.
7. http://www.lambdalegal.org/sites/default/files/publications/downloads/hospital-policies-2016_5-26-16.pdf.
8. Steensma TD, Cohen-Kettenis PT. More than two developmental pathways in children with gender dysphoria? J Am Acad Child Adolesc Psychiatry. 2015;54(2):147–8.
9. Aparicio-García ME, Díaz-Ramiro EM, Rubio-Valdehita S, López-Núñez MI, García-Nieto I. Health and well-being of cisgender, transgender and non-binary young people. Int J Environ Res Public Health. 2018;15(10):pii: E2133. https://doi.org/10.3390/ijerph15102133.
10. Turban JL, Keuroghlian AS. Dynamic gender presentations: understanding transition and "de-transition" among transgender youth. J Am Acad Child Adolesc Psychiatry. 2018;57(7):451–3.
11. Turban JL, Carswell J, Keuroghlian AS. Understanding pediatric patients who discontinue gender-affirming hormonal interventions. JAMA Pediatr. 2018;172(10):903–4.
12. Birkett M, Newcomb ME, Mustanski B. Does it get better? A longitudinal analysis of psychological distress and victimization in lesbian, gay, bisexual, transgender, and questioning youth. J Adolesc Health. 2015;56(3):280–5. https://doi.org/10.1016/j.jadohealth.2014.10.275. Epub 2015 Jan 10.
13. Bojarski E, Qayyum Z. Psychodynamics of suicide in lesbian, gay, bisexual, or transgender youth. J Infant Child Adolesc Psychother. 2018;17(3):178–86.

Psychotherapy: A Clinical Perspective 12

Teresa Daniels and Micaela Condon

Introduction

Psychotherapy is central to comprehensive, affirmative care for adolescents with diverse gender identities. Mental health providers can support their TGD clients through a broad range of services. In this chapter, we provide a brief overview of various modalities and considerations, supported by insights from clinical practice and evidence from a growing body of literature. Whereas this segment of the population is historically underrepresented and under recognized in the vast majority of mental and public health research, the increasing need for gender-competent providers and an evidence basis for their practice has led to a sea change in the professional community's understanding of gender and its diverse range of expression. With continued investigation, reflection, and, most importantly, openness to the voices of TGD people, systems of mental health care will move toward a model that affirms the identities of the individuals it seeks to support.

Treatment begins by understanding the individual needs of each unique TGD youth that presents to the office. Clarifying with the adolescent (and their family, whenever possible) what specifically brings them to you will set the framework for your work together. Whether it is to explore their individual gender identity and expression, find support in the process of coming out and affirming their identity, address requirements for medical and surgical interventions, or ameliorate the psychosocial difficulties that may or may not be related to their gender experience, there are core principles that can be used to drive compassionate, affirmative gender care through psychotherapy.

T. Daniels (✉)
Brown University, Providence, RI, USA
e-mail: teresa_daniels@brown.edu

M. Condon
Butler Hospital, Providence, RI, USA
e-mail: mcondon@butler.org

M. Forcier et al. (eds.), *Pediatric Gender Identity*,
https://doi.org/10.1007/978-3-030-38909-3_12

In the gender affirmative model, gender health is described as the opportunity for an individual to live in the gender that "feels most real" and to express their unique gender "without experiencing restriction, criticism, and ostracism" [1]. It asserts that variations in gender are indeed normative and non-pathological. As gender identities are diverse, they reflect a tapestry of biology, development, culture, and context, and may change over time. Societal messaging, however, reinforces gender binary constructs. Consequently, the psychological pain we often encounter in our clients results from chronically invalidating interpersonal and cultural reactions [1–3]. A growing evidence basis supports a practice that communicates respect, inclusion, and affirmation for improved gender health and overall health outcomes [1–5].

An affirming model calls for providers to utilize the same practices as they would in any other setting, namely providing a safe environment, developing a strong therapeutic alliance, allowing for pain and suffering to be voiced, with themes of neutrality, empathy, and interpretation to enhance self-understanding. In this chapter, we will explore how these principles inform an approach to psychotherapy.

Exploration of Gender Identity and Expression

There is no singular narrative that underlies the experience of a TGD adolescent. One element that is unifying, however, is that their sense of self is distinct from the gender assumed to correspond to their sex assigned at birth. In keeping with an affirmative model, this sense of self has biological, developmental, cultural, and contextual influences. It can be clarified and better understood through work with a psychotherapist, but notably comes from within. Thus, therapists working with TGD clients are tasked with joining, rather than leading, their clients in the exploration of their unique gender experience, identity, and expression. In this collaborative approach, it is important to recognize that each individual is the authority on their own gender identity and in doing so, the provider powerfully affirms and validates the agency of their client.

Therapists, clients, and their families can explore gender experiences from the perspective of relation to self, relation to one's body and relation to others. More frequently than not, the history gathered does not follow the pattern of a persistent, insistent, and consistent declaration that is traditionally thought to underlie the TGD experience. Rather, adolescents will report knowing that something was "different" over time, whether it is through an escalation in these feelings in the context of puberty or through psychosocial stress from negative reactions of family or society. This dissonance will declare itself as a gender that is liberated from the sex assigned at birth. The way in which the patient has expressed gender, in the form of appearance and interests, may continue to change.

The experience of gender is iterative and in a perpetual state of becoming. In *The Lives of Transgender People*, Beemyn and Raskin interviewed more than 3500 individuals with diverse gender identities and gender expressions, and found these individuals described their gender with more than 200 distinct descriptions [5].

Psychological Support from Family Members

The support of one's family is a particularly important prognostic indicator for TGD adolescents. For this reason, whenever possible, it is critical to involve the client's family during the course of psychotherapy treatment. Including the family from the first intake interview serves to provide a better understanding of the environment in which the adolescent is thriving or not. Across a treatment course, family sessions can be utilized to follow the changing dynamics within the client's environment and to provide support, reassurance and education where needed. Depending on the relative levels of support and stress offered by the family dynamic, a referral to an independent family therapist, preferably with a background in working with TGD populations, may be necessary. Additionally, group therapy and support groups for parents and siblings can serve to address needs within TGD families and referrals should be made as appropriate, and available.

Assessing for Related Difficulties

While a gender-competent provider seeks to affirm a TGD adolescent's gender experience, identity, and expression, they should also evaluate for and treat the psychological concerns that may also be present. TGD youth are a heterogenous group, and many may not experience significant psychological distress. However, compared to cisgender adolescents, TGD adolescents appear to experience disproportionately high rates of psychological distress, with increased risk of depression, anxiety, and suicidal thoughts [6–8]. Further, accumulating evidence demonstrates a clear need to improve mental health treatment for TGD individuals – especially among adolescents. According to the 2015 United States Transgender Survey (USTS), more than half of respondents reported "current serious psychological distress." It is important to recognize that conditions may or may not be related to the client's gender experience. As described further in the section on minority stress below, external societal stressors may or may not contribute to the psychological turmoil experienced by TGD individuals [4]. The broad range of experiences of TGD adolescents underlies the need for a thorough gender and mental health history, review of symptoms, as evaluation of chronic minority stress.

Providers may encounter a variety of symptomatology in their evaluations. Chronic minority stress and "massive gender trauma" may lead to constellations of symptoms commonly associated with Post-Traumatic Stress Disorder (PTSD) [9, 10]. Careful screening for a history of abuse and neglect is essential as well, though many related psychological concerns may include anxiety, depression, self-injury, thoughts of suicide, compulsivity, substance use, sexual concerns, personality disorders, eating disorders, psychotic symptomatology, and autism spectrum disorders. Co-occurring mental health issues do not preclude changes in gender role or access to gender-affirming hormones or surgery; rather, they should be optimally managed concurrently with gender-affirming treatment.

Providers of adolescents find that their patients are highly resourceful, using the plethora of information available on the internet to seek answers to their circumstances. Clients may present asking whether psychological symptoms are related to various diagnoses, such as Autism Spectrum Disorder (ASD). While there is some preliminary evidence suggesting a higher prevalence of ASD among TGD youth compared to their cis-gender counterparts, there is no known developmental etiology for this relationship [11, 12]. As with any patient, we find the best approach is to evaluate whether the collection of symptoms meet criteria for a specific diagnosis and provide treatment accordingly. In cases where the symptoms do not meet diagnostic criteria, the clinician can provide validation and introduce therapeutic skills that the client may utilize to reduce associated distress.

Overview of Modalities

When developing a treatment plan with a TGD adolescent, the client and provider consider the individual strengths and needs of the client. As discussed throughout this chapter, understanding of individual's gender narrative is key to their experience and is obtained through a narrative approach. By using this approach, both clients and clinicians are able to identify and gain insight into the multidimensionality of the TGD youth's individual identity and recognize its role in their story. Narrative therapy aims to empower the client as an individual with external difficulties that they have the power to address with a complement of resilience-building skills. This intervention reduces the internal narrative of being a problem that can stem from internalized stigma [13].

As clinicians develop an understanding of the TGD client's story, they can better understand the negative cognitions and core beliefs that developed through their journey. Transgender Affirming Cognitive Behavioral Therapy (TA-CBT) is one modality by which the therapist challenges and reframes these cognitions to improve the client's sense of self. Adapted from traditional Cognitive Behavioral Therapy (CBT), it aims to provide an affirming stance toward gender diversity, recognition of gender-specific sources of stress, and the delivery of CBT within an affirming and trauma-informed framework. The cornerstone of this modality rests upon the therapist's unconditional positive regard for the diversity of gender expression and requires that the provider engage in diligent exploration of their own gender-related attitudes, beliefs and biases. Together, the clinician and client seek to better understand gender-specific sources of distress, with the provider imparting psychoeducation, strategies for self-regulation, and cognitive restructuring around negative patterns of thought [14].

As TGD youth often experience socialization in a gender that is not their own, they are at increased risk of both direct and inadvertent invalidation throughout social development. Together with the continuous concern for safety and hypervigilance associated with chronic minority stress (discussed further below), TGD individuals may be at particularly high risk for inhibited maturation of interpersonal skills. For this reason, the interpersonal effectiveness skills of Dialectical Behavioral

Therapy (DBT) can be effective in fostering social connection. While there remains limited peer-reviewed evidence on this modality in TGD adolescents, DBT concepts of mindfulness, distress tolerance, and emotion regulation may provide important skill-building in this population, as they navigate a potentially invalidating and stressful social environment.

Ego psychologists characterize adolescence by the psychosocial development of fidelity, or the ability to accept others despite differences. In this developmental stage, adolescents engage in questions of identity vs. role confusion [15]. Clinicians working with TGD youth may utilize this critical developmental period to explore identity in ways that may not be specific to gender. The clinician can support this process by encouraging teens to use their values as a guide for the practice of self-acceptance. These skills can be taught using the framework of Acceptance and Commitment therapy (ACT). Again, while evidence in this population is limited, the concept of acceptance is not only beneficial in relation to self, but also supportive of empowering youth who are struggling with a mental health condition to achieve their goals.

Here, it is important to acknowledge the ongoing detrimental practice of "reparative" therapy. "Reparative" or "conversion" therapy is a pseudoscientific practice characterized by an active attempt to change an individual's gender identity or sexual orientation. It is shown to be gravely harmful to the individuals it intended to serve and has been rejected by all the major professional societies for many years [16–19]. At this time, it is legislatively prohibited in 14 states and the District of Columbia [20], but unfortunately continues to be practiced in various settings to the detriment of those who encounter it. It is important to provide psychoeducation to families inquiring about these practices, emphasizing its deleterious effects, and to encourage affirming forms of therapy to process these experiences with survivors.

Further investigation is needed regarding the efficacy of various therapeutic modalities in working with treatment of TGD adolescents [21]. The models suggested here approach some of the common difficulties faced by TGD youth seeking support from a psychotherapist. As in any clinical scenario, the client's presenting symptomology and circumstances will guide the evidence-based practices to address their unique needs.

Minority Stress

Minority stress, more thoroughly discussed in Chap. 5: "Minority Stress and the Impact of Acceptance", encompasses the chronic psychosocial and structural stress experienced by stigmatized groups. Briefly, it is a process that consists of daily exposure to prejudice, the development of discrimination, and results in an internalized sense of stigma [22]. These experiences can lead to social isolation, the inhibition of an individual's ability to connect with others, and diminished opportunities for validation.

Most TGD adolescents exist within a societal structure that communicates pervasive binary, cis-gendered expectations in daily social interactions and media. This messaging often occurs through microaggressions, which are brief and commonplace signals that may be verbal, behavioral, or environmental. Whether intentional or unintentional, microaggressions ultimately communicate hostile, derogatory, or negative perspectives and serve to undermine a TGD individual's sense of identity [23].

The client may experience discomfort with their own TGD identity, stemming from conflict with normative gender expectations and resulting in an internalized sense of transphobia [10]. Psychosocial development with transgender identity may foster an internal challenge to the individual – inner feelings that do not match external expectations of sex assigned at birth may be suppressed. The division of one's identity into a private and public self may subsequently serve as a source of distress, contributing to the development of anxiety, depression, substance abuse, and personality disorders. Such experiences can impede healthy ego development and drive a distorted valuation of self-worth.

While the body of evidence describing the effects of chronic minority stress in TGD youth is limited, recent studies demonstrate increased prevalence of PTSD symptoms in TGD individuals with chronic, daily stress associated with their asserted gender independent of prior trauma [9]. The 2015 USTS demonstrated high rates of harassment across public environments – from educational, health care, and employment settings to places of public accommodation, such as hotels and restaurants. Interactions with police, governmental agencies, and even air travel pose an increased risk of harassment. Thirty-nine percent identified "serious psychological distress" in the month prior to completing the survey, compared to only 5% in the general U.S. population. The effect of chronic minority stress on this population is not subtle, with 40% of TGD respondents reporting at least one lifetime suicide attempt [4].

With this background in mind, the clinician is able conduct a thorough assessment of their clients' individual experience of environmental stressors, thus better understanding the lens through which their client perceives and interprets the world around them. The therapeutic goals of building alliance and providing a safe space for healing rely on the clinician's ability to consider the effects of minority stress in relation to their client's individual gender narrative. This begins by understanding the role of minority stress in the client's life and the potential for deleterious effects of this stress on an individual's health and mental health. The therapist should empathically seek to understand the circumstances in which the youth is thriving, or otherwise. Together with the client, the provider can then identify and process sources of stress and strengthen sources of support. Affirmative gender treatment, consistent with WPATH Standards of Care and the American Academy of Pediatrics guidelines, as well as supportive peer relationships, can aid in the process of self-acceptance and identity integration.

Assessment and Referral for Feminizing/Masculinizing Medical and Surgical Interventions

The WPATH Standards of Care version 7, released in 2011, provide recommendations for the assessment and referral for gender-affirming medical and surgical interventions. It is important to be aware that these are recommendations and not requirements, though providers may find that many physicians and surgeons request these prior to initiating gender-affirming treatment both because they are less familiar with the patient as well as for insurance criteria for reimbursement. Additionally, it is important to remember that these, mostly arbitrary, recommendations have changed significantly over each iteration of the Standards of Care (with previous versions recommending living for one year "full time" as one's identified gender in order to meet criteria for affirmative surgical interventions). At the time of this writing, the working group responsible is revising and updating the document. Notably, there is no evidence base that the fulfillment of these recommendations leads to improved health outcomes in this population.

That said, it is important to be familiar with these recommendations when a TGD adolescent presents for care, or merely for a pre-operative letter of support. The most recent recommendations include one letter from a healthcare provider for medical interventions and two for surgical interventions. Briefly, these letters typically include psychological assessment with complete gender and sexual history, including sex assigned at birth, gender identity, social gender role and sexual orientation, and the patient's experience of gender within a detailed biopsychosocial and developmental history [24].

Additionally, among various power differentials that may be present in the provider–client relationship, clinicians should be particularly mindful of the "gatekeeper" role generated by the need for these letters in order to access interventions that are life-saving in many cases. Nevertheless, by acknowledging these requirements as somewhat arbitrary, a provider that is well-informed in these processes and supportive of their clients' goals can facilitate an empowering experience in the patient's pursuit of gender-affirming treatment [25].

Connecting TGD Youth to Community-Based Resources

Psychotherapists are a critical source of support in the affirmation process. This work does not occur solely in therapy sessions, but requires a broad knowledge of community resources to connect individuals with safe, supportive, and reliable professionals. It is important that psychotherapists take care to familiarize themselves with community providers and resources for this reason. This knowledge is crucial in all stages of gender identity development, from the first stages of creating a connection with the community, to assisting with documentation, and supporting those who choose affirmation through medical and surgical means.

This knowledge base should include familiarity of support group and community organizations related to gender identity and expression. These resources help clients engage in community as part of their affirmation process. The clinician should also have the ability to provide information on affirming healthcare providers in the area. The therapist may be the first connection the client has to the affirmation process and thus should be prepared to refer clients who are seeking gender-affirming hormones (GAH) to providers who offer it. Other resources the therapist may provide referrals for include voice coaching, electrolysis, and surgeons.

To that end, the clinician should also have knowledge of their state practices in offering changes in name and gender-marker documentation, so they can assist the client with overcoming any potential barriers. The clinician should have a general understanding of state laws with regard to rights, protections, access to care, and documentation changes for TGD individuals. With a base knowledge of state laws, the clinician may be able to offer insight into whether a client's insurance covers both GAH and gender-affirming procedures such as electrolysis or various affirming surgeries.

In the clinician's role as a sounding board for pain and a vessel for empowerment, the clinician may be the first person with which the client shares an episode of discrimination. Not only should the clinician engage with the client to process and validate their emotional experience, they should also connect the client with community advocates and legal resources to support the client through their experience. Gathering these resources requires time to develop a network within the community of practice and is an important part of the commitment to the work. Further, clinicians can serve to optimize patient's comprehensive care via thoughtful referrals if clients experience common comorbidities such as eating disorders, substance abuse, and trauma [26].

Considerations and Affirmative Practices

Epidemiological data describing the health needs of TGD individuals reveal a profound need for improved quality of care in several domains. While not specific to adolescents, the 2015 USTS demonstrated one-third of respondents reported having at least one negative gender-related experience with a healthcare provider, including having to provide gender-related education in order to receive appropriate services (24%), invasive or unnecessary questions about gender (15%), or being refused transition-related treatment (8%). Nearly one quarter acknowledged needing health care over the past year, but did not seek it due to concerns of maltreatment or disrespect related to gender [4]. Thus, as healthcare providers, we are charged with the responsibility to address these damaging tendencies within our field.

In caring for TGD youth, the clinician must be familiar with their own gender narrative, biases associated with gender, and recognize the diversity of gender identity and expression. The influence of the provider's socialization within a binary gender system requires thoughtful self-examination when treating TGD youth. The safety of the therapeutic environment and the alliance with the youth can be reinforced or undermined by the provider's ability to reflect on their own biases. Processing the countertransference that arises may reveal feelings of alienation, powerlessness, helplessness, cluelessness, and confusion [27].

A youth's early experiences in therapy can influence their identity development and sense of validation. It is important that the clinician is mindful not to make assumptions about the client's gender narrative, but rather listen and validate their experiences. Clinicians must further recognize their own degree of knowledge and experience in working with TGD youth. Critically, they must acknowledge their limits. If the clinician's limitations in training or experience detract from the treatment goals, the clinician is responsible to refer to a provider with experience specializing in gender or seek further education or supervision in this area. According to WPATH SOC version 7, it is recommended that therapists have knowledge of variations in gender and related psychosocial concerns and engage in continuing education regarding gender when working with TGD clients [24].

Throughout the course of treatment, clinicians are responsible to reflect on whether their prompting serves the needs of the client or their own motivation to further their education. In these moments, acknowledging deficits in exposure or knowledge and seeking to address them between sessions through training or gender expert supervision serve to focus the therapy and bolster the therapeutic alliance. This will preserve the therapy session as a place for the patient to voice their own narrative and not provide education on gender.

Conclusion

In closing, gender affirmative care requires that clinicians be knowledgeable about their own lens as well as recognize their duty to meet the client where they are and join them on their gender journey. The role of the psychotherapist in working with the TGD youth is multidimensional and requires careful listening to the client's reasoning for seeking support and collaborating on a plan to assist the client in their process. The clinician's ability to provide affirming care is paramount to the client's treatment in that the provider may be the client's first experience with mental health treatment and set the tone moving forward.

References

1. Keo-Meier C, Ehrensaft D. The gender affirmative model: an interdisciplinary approach to supporting transgender and gender expansive children. Washington, DC: American Psychological Association; 2018.
2. Hidalgo MA, Ehrensaft D, Tishelman AC, Clark LF, Garofalo R, Rosenthal SM, et al. The gender affirmative model: what we know and what we aim to learn. Hum Dev. 2013;56(5):285–90.
3. Ehrensaft D, Spack N. The gender creative child: pathways for nurturing and supporting children who live outside gender boxes. Mulgrave: Simon & Schuster Australia; 2017.
4. James SE, Herman JL, Rankin S, Keisling M, Mottet L, Anafi M. The report of the 2015 U.S. Transgender survey. Washington, DC: National Center for Transgender Equality; 2016.
5. Beemyn G, Rankin S. The lives of transgender people. New York: Columbia University Press; 2011.
6. Aitken M, Vanderlaan DP, Wasserman L, Stojanovski S, Zucker KJ. Self-harm and suicidality in children referred for gender dysphoria. J Am Acad Child Adolesc Psychiatry. 2016;55(6):513–20.
7. Olson-Kennedy J. Mental health disparities among transgender youth. JAMA Pediatr. 2016;170(5):423.
8. Millet N, Longworth J, Arcelus J. Prevalence of anxiety symptoms and disorders in the transgender population: a systematic review of the literature. Int J Transgenderism. 2016;18(1):27–38.

9. Reisner SL, Hughto JMW, Gamarel KE, Keuroghlian AS, Mizock L, Pachankis JE. Discriminatory experiences associated with posttraumatic stress disorder symptoms among transgender adults. J Couns Psychol. 2016;63(5):509–19.
10. Saketopoulou A. Mourning the body as bedrock. J Am Psychoanal Assoc. 2014;62(5):773–806.
11. Glidden D, Bouman WP, Jones BA, Arcelus J. Gender dysphoria and autism spectrum disorder: a systematic review of the literature. Sex Med Rev. 2016;4(1):3–14.
12. Strang JF, Kenworthy L, Dominska A, Sokoloff J, Kenealy LE, Berl M, et al. Increased gender variance in autism spectrum disorders and attention deficit hyperactivity disorder. Arch Sex Behav. 2014;43(8):1525–33.
13. Drutchas A, Rafferty J. The impact of narrative medicine on gender care: learning to "see" our patients' stories. In: Forcier M, Brown JD, Brown RT, editors. AM:STARs LGBTQ youth: enhancing care for gender and sexual minorities. Itasca: American Academy of Pediatrics; 2018. p. 168–84.
14. Austin A, Craig S, Alessi E. Affirmative cognitive behavior therapy with transgender and gender nonconforming adults. Psychiatr Clin N Am. 2017;40(1):141–56.
15. Erikson E. Childhood and society. New York: Norton; 1950.
16. Report of the American Psychological Association Task Force on Appropriate Therapeutic Responses to Sexual Orientation [Internet]. Washington, DC: Task Force on Appropriate Therapeutic Responses to Sexual Orientation. 2009 [cited 20 August 2018]. Available from: http://www.apa.org/pi/lgbc/publications/therapeutic-resp.html.
17. Substance Abuse and Mental Health Services Administration, Ending Conversion Therapy. Supporting and affirming LGBTQ youth. HHS publication no. (SMA) 15-4928. Substance Abuse and Mental Health Services Administration: Rockville; 2015.
18. Conversion Therapy [Internet]. Aacap.org. 2018 [cited 11 August 2018]. Available from: https://www.aacap.org/AACAP/Policy_Statements/2018/Conversion_Therapy.aspx.
19. Position Statement on Conversion/Reparative Therapy [Internet]. Council on social work education. 2018 [cited 20 August 2018]. Available from: https://www.cswe.org/getattachment/Centers-Initiatives/Centers/Center-for-Diversity/About/Stakeholders/Commission-for-Diversity-and-Social-and-Economic-J/Council-on-Sexual-Orientation-and-Gender-Identity/CSOGIE-Resources/CSWEPositionStatementonConversion-ReparativeTherapy(003).pdf.aspx.
20. Movement Advancement Project | Home [Internet]. Lgbtmap.org. 2018 [cited 25 July 2018]. Available from: http://lgbtmap.org/.
21. Spivey A, Edwards-Leaper L. Future directions in affirmative psychological interventions with transgender children and adolescents. J Clin Child Adolesc Psychol. 2019;00(00):1–14.
22. Meyer I. Minority stress and mental health in gay men. J Health Soc Behav. 1995;36(1):38.
23. Sue DW, Capodilupo CM, Torino GC, Bucceri JM, Holder AMB, Nadal KL, et al. Racial microaggressions in everyday life: implications for clinical practice. Am Psychol. 2007;62(4):271–86.
24. Standards of Care – WPATH World Professional Association for Transgender Health [Internet]. Wpath.org. 2011 [cited 5 July 2018]. Available from: https://www.wpath.org/publications/soc.
25. Budge S. Psychotherapists as gatekeepers: an evidence-based case study highlighting the role and process of letter writing for transgender clients. Psychotherapy. 2015;52(3):287–97.
26. Krieger I. Counseling transgender and non-binary youth: the essential guide. London: Jessica Kingsley Publishers; 2017.
27. Güldenring A. A critical view of transgender health care in Germany: psychopathologizing gender identity – symptom of 'disordered' psychiatric/psychological diagnostics? Int Rev Psychiatry. 2015;27(5):427–34.

Treatment Paradigms for Prepubertal Children

13

Diane Ehrensaft

Introduction

A parent places a call to a mental health gender specialist recommended by the child's pediatrician. Alex, their five-year-old child, has been playing with dolls and imagining himself to be a famous ballerina since the age of three. The parents have both been fine with this, believing that children should not be bound by gender norms in what they do and what roles they imagine themselves taking. Recently, however, the parents have run into a snag with Alex. He is about to start kindergarten and has grown increasingly anxious as the fall semester grows near. He expresses no worries about leaving home or facing the academic expectations in grade school. Rather, Alex breaks down sobbing that he will no longer be able to play with his dolls and his tutus, that everyone will always think he's a boy, but he thinks maybe he's actually a girl. For the next week, he vacillates between listless ennui and anxious agitation. He finds himself better able to articulate more of his upset: he does not like his body, particularly his penis; he wishes he could trade it in for a vagina; he only likes to play with girls; children in his preschool had started teasing him for liking "girl" things; he wants to grow up and be able to get pregnant and be a mommy. The tipping point for Alex's parents came when he moaned that he wished he had never been born and that he wanted to die because he was a strange kind of boy who wanted to change into a girl. The parents' growing concern prompted the call to Alex's pediatrician.

This vignette is just one variation on a theme that would bring parents to seek out psychological services for a child who is demonstrating gender stress or distress, meaning the anxiety, discomfort, or confusion emanating from the child's present gender status or explorations. The impetus for treatment might come from the parents or family, the child's school, the primary care physician, or the child. The stress or distress may be related to the child's gender identity, the child's gender

D. Ehrensaft (✉)
University of California, San Francisco, CA, USA

M. Forcier et al. (eds.), *Pediatric Gender Identity*,
https://doi.org/10.1007/978-3-030-38909-3_13

expressions, or both. The discomfort may be situated in the child's body, psyche, relations with the outside world, or any combination thereof. Alternatively, the child may be feeling just fine, but the parents grow worried about their child's seeming gender confusion or refusal to abide by societal gender norms. Whatever the domain or locus of concern, if working within a gender affirmative approach, the treatment goal will remain the same: to promote the child's gender health, defined as the opportunity for the child to live in the gender that feels most authentic and comfortable for that child [11, 12, 17]. As no child is an island, this treatment goal will be accomplished only by taking into account the child, the family, and the social environment in which that child resides.

Until very recently, knowledge about the treatment of children who digressed from gender expectations or norms was limited to modalities that perceived such digressions as anomalies or pathologies in need of cure (cf. for example, [32], or [15]). The past quarter century has seen a radical transformation in the approach to treating children who deviate from societal gender norms, along with an explosion in the numbers of children seeking out services related to their gender identity and/or expressions [1, 5, 38] and the numbers of clinics providing services to these children and their families [18]. This expansion has been accompanied by active efforts on the part of mental health and medical practitioners to define a model of care that would be optimal for children who either indicate that they are feeling out of sync with the gender that matches the sex designated to them at birth or are troubled by the social demands of gender behaviors and presentations in the culture in which they are growing, or both. At this moment in history, the prevailing model being adapted in clinics across the globe is most commonly known as the gender affirmative model. This chapter will bring this model to life and contrast it to earlier conceived models of practice, the reparative models, and the watchful waiting approach. Focus will be on children before they arrive at the stage of puberty; therefore, the terms "child" and "children" used throughout will refer to youth who have not yet reached the early stages of puberty.

What Do Standards of Care and Clinical Guidelines Tell Us?

Only recently has the gender treatment of young children been addressed as a separate consideration in major professional organizations' standards and guidelines. For the first time, the World Professional Association for Transgender Health, the most internationally recognized organization addressing the care of transgender and gender diverse (TGD) individuals, will have a separate chapter on childhood when it releases the 8th version of its standards of care. Presently, the 7th edition provides the following guidelines specific to or applicable to gender diverse prepubertal children [39]:

1. Psychological treatment:
    - Changes in gender expression and role (which may involve living part time or full time in another gender role, consistent with one's gender identity).
    - Psychotherapy for purposes such as exploring gender identity, role, and expression; addressing the negative impact of gender dysphoria and stigma on

mental health; alleviating internalized transphobia; enhancing social and peer support; improving body image; or promoting resilience.

2. Social support options to alleviate gender dysphoria, for example:
   - Offline and online peer support resources, groups, or community organizations that provide avenues for social support and advocacy.
   - Offline and online support resources for families and friends.
3. Required competencies for mental health professionals:
   - Training in childhood and adolescent developmental psychopathology.
   - Competence in diagnosing and treating the ordinary problems of children.
4. Roles of mental health professional:
   - Directly assess gender dysphoria in children and adolescents.
   - Provide family counseling and supportive psychotherapy.
   - Assess and treat any co-existing mental health concerns of children.
   - Educate and advocate on behalf of children and their families in their community.
   - Provide children and their families with information and referrals for peer support.
5. Psychological Assessments.
   - Assessment of gender dysphoria and mental health should explore the nature and characteristics of a child's gender identity.
   - A psychodiagnostic and psychiatric assessment – covering emotional functioning, peer/social relationships, and intellectual functioning/school achievement.
   - Assessment should include an evaluation of the strengths and weaknesses of family functioning.
6. Psychological and Social Interventions.
   - Mental health professionals should help families to have an accepting and nurturing response to the concerns of their gender diverse child.
   - This also applies to peers and mentors from the community.
   - Psychotherapy should focus on reducing a child's distress related to the gender dysphoria and on ameliorating any other psychosocial difficulties.
   - Treatment aimed at trying to change a person's gender identity and expression to become more congruent with sex assigned at birth has been attempted in the past without success. Such treatment is no longer considered ethical.
   - Families should be supported in managing uncertainty and anxiety about their child's psychosexual outcomes and in helping children to develop a positive self-concept.
   - Mental health professionals should not impose a binary view of gender. They should give ample room for children to explore different options for gender expression.
   - Children and their families should be supported in making difficult decisions regarding the extent to which children are allowed to express a gender role that is consistent with their gender identity, as well as the timing of changes in gender role and possible social transition.
   - Health professionals should support children and their families as educators and advocates in their interactions with community members and authorities such as teachers, school boards, and courts.

- Mental health professionals should strive to maintain a therapeutic relationship with gender diverse children and their families throughout any subsequent social changes.

7. Early social transitions (defined as a child transitioning from one gender to another, either everywhere, or in select situations which may be expanded over time).
   - The current evidence base is insufficient to predict the long-term outcomes of completing a gender role transition during early childhood.
   - Regardless of a family's decisions regarding transition (timing, extent), professionals should counsel and support them as they work through the options and implications.

In sum, the WPATH standards of care designate the mental health professional as a key figure in the gender care of all gender diverse young children, are cautionary about early social transitions, and advocate for a systemic approach in which the social context and institutions surrounding the child are recognized as key ingredients in the care and support of the children and their families.

In 2015, a task force of the American Psychological Association drew up their own guidelines for the treatment of TGD children [3]. As with the WPATH standards of care, specific attention to the needs of prepubertal children was minimal in contrast to the emphasis on postpubertal youth. Consistent with the WPATH standards of care in almost all respects, the APA guidelines go further in stressing the necessity of understanding that not all youth will persist in a TGD identity into adulthood, coming to the conclusion: "Due to the evidence that not all children persist in a [TGD] identity into adolescence or adulthood, and because no approach to working with [TGD] children has been adequately, empirically validated, consensus does not exist regarding best practice with prepubertal children" ([3], p. 841). This statement becomes the cornerstone around which the APA guidelines are organized, directing psychologists to understand the varying approaches with gender diverse children and emphasizing the importance of letting children know that they have the freedom to return to a previous gender identity or evolve into a wholly different one. The most recent policy statement supporting the gender affirmative care of transgender and gender diverse youth, issued by the American Academy of Pediatrics in 2018 [28], also makes reference to the lack of clear guidelines in directing pediatric practices with TGD pre-pubertal children.

Evident in both WPATH and APA's directives, although not expressed in the AAP guidelines, is the concern about lack of knowledge and potential risks in allowing a prepubertal child to engage in a social transition from one gender to another. Shortly, it will be seen how the gender affirmative model has addressed this concern, in contrast to the other two models of care for TGD children. First, it will be helpful to review the most recent standards of care for TGD children, released in Australia in 2018 [33]. Again, the section on prepubertal children is relatively brief when compared to the extensive articulation of standards for postpubertal youth, with specific attention to early social transitions. Yet, unlike both the WPATH and APA documents, the Australian Standards of Care are far less cautious, with a more positive bent on social transitions in young children, stating: (1) Social transition should be led by the child and does not have to take an all or nothing approach; (2) Social transition can reduce a child's distress and improve their emotional functioning; (3) If the child is expressing a desire to live in a role consistent with their asserted gender identity, the mental health practitioner tasks include providing psychological support and practical assistance to the child and their family to facilitate a social transition. The guidelines state specifically that a TGD child may not need mental health services if they are doing well within a supportive environment; lastly, in contrast to the WPATH standards of care, no mention is made of the need for extensive psychometric evaluations.

Whether it is the composition of the organizational entities themselves, or the passage of time, the four sets of guidelines, overlapping in many areas, part ways regarding social transitions and the need for intensive mental health involvement with prepubertal TGD children. In review, it can be said that the Australian standards of care most accurately represent the gender affirmative model for supporting prepubertal children.

The Gender Affirmative Model

Let us return to Alex. By all definitions, Alex is exhibiting gender stress. By diagnostic criteria, Alex may well qualify for a DSM 5 diagnosis of Gender Dysphoria in Children or ICD diagnosis of Gender Incongruence (DSM V 302.6 or ICD-10 F64.2). To qualify for the DSM diagnosis, he will need to meet six of the nine diagnostic criteria and fit the definition of a child experiencing a significant incongruence between the gender the child identifies with and the sex designated to that child at birth, an experience that must last a minimum of six months [2]. Applying that diagnosis to Alex may be controversial and repudiated by a mental health professional concerned about pathologizing a natural variation in gender development and stigmatizing a child who goes against the grain of social gender norms [37]. Another mental health professional not sharing that concern may use the diagnosis as a roadmap to help Alex's parents get Alex in focus psychologically, i.e., have a clear vision of who their child is both in terms of gender expressions and gender identity, and determine what Alex will need in terms of psychological supports. With or without diagnosis, Alex is distressed and the questions remain: What does Alex need therapeutically? How should a clinician go about offering supports to Alex and his family? The answer to those questions depends on the model by which the professional practices. The gender affirmative model, the ascendant approach to care for TGD children internationally, and the one emphasized in this volume, would go to work in the following fashion.

This model of care might also be labeled "listen and act," meaning that the role of the provider is to listen to the child and act in the child's best interest, running the gamut from authenticating the child's gender to facilitating gender affirming interventions, such as social transitions. The underlying premise in this model is that an individual at any age is capable of articulating their authentic gender, and the role of the clinician is to listen to the child, assess what the child is expressing about their gender, and facilitate the child's exploration of gender in safe and loving home and social settings [10, 17]. No attempts are made on the part of either clinician or parents to change a child's gender behaviors or invalidate a child's feelings. Instead, the provider listens carefully and assists the child as they move through a variety of expected developmental processes necessary to assuming an adult gender identity and or presentation. The model of care is based on stages, not ages, meaning there is no set age for gender affirmation, only each individual person's process as they move toward gender congruence, i.e., the integration of body, identity, and expressions. Within the perspective that gender exploration and consolidation are evolutionary, life-long processes, the gender affirmative model applied to children acknowledges what is also seen in adult and mature patients – that social transitions may occur and are just as "valid" at any age or stage of life.

Practitioners who adopt this gender affirmative model vary in their evaluative procedures, but all act under the underlying premise that gender diversity signifies healthy variations, rather than anomalies, and that the goal is to facilitate a child living in their authentic gender. Some administer formal evaluations to determine a child's gender status and any co-occurring psychological issues [4]. Others, adhering to the tenet that gender diversity is a healthy variation of development, not necessarily subject to mental health diagnosis, a tenet supported by the ongoing research of Dr. Kristina Olson and her associates at The University of Washington [26, 9, 27], prefer to forego formal psychological assessments and replace them with a model of child and parent consultations. Increasingly, ongoing psychotherapy is introduced only if the child is demonstrating signs of gender stress or distress or desiring or in need of a "room of their own" to further explore their gender [12]. Emphasis may instead be put on an ecological approach, evaluating the systems in which the child is growing, including family, day care, school, religious institutions, and striving to institute plans in each of those domains to assure support and acceptance of the child as they express their gender in the manner that feels most authentic to them [20]. The gender affirmative model advocates interdisciplinary teams of mental health and medical providers; the child, parents, and allied professionals are also considered critical members of the care team [30].

Attention is also paid to siblings, grandparents, and other extended family members, under the rubric that family acceptance is a key ingredient to a child's gender health and that all family members from siblings to grandparents may need their own supports as they adjust to a child's newly articulated gender self [22]. A growing body of research is resounding in demonstrating the critical importance of family support, beginning with the research of Caitlin Ryan and her associates, followed by the research of Trans PULSE [34] and Sabra Wise-Katz and her research team at Harvard [19]. For example, in the Trans PULSE findings, suicidality in trans youth was 4% when parental support was in place versus 57% when youth faced parental rejection, a remarkable contrast.

The gender affirmative model evolved in reaction to the first and on the foundation of the second of the two other prevalent models developed to treat gender diverse children, both of which continue to be practiced nationally and internationally. With that said, it will be helpful to understand how the gender affirmative model stands in contrast to these two other models – the "live in your own skin" and the "watchful waiting" model, to which we will now turn.

The "Living in Your Own Skin" Model

Traditionally, prevailing models for treating gender expansive children involved some form of what has come to be known as "reparative therapy" for gender identity [24]. Applied to children, this model involved therapeutic efforts to change the gender behaviors and identities of children to conform to the prevailing standards for gender, within a binary model of gender-divided "appropriateness" for males and females [15]. Although illegal in several states in the U.S. and one province in Canada (Ontario) [14], the model of care is still used, especially in church-based counseling programs and more conservative mental health institutions [16]. While argued by its developers not to be a reparative technique (though description of their intervention techniques speaks otherwise), the treatment model for pre-pubescent children that had as its goal a change in the gender presentations of a young child became best known in the work of Drs. Susan Bradley, Kenneth Zucker and their colleagues at the Center for Addiction and Mental Health in Toronto [40, 41]. This model has become known as the "living in your own skin" approach. The goal of the treatment is to facilitate young children accepting the gender that matches the sex designated to them at birth. The underlying premise is that young children have a malleable gender brain and can be influenced to achieve psychological congruence between their sexed body and the gender identity that would match that body according to social expectations. The rationale for implementing this treatment was that living life as a cis- rather than a transgender individual relieves the child both of the burdens of the stigmatization of being a transgender person and the added medical interventions (hormones, surgeries) that might accompany a transgender identity [7]. With the requisite that the parents consent to the treatment, the "living in your own skin" interventions include removing "cross-gender" toys and activities, replacing them with toys and activities more "gender-appropriate", introducing same-gender playmates to replace opposite-gender playmates, encouraging same-gender parent to become more active in the child's life while asking the opposite-gender parent to step back, and involving both parents and child in ongoing psychotherapy [23].

If, however, such efforts are not implemented or a child is still expressing a desire to live in the opposite gender by adolescence, the sensitive period for gender malleability is over, and therefore it is too late to employ "living in your own skin" methods. In those instances, every effort is made to help a youth socially transition and receive medical interventions (hormones, surgery) to achieve gender congruence. In sum, the "living in your own skin" model, which got its name from Dr. Zucker's explanation of his treatment program as helping pre-pubertal children to live in the gender that matches the sex designated at birth and the body accompanying that designation, ergo, their own skin, synthesized behavior modification, social engineering, and psychodynamic psychotherapy to achieve the set goals of gender congruence between designated sex at birth and child's gender identity. The "living in your own skin" approach is in part informed by the extant research indicating that the majority of young children referred for gender-related care and receiving a gender diagnosis (Gender Identity Disorder in the past, Gender Dysphoria more recently) do not continue to identify as TGD at puberty (see Chap. 2 and [31]). It is therefore assumed that a young child may be still be flexible and able to conform to others' expectations for their gender. As will be discussed shortly and is discussed in earlier chapters of this text, this underlying assumption is problematic in light of the critiques of the "persistence" research for its problematic methods and conclusions [13].

The Watchful Waiting Model

The second form of treatment was developed in the Netherlands at the Vrije Universiteit Medical Center [6, 8]. In this model, children brought to their clinic at a young age are first psychologically evaluated, as in the above model, to determine whether they exhibit gender dysphoria and to identity co-occurring psychological issues. Those children who are identified as having gender dysphoria are offered ongoing psychotherapy, along with psychological supports for their parents. Parents are encouraged to allow their children to explore and express their gender as the child desires at home or in specific protected environments. However, for those children who at an early age express a strong desire to live in the other gender, a watchful waiting approach is recommended: allowing a child-free rein in their gender expressions but holding off on facilitating a full social transition from the gender matching their designated sex at birth until adolescence [8]. The rationale for the waiting period is based on three assumptions: (1) On the basis of their own research in their program, only a small percentage of the children receiving a diagnosis in early childhood maintain that diagnosis in adolescence, so best to wait until adolescence and the beginning stages of puberty to be able to better discern a child's stable gender status; (2) Even for the child who may appear quite clear in their affirmed gender identity, having them switch genders early in life might cognitively pigeonhole them prematurely into a gender identity that had not yet been established, depriving them of the opportunity for perhaps needed further exploration of their gender identity; (3) premature social transition may prevent a child from being realistic about the phenotypic features of their body based on their chromosomal sex.

Relying on codified diagnostic categories, if by adolescence the youth still, in the watchful waiting model qualifies for a diagnosis of gender dysphoria and is articulating a transgender identity, a youth will then be afforded the opportunity for a social transition and for medical interventions that will allow the youth greater gender congruence, with certain age requirements set for puberty blockers, gender affirming hormones, and surgeries, as outlined in subsequent chapters. In sum, the watchful waiting approach supports a child in evolving into the gender identity that is most authentic to them, without attempting to change them, but also takes a cautious approach with prepubertal children regarding changes in their gender identity roles. Unless a prepubertal social transition has already occurred prior to presentation to the clinical team, this model postpones social transitions until adolescence.

Recall that, like in the living in your own skin model, the research on which this model for treatment of prepubertal children is based is the findings about persistence and desistance of gender dysphoria in young children, with the presupposition that the majority of children will "desist" by adolescence. One of the main problems with this research is that it relied on psychiatric classification and failed to measure the main variable that would determine if a young child would be a good candidate for social transition. That would be their gender identity. In this research, no differentiation is made between gender identity and gender expressions, and thus the baby gets thrown out with the bathwater when little children who are clear about their gender identity in insistent, consistent, persistent fashion are lumped together with children who are exploring gender expressions but not an alternative gender identity [12, 13, 21]. It should also be mentioned that linguistically the term "desistance" most often refers to a phenomenon that would best be halted or extinguished, which can very well send a message to clinicians that gender diversity, when it appears in childhood, should be taken with a grain of salt, as it might just disappear, a potentially "good outcome." Unwittingly, this message to a clinician may then subliminally communicate to parents or to a prepubertal child who wishes to socially transition that a more conforming gender outcome would be preferred over the child's asserted gender identity.

Circling back to the gender affirmative model, the main arena in which this model parts ways with the watchful waiting model is around the issue of social transitions. The gender affirmative model starts with the dictum that gender health is defined by the opportunity of the child to live in the gender that feels most authentic to them with no rejection or aspersion. Following that rubric, to prevent a child who has been insistent, consistent, and persistent in their articulated gender identity from expressing their gender identity as they experience it is perceived as unnecessary and possibly harm-inducing, rather than risk-aversive [13, 21]. Further, since gender is considered a lifelong developmental process, rather than being fixed at a certain age, there is less concern than in the watchful waiting model that a premature social transition might lock a child into a gender identity from which they cannot exit. Instead, every effort is made to leave all gender pathways open, with supports offered if the child finds themself evolving into a different gender, either in expression or identity, over the course of time. Lastly, the assumption that a child will be cognitively constricted by potentially losing track of their own body parts and phenotypic sex has no evidence base. Quite to the contrary, socially transitioned young children remain all too aware of their body parts. Recently, gender affirmative practitioners have witnessed the stress that can accompany this realization profoundly minimized by new social narratives in which children grow to understand that most girls have vaginas, but some have penises, and most boys have penises, but some have vaginas, allowing gender diverse children to experience themselves not as an anomaly but a variation on a theme.

Alex Through the Looking Glass

Let us return to Alex, introduced at the beginning of this chapter. Having laid out the parameters of the gender affirmative model and contrasted the model to the other two extant models – living in your own skin and watchful waiting, it is now time to take a look at how Alex might have fared in each of the three programs. To review: Alex is five, feminine in his gender expressions, articulating a wish to be a girl, and growing increasingly anxious as he is about to enter kindergarten, demonstrating signs of gender stress. His parents are seeking professional help.

If Alex were to be brought to a clinic practicing the living in your own skin model, his parents would be interviewed to uncover how they had been handling Alex's gender behaviors to date. The provider would explore influences they may have had, if any, on his gender dysphoria. A battery of psychometric tests would be administered to determine if Alex qualified for a diagnosis of gender dysphoria and to identify any co-occurring psychological issues. A program might be instituted to spend more time with Dad doing "boy-like things," substituting a mini-basketball net for tutus (with tutus removed), and encouraging playdates with other boys in his new kindergarten class. Psychotherapy would also be offered to Alex to address his distressed feelings and facilitate Alex being content living in his own skin as a boy. Supportive therapy would also be offered to the parents. However, if Alex's family lived in the state of California, for example, this form of treatment would be prohibited and a practitioner employing this form of treatment would be at risk for being reported to their licensing board for engaging in harmful, unethical practices, this in line with the directives of major health and mental health organizations, as outlined above.

If Alex's parents were to make an appointment at a clinic following the watchful waiting approach, Alex's parents would be interviewed about their child's gender history, Alex would receive a formal psychological evaluation, as in the living in your own skin model, and Alex would be eligible for psychological services, which would be recommended to afford Alex the opportunity to continue to explore his gender and to address psychological stressors, such as his reluctance to go to school and expressed wishes never to be born. Until Alex reached puberty, Alex's parents would be encouraged to continue to support his gender at home with no interference in his play choices, presentation, or playmates. However, they would be cautioned against a full social transition, as it would be too early to determine if Alex was a "persister," and what would be considered in this model as a premature gender transition might back Alex into a corner of feeling stuck in a gender identity that eventually may end up not being his authentic one. As puberty approached, Alex would be re-evaluated. Once he had experienced the first stages of puberty, he could be considered for puberty blockers to allow more time for gender exploration, along with a full social transition if a transgender identity was evident, followed by gender affirming hormones and surgical interventions, if desired.

If Alex's parents contacted a clinic using the gender affirmative approach, their experience in many ways would be similar to having made an appointment with a program adopting the watchful waiting model. The main difference would be that the gender affirmative clinician would begin from the assumption that a young child is capable of articulating an authentic gender identity. This model, also supported by the 2018 AAP policy statement, suggests that listening to our patients, including prepubertal children, is an important aspect of support and care. This does not translate, as some critics of the gender affirmative model impute, into a clinician simply rubber stamping whatever the young child says about their gender on their first visit. Listening is a process, and for young Alex, the listening would mean taking as much time as was needed for Alex's gender story to unfold and for the adults around him to understand that story. If, upon evaluation, it was determined that Alex was insistent, persistent, and consistent in articulating a female identity and a desire to live full-time as a girl, and if parents were in support of a social transition, the clinician would help facilitate that transition, either in all settings, or in more limited settings that felt comfortable to Alex and Alex's family. If, alternatively, Alex's gender journey took him to a place where he experienced himself as a girl-boy or a rainbow kid, or some other gender-nonbinary sense of self, that pathway would be supported as well. If, as Alex grew older, Alex exhibited anxiety about continued development into a more masculine or male phenotypic puberty, or if Alex was unclear on how masculine or feminine their growing gender identity might be, Alex would be offered puberty blockers at the onset of puberty and continued resources to explore an authentic individual gender identity.

In contrast to the watchful waiting model, holding back on a gender transition until later, if it was discovered that Alex was clear in an articulation of a female gender identity, would seem counter-indicated, under the premise that gender health equates with allowing a child the opportunity to live in their authentic gender when and as they know it, no matter the age of the child. Within the gender affirmative model, the clinician seeing Alex's family would be informed by the premise that delaying what the child reports is their current state of gender expression and identity has the risk of sending a message of lack of acceptance, disapproval, or invalidation of Alex's authentic gender. As mentioned early, there is growing evidence that gender diverse youth supported by their parents have improved psychological functioning compared to youth who are not supported [29, 34], and one could easily hypothesize that facilitating a gender transition would be a significant form of parental support.

At the same time, under the care of a gender affirmative practitioner, Alex's parents would be assured that if Alex was to discover later in childhood that Alex's articulated gender self was no longer a good fit, this would not represent a risk factor, but rather an opportunity to evolve into Alex's next iteration of gender, be it moving back to the original gender identity or a new one (e.g., gender nonbinary). This assurance would be predicated on the assumption that gender pathways would always remain open, that there is no one desired outcome, other than what is authentic and true for Alex. In sum, the gender affirmative model would offer supports and opportunities for Alex to live in their authentic gender at present while simultaneously continuing to explore their gender in the evolutionary unfolding of gender that may occur over time.

Where Do We Go from Here?

Of the three treatment models, the gender affirmative model is the newest approach, but the approach with the most evidence to support its potential benefit and reduction of harm in TGD children. To date, there are ongoing longitudinal studies creating a growing body of evidence to support the gender affirmative model, and increasing documentation that for some young children, early social transition may be in their best interest and with no evidence of harm [35]. More specifically, the research of Dr. Kristina Olson and associates at the University of Washington TransYouth Project provides evidence that children who have socially transitioned at an early age are doing as well mental healthwise as a matched group of cisgender children, indicating normative levels of anxiety and depression in both groups [9, 25–27]. The ongoing TransYouth Project research involves a longitudinal cross-sectional study evaluating the children on a limited number of psychological variables, but does not yet provide information about long-term outcomes, nor does it provide a comparison to children who are gender diverse but do not socially transition at young ages. Looking toward the future, more evidence-based studies are needed to document long-term outcomes for children who have socially transitioned at an early age and also for children claiming a nonbinary or alternative gender identity, with at least one such study presently being launched in a four-site NIH research project investigating gender pathways in prepubertal children. Such research will provide the means for testing the basic premises of the gender affirmative model: that listening to the child, providing parental and social acceptance, facilitating social transitions, and adopting a developmental, evolutionary, rather than static concept of gender generates well-being and positive mental health among TGD children.

The field of gender care for TGD children is in many ways in its own childhood stage. The gender affirmative model of care has been presented as the optimal model of care for TGD children, with comparison to the two other extant models of care – the living in your own skin and watchful waiting approaches. The former falls within the category of reparative forms of treatment that have now been rejected by major professional societies as unethical and harmful. Yet, the living in your own skin model continues to be practiced in certain settings that view a TGD or gender fluid/nonbinary outcome as problematic and undesirable. Some of the work ahead is to continue to educate professionals and parents alike about reparative modes of treatments' harmful effects on children [36] and their contribution to transphobic attitudes and behaviors within the world at large.

The watchful waiting and gender affirmative models live in creative tension with each other, sharing many basic premises but respectfully questioning each other in domains where they differ, particularly the advisability of early social transitions and reliance on "persistence" data that comes with its own inherent flaws and has been systematically critiqued for failing to differentiate their young subjects who were exploring their gender expressions from those who were exploring their gender identities and making the false assumption that children who dropped out of their studies could be counted as desisters because they no longer came for care at the clinic. As the gender affirmative model becomes more ascendant as the optimal model of care, we witness gender care evolving to incorporate a more dynamic and fluid understanding of gender in which gender multiplicity replaces the gender binary. The individuals taking the lead in this evolution are not the professional experts, but the children themselves, as they demonstrate the beauty of gender in its infinite iterations. With the children to guide us, the task before us is to reach at least the adolescence of our pediatric gender care – to continue to explore, evaluate, and execute evolving models of care that consider the best interests of the child, the social milieus in which the children live, and the emerging scientific evidence and longitudinal outcome studies that will contribute to all children having a fulfilling life in their authentic genders.

References

1. Aitken M, Steensma TD, Blanchard R, VanderLaan DP, Wood H, Fuentes A, Spegg C, Wasserman L, Ames M, Fitzsimmons CL, Lishak V, Reim E, Takagi A, Vinik J, Wreford J, Cohen-Kettenis PT, de Vries AL, Kreukels BP, Zucker KJ, Leef JH. Evidence for an altered sex ratio in clinic-referred adolescents with gender dysphoria. J Sex Med. 2015;12:756–63.
2. American Psychiatric Association. Diagnostic and statistical manual of mental disorders. 5th ed. Arlington: American Psychiatric Publishing; 2013.
3. American Psychological Association. Guidelines for psychological practice with transgender and gender nonconforming people. Am Psychol. 2015;70(9):832–64.
4. Berg D, Edwards-Leeper L. Child and family assessment. In: Keo-Meier C, Ehrensaft D, editors. The gender affirmative model. Washington, DC: American Psychological Association Publications; 2018. p. 101–24.
5. Chen M, Fuqua J, Eugster EA. Characteristics of referrals for gender dysphoria over a 13-year period. J Adolesc Health. 2016;58:369–71.
6. Cohen-Kettenis PT, Pfaffian F. Transgenderism and intersexuality in childhood and adolescence. London: Sage; 2003.
7. Cross JS. Outcry prompts CAMH to review its controversial treatment of trans youth. Metro News, Toronto. 2015. March 18, 2015, metronews.ca.
8. De Vries ALC, Cohen-Kettenis PT. Clinical management of gender dysphoria in children and adolescents: the Dutch approach. J Homosex. 2012;59(3):301–20.
9. Durwood L, McLaughlin KA, Olson KR. Mental health and self-worth in socially transitioned transgender youth. J Am Acad Child Adolesc Psychiatry. 2017;56:116–123. e2.
10. Ehrensaft D. Gender born, gender made. New York: The Experiment; 2011.
11. Ehrensaft D. From gender identity disorder to gender identity creativity: true gender self child therapy. J Homosex. 2012;59(3):337–56.
12. Ehrensaft D. The gender creative child: pathways for nurturing and supporting children who live outside gender boxes. New York: The Experiment; 2016.
13. Ehrensaft D, Giammattei SV, Storck K, Tishelman AC, Keo-Meier C. Prepubertal social gender transitions: what we know what we can learn—a view from a gender affirmative lens. Int J Transgenderism. 2017;19(2):251–68.
14. Frankel J. More and more states are outlawing gay-conversion therapy. Atlantic. 2017. https://www.theatlantic.com/health/archive/2017/07/states-outlawing-conversion-threapy/533121.
15. Green R. The "Sissy boy" syndrome and the development of homosexuality. New Haven: Yale University Press; 1987.
16. Greenough D. Some Christian groups still promote 'gay conversion therapy' – but their influence is waning. Conversation. 2018. http://theconversation.com/some-christian-groups-still-promote-gay-conversion-therapy-but-their-influence-is-waning-91523.

17. Hidalgo MA, Ehrensaft D, Tishelman AC, Clark LF, Garofalo R, Rosenthal SM, Spack NP, Olson J. The gender affirmative model: what we know and what we aim to learn. Hum Dev. 2013;56:285–90.
18. Hsieh S, Leininger J. Resource list: clinical care programs for gender-nonconforming children and adolescents. Pediatr Ann. 2014;43:238–44.
19. Katz-Wise SL, Ehrensaft D, Vetters R, Forcier M, Austin SB. Family functioning and mental health of transgender and gender nonconforming youth in the trans teen and family narratives project. J Sex Res. 2018;55:582. https://doi.org/10.1080/00224499.2017.1415291.
20. Kaufman R, Tishelman A. Creating a network of professionals. In: Keo-Meier C, Ehrensaft D, editors. The gender affirmative model. Washington, DC: American Psychological Association Publications; 2018. p. 173–88.
21. Keo-Meier C, Ehrensaft D, editors. The gender affirmative model. Washington, DC: American Psychological Association Publications; 2018.
22. Malpas J, Glaeser E, GiamThemattei SV. Building resilience in transgender and gender expansive children, families, and communities: a multidimensional family approach. In: Keo-Meier C, Ehrensaft D, editors. The gender affirmative model. Washington, DC: American Psychological Association Publications; 2018. p. 141–56.
23. Meyer-Bahlburg HF. Gender identity disorder in young boys: a parent-and peer-based treatment protocol. Clin Child Psychol Psychiatry. 2002;7(3):360–76.
24. Nicolosi J. Shame and attachment loss: the practical work of reparative therapy. Westmont: IVP Academics; 2016.
25. Olson KR, Key AC, Eaton NR. Gender cognition in transgender children. Psychol Sci. 2015a;26:467–74.
26. Olson J, Schrager SM, Belzer M, Simons LK, Clark LF. Baseline physiologic and psychosocial characteristics of transgender youth seeking care for gender dysphoria. J Adolesc Health. 2015b;57:374–80.
27. Olson KR, Durwood L, DeMeules M, McLaughlin KA. Mental health of transgender children who are supported in their identities. Pediatrics. 2016;137:1–8.
28. Raferty J, Committee on Psychosocial Aspects of Child and Family Health, Committee on Adolescence, Section on Lesbian, Gay, Bisexual and Transgender Health and Wellness, American Academy of Pediatrics. Ensuring comprehensive care and support for transgender and gender-diverse children and adolescents. Pediatrics. 2018;142(4):e20182162. http://pediatrics.aappublications.org/content/142/4/e20182162.
29. Ryan C, Russell ST, Huebner D, Diaz R, Sanchez J. Family acceptance in adolescence and the health of LGBT young adults. J Child Adolesc Psychiatr Nurs. 2010;23(4):205–13.
30. Sherer I, Rosenthal SM, Ehrensaft D, Baum J. Child and adolescent gender center: a multidisciplinary collaboration to improve the lives of gender nonconforming children and teens. Pediatr Rev. 2012;33:273–5.
31. Steensma TD, Biemond R, de Boer F, Cohen-Kettenis PT. Desisting and persisting genderdysphoria after childhood: a qualitative follow-up study. Clin Child Psychol Psychiatry. 2011;16(4):499–516. https://doi.org/10.1177/1359104510378303.
32. Stoller RJ. Presentations of gender. New Haven: Yale University Press; 1985.
33. Telfer MM, Tollit MA, Pace CC, Pang KC. Australian standards of care and treatment guidelines for trans and gender diverse children and adolescents version 1.1. Melbourne: The Royal Children's Hospital; 2018.
34. Travers R, Bauer G, Pyne J. Impacts of strong parental support for trans youth: a report prepared for Children's Aid Society of Toronto and Delisle Youth Services. Toronto: Trans Pulse; 2012.
35. Turban JL, Ehrensaft D. Research review: gender identity in youth: treatment paradigms and controversies. J Child Psychol Psychiatry. 2017;59:1228. https://doi.org/10.1111/jcpp.12833.
36. Wallace R, Russell H. Attachment and shame in gender non-conforming children and their families: toward a theoretical framework for evaluating clinical interventions. Int J Transgenderism. 2014;14(3):113–26.

37. Winters K. Gender madness in American psychiatry: essays from the struggle for dignity. Dillon: GID Reform Advocates; 2008.
38. Wood H, Sasaki S, Bradley SJ, Singh D, Fantus S, Owen-Anderson A, Di Giacomo A, Bain J, Zucker KJ. Patterns of referral to a gender identity service for children and adolescents (1976–2011): age, sex ratio, and sexual orientation. J Sex Marital Ther. 2013;39:1–6.
39. World Professional Association for Transgender Health. Standards of care for the health of transsexual, transgender, and gender nonconforming people (version 7). Minneapolis: WPATH; 2011.
40. Zucker KJ, Bradley S. Gender identity disorder and psychosexual problems in children and adolescents. Guilford: Guilford Press; 1995.
41. Zucker KJ, Wood H, Singh D, Bradley SJ. A developmental, biopsychosocial model for the treatment of children with gender identity disorder. J Homosex. 2012;59(3):369–97.

Treatment Paradigms for Adolescents: Gender-Affirming Hormonal Care

14

Kathleen Chung, Sarah Rhoads, Alicia Rolin,
Andrew C. Sackett-Taylor, and Michelle Forcier

Abbreviation

AYA	Adolescents and young adults
GAH	Gender-affirming hormones
GAS	Gender-affirming surgery
GD	Gender dysphoria
GnRHA	Gonadotropin-releasing hormone analogs
HPG	Hypothalamic–pituitary–gonadal
TGD	Transgender and gender diverse

Introduction

In recent years, health and social issues related to a broader understanding of gender diversity have gained greater visibility. As a result, an increasing number of transgender and gender diverse (TGD) individuals are presenting to healthcare settings at younger ages [1] with significant diversity in gender presentation and desired

K. Chung (✉) · A. Rolin
Warren Alpert Medical School of Brown University, Providence, RI, USA
e-mail: kathleen_chung@brown.edu

S. Rhoads
Medicine-Pediatrics Residency Program, Brown University, Providence, RI, USA

A. C. Sackett-Taylor
Gándara Mental Health Center, Springfield, MA, USA

M. Forcier
Department of Pediatrics, Brown University, Providence, RI, USA

M. Forcier et al. (eds.), *Pediatric Gender Identity*,
https://doi.org/10.1007/978-3-030-38909-3_14

transition goals. Some patients may present reporting gender dysphoria (GD), which is defined within The Diagnostic and Statistical Manual of Mental Disorders, Fifth Edition (DSM-5) as the distress that may accompany the incongruence between one's experienced or expressed gender and one's assigned gender. Other patients may not experience significant dysphoria or may have transition goals that lie outside the traditional gender binary [2].

Gender-affirming hormones (GAH) are one option for care that help patients physically and phenotypically affirm their asserted gender. Hormones can play a significant role in a greater plan for gender care that may include social, legal, and surgical interventions, all together known as "affirmation" (a process formerly known as "transition"). The goals of GAH therapy are to suppress endogenous hormone production and replace it with exogenous hormones corresponding to the patient's asserted gender identity with goals of masculinization, feminization, or other gender diverse presentation. Management of GAH therapy should be driven by the patient's gender goals and response to the medication(s).

Pre-hormone Assessment

As with any new patient or medical encounter, it is important to take a comprehensive history. Thorough understanding of the patient's gender experience is key to providing appropriate information, support, and options for care. Providers can create a safe and respectful clinical environment by avoiding assumptions and inviting the patient to tell their unique gender story in their own words. Taking a gender history involves exploring thoughts, feelings, and expressions of gender in the context of overall development from childhood to puberty with the patient and any involved parent or guardian. See Table 14.1 for suggested questions. Providers should remember that there is significant diversity in the gender histories of patients, with some individuals experiencing GD since early childhood, and others who first experience GD with the onset of puberty or even later in life. Regardless, each gender experience is valid and worth exploring using a gender-affirming model.

When working with adolescents, it is important to have protected time to interview them alone to gain a clear sense of their identity and goals. In addition to establishing their asserted name and pronouns, aspects of social disclosure and affirmation planning can be discussed during this time. It is particularly important to assess family support and acceptance, as gaining guardian consent can be a barrier to treatment for adolescents under 18 years old. This can be especially challenging for patients who are under the care of the state. For younger patients, it may take time to build enough trust and rapport for them to feel comfortable without their parents present. Regardless of the child's age, incorporating a plan for safe and healthy exploration of gender, while engaging relevant guardian and community supports, is a critical step that is both protective and respectful of the patient [3].

As part of the initial evaluation, exploring goals regarding social, legal, medical, and surgical affirmation provides a framework for next steps and options for care

Table 14.1 Age-appropriate gender history

Developmental stage	Suggested questions for a gender history	Affirmative medical provider responses
Pre-puberty	How do you like being a boy/girl? Do you feel like a boy/girl on the inside? Do you feel more like yourself when you dress like a boy/girl? Do you want people to see you like a boy/girl?	Sometimes people feel more like a boy or a girl, sometimes people feel like both, and sometimes people feel like they don't quite fit with either.
Peri-puberty	What was your childhood like? Did you ever feel like a boy/girl before puberty? How do you feel about the changes in your body during puberty? How did you feel when you started your period? How do you feel about your body hair? Are there body changes that you are dreading? Are there parts of your body that you like? Are there parts that cause you distress? Does anyone around you know how you feel? How do you want other people to see you?	Puberty can be very difficult for a lot of people. Many patients feel like there are parts of their body that don't fit with who they are. There are lots of things we can work on together in order to help you feel better about your body's changes. Sometimes people find it helpful to talk to someone who understands what they're going through.
Post-puberty	What was your childhood like? How did puberty affect you? Are there parts of your body that cause you distress? Does anyone around you know how you feel? Have you tried to transition previously (medical/social/legal)? How do you want other people to see you?	It can be really hard to talk to people about how you're feeling – we can work together on what makes the most sense for you to accomplish your goals. Everyone has a different way of reaching their goals. My goal is to help make your affirmation work for you.
Parents	Are you aware of your child's feelings toward his/her gender? Did you ever notice your child experimenting with gender? How did your child tell you about his/her gender identity? How do you feel about your child being transgender/gender diverse?	It's often difficult for parents to think about their lives and their child's life changing so much. By being here and supporting your child, you've already taken a huge step in helping them on this journey. I'm here to help answer questions and support you both.

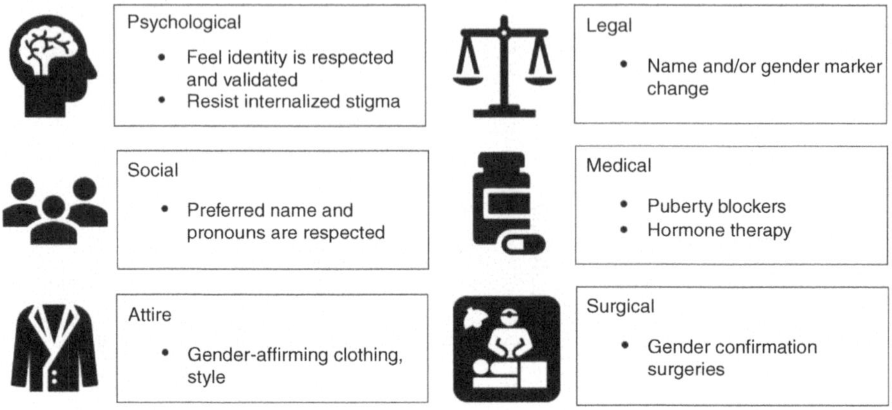

Fig. 14.1 Gender-affirming care

(Fig. 14.1). Assessing the patient's understanding and goals regarding fertility and future family building is a crucial part of the discussion prior to starting hormones. If the patient has a strong desire to have biological children, referrals for egg, sperm, and fertility preservation may be offered before hormonal interventions begin (see Chap. 15).

There is some controversy surrounding the degree and type of assessment required prior to initiating medical interventions, including who should perform the psychosocial interview. There is also debate around whether or not gender dysphoria can be diagnosed in a single visit or if patients should be followed for a period of time. As our understanding of gender diversity and nonbinary presentations broadens, use of a developmental model rather than basing care solely on diagnostic criteria may offer additional room to understand patient experiences.

There is little utility in delaying care for further observation of patients who present with insistent, consistent, and persistent gender dysphoria over time. Beginning earlier social transition offers a clearer pathway for patients, parents, and providers. Delaying treatment in this population may cause additional harm, considering the time-sensitive nature of initiating puberty blockers or GAH therapy in adolescents. The risks of delaying treatment include progressing through the wrong puberty and developing irreversible secondary sex characteristics, prolonged gender dysphoria, and development on a delayed timeline relative to peers.

To understand patients in a holistic sense, within the context of their sense of self, family, and community, the adolescent HEADSS examination can provide a helpful framework for determining factors of resiliency and risk within this age group as part of a robust medical, family, social, and gender history. In conducting a comprehensive medical and psychosocial interview, patients and guardians alike can be reassured that the patient's overall well-being is an important part of decision-making within a gender-affirming, patient-centered care model. See Fig. 14.2 for a GAH consent-based care summary.

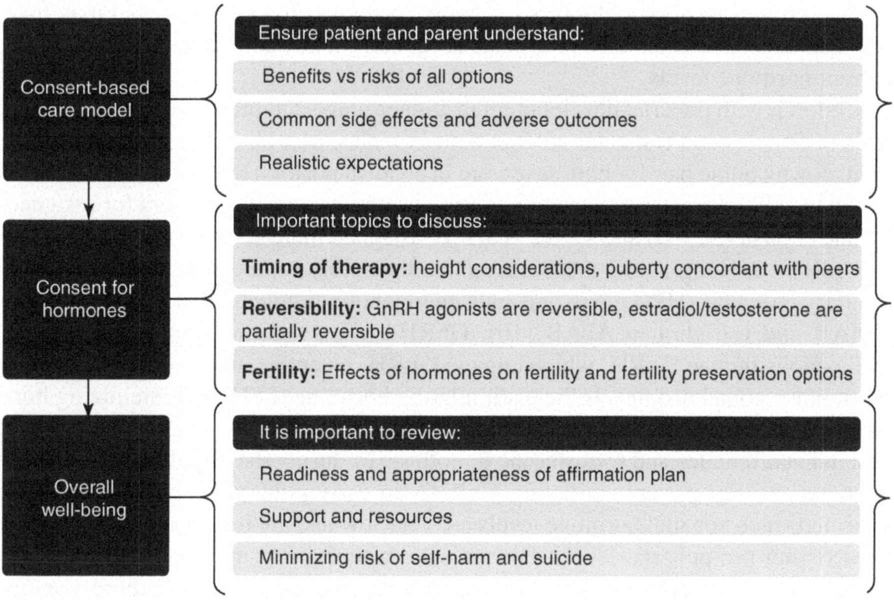

Fig. 14.2 GAH consent-based care model

Pre-puberty

The Endocrine Society, the World Professional Association for Transgender Health (WPATH), and the UCSF Center of Excellence for Transgender Health publish helpful information and guidelines for hormone initiation and management based on recent literature and expert opinion [4–6]. However, the majority of clinic visits for pre-pubertal children do not address GAH therapy in more than a peripheral sense, but instead focus on the youth's gender exploration and parental support. During these visits, one might discuss how the child views and expresses their gender (e.g., clothes, hair, makeup, jewelry, play activities, friends, name, and pronouns). Some children may present to a medical visit having already socially transitioned. As with any pediatric visit, it is appropriate to ask about support at school, peer relationships, and if extended family or other support persons are involved. TGD youth are at higher risk for bullying and mental health issues such as anxiety and depression; therefore, early and frequent assessment for these potential risks is important [7].

Early Puberty

Conversations about puberty-blocking options may begin before puberty to both establish timing and address patient and parental concerns. Adolescents who have started puberty may consider gonadotropin-releasing hormone analogs (GnRHA), commonly referred to as puberty blockers, prior to starting GAH. Determining the starting point for puberty blockers is largely based on physical exam, but may take into account patient anxiety and distress, genetic and familial development, and current hormone levels.

Children with pubertal development in Tanner Stage 2, typically defined by breast buds in females and testicular enlargement in males, as well as the development of light, downy pubic hair for both sexes, are in an ideal position to begin puberty blockers. In the USA, the average age of puberty onset is usually 10–11 years for assigned female at birth (AFAB) and 11–12 years for assigned male at birth (AMAB) [8, 9].

GnRHA are long-acting medications that reversibly suppress the hypothalamic–pituitary–gonadal (HPG) axis and halt endogenous production of testosterone in AMAB and estradiol in AFAB [10]. GnRHA are synthetic peptides similar to endogenous human GnRH, which engage GnRH receptors and modify the release of pituitary gonadotropins, follicle stimulating hormone (FSH) and luteinizing hormone (LH). All GnRHA cause a transient increase in serum concentrations of estradiol in natal females and testosterone in both sexes during the initial one to 2 weeks of treatment. For patients initiating GnRHA in early puberty, side effects are not expected since gonadal hormone levels are very low and are being suppressed to the pre-existing pre-pubertal levels. For patients farther along in puberty with higher baseline levels of gonadal hormones, GnRHA might precipitate temporary menstruation, menopausal symptoms such as hot flashes, or mood changes in AFAB and increased erectile function or mood changes in AMAB. These changes generally resolve quickly and are not terribly distressing to youth who are well prepared for potential side effects. By week four, suppression of gonadal hormones will occur, and puberty is temporarily halted. See Table 14.2 for a summary of GnRHA and other GAH medications.

Patients and parents must understand that these medications do not alter the patient's pubertal development, but instead temporarily halt the progression of puberty. They are completely reversible and are often considered a "pause button," allowing patients and their families time for further exploration of gender identity and care options without committing to the semi-reversible effects of GAH therapy or the largely irreversible changes of endogenous puberty. As with many medications in pediatrics, the uses are considered off-label by the Food and Drug Administration (FDA). While there is limited data on the long-term effects, existing literature supports their use and safety [3]. While it is ideal to initiate blockers at early Tanner Stage 2, it can be used in all stages of puberty for various purposes. These may include stopping menses, halting puberty reversibly to allow the youth and family time process and form a plan, and preventing further development of secondary sex characteristics.

Peri-puberty

The decision of when to start GAH therapy should be based on careful discussion with the patient, family, and care team. WPATH and the Endocrine Society guidelines recommend initiating GAH at the age of majority or at 16 years of age, respectively, 14 in selected cases [4, 5]. This is primarily based on expert opinion and it is the age at which adolescents are deemed to have the capacity to consent to

Table 14.2 Gender-affirming hormone therapy

Medication	Administration	Typical dosing	Reversible changes	Permanent changes	What won't change	Common side effects
Puberty-blocking GnRH analogs						
Leuprolide	Intramuscular (IM) injection	11.25–30 mg IM every 3–6 months	Prevention of puberty progression, breast bud regression in early Tanner Stage 2	None	Aside from breast buds, no reversal of secondary sex characteristics	Changes in mood (may include improved mood/ affect as well as irritability), change in libido, erectile dysfunction, amenorrhea
Histrelin	Subcutaneous implant	50 mcg 2 years				
Feminizing medications						
17B Estradiol	Sublingual, oral tablet, patch	Daily (sublingual, oral) 2–8 mg, Patch 100–400 mcg once weekly	Softened less oily skin, fat and muscle redistribution toward a female pattern habitus	Breast growth	Adam's apple, facial and skeletal structure, vocal tone	Changes in mood (may include improved mood/ affect as well as irritability), change in libido, erectile dysfunction
Spironolactone (Androgen receptor antagonist)	Oral tablet	1–2 times daily, 1–100 mg twice daily oral	Breast growth (usually reversible 6–12 months), decreased hirsuitism			Increased urinary frequency, potential hypotension, and mild hyponatremia, hyperkalemia
Finasteride (5α-reductase inhibitor)	Oral tablet	Daily, 1–5 mg	Decreased virilization, hirsutism	No reversal of previous male pattern hair loss		Decreased libido, erectile dysfunction

(continued)

Table 14.2 (continued)

Medication	Administration	Typical dosing	Reversible changes	Permanent changes	What won't change	Common side effects
Progesterone	Medroxyprogesterone oral tablet Depo Medroxyprogesterone injection Progesterone oral tablet	10 mg daily 150 mg IM q 3 months 100–200 mg daily	Feminization (breast development)			Bloating, breast pain, appetite increase, mood changes, sedation
Masculinizing medications						
Testosterone	Intramuscular injection Subcutaneous injection Transdermal Subdermal implants	40–100 mg weekly; 60–200 mg every 2 weeks Weekly 20–100 mg Daily 2–8 mg Every 2–900 mg pellets placed q3–6 months, 750 mg IM	Coarser, oily skin, muscle and fat redistribution to male pattern habitus, amenorrhea	Lower voice, male pattern hair, clitoromegaly	Facial and bone structures, loss of breast mass	Loss of menstrual period, increased libido, mood changes (early irritability, later improved mood)

partially irreversible therapy. These recommendations have changed over time as we learn more about our TGD youth, and we expect that future evidence may precipitate further changes in recommendations and guidelines. It is important to note that withholding GAH in the setting of prolonging gender dysphoria or progressing into an undesired puberty may cause harm. It is important for parents to understand that in terms of consequences and outcomes, choosing to not provide care is as much of an active decision as deciding to start care. A delay in treatment may result in developing irreversible pubertal changes that would later require surgical intervention and psychological consequences of prolonging GD, such as depression, anxiety, and suicidal ideation. These factors may justify initiating puberty-blocking and GAH therapy earlier as appropriate to the patient and clinical indications. Initiation of GAH may depend on patient and parent readiness, articulation of a safe and realistic affirmation plan, patient age relative to average age of puberty onset in cisgender peers, and continued growth considerations. See Table 14.3 for common sources of gender dysphoria and related goals.

Table 14.3 Common causes of dysphoria

Masculinizing interventions	Common sources of distress	Feminizing interventions
GAH therapy	Facial structure (too masculine/feminine, bone structure)	Facial feminization surgery, tracheal shave, GAH therapy
GAH therapy, finasteride	Hair (too little/too much,)	Wigs, anti-androgen medications, GAH therapy, electrolysis/shaving (hair removal)
Voice training (post-pubertal), GAH therapy if pre/peri-pubertal	Voice (too masculine/feminine)	Voice training (post-pubertal), GAH therapy if pre/peri-pubertal, vocal cord surgery
GAH therapy, mastectomy, chest binding	Chest (breast absence/presence)	GAH therapy, breast augmentation, padded bras, and pectoral exercises
GAH therapy, clothing	Hips (too masculine/feminine)	GAH therapy, clothing
Phalloplasty, metoidioplasty, hysterectomy/oophorectomy, packing	Genitals (absence/presence)	Orchiopexy, Vaginoplasty, tucking
Hormonal contraceptives, GAH therapy, hysterectomy/oophorectomy	Menstruation	—
Options for legal gender marker change, develop tools for responding to misgendering	Misgendering	Options for legal gender marker change, develop tools for responding to misgendering
Options for legal name change/identity change (national database for patients: https://transequality.org/documents)	Birth name	Options for legal name change/identity change (national database for patients: https://transequality.org/documents)

Note: Transgender adolescents may get surgery according to need, just as minors assent to surgery with parent support and consent for other medically indicated procedures

Table 14.4 Effects of hormone therapy

Masculinizing hormone effect	Time of onset	Maximum effect	Feminizing hormone effect
Fat redistribution	3–6 months	2–5 years	Fat redistribution
Increased muscle mass	6 months	2–5 years	Decreased muscle mass
Acne	1–6 months	1–2 years (male)	Softer skin
Increased libido	1–3 months	1–2 years	Decreased libido
Clitoral enlargement (irreversible)	1–6 months	1–3 years	Breast growth (irreversible)
Cessation of menses	1–6 months	—	Decreased erections
Facial/body hair (irreversible)	6–12 months	4–5 years	No regrowth of male pattern baldness
Voice deepening (irreversible)	1–12 months	1–2 years	—

For those youth who have been on puberty-blocking therapy, low-dose GAH is typically started in a way that mimics endogenous hormone secretion. Patients will typically continue puberty blocker use while estradiol or testosterone is added at progressively increasing doses consistent with endogenous pubertal development to achieve levels consistent with adult hormone levels. Exogenous puberty for TGD patients requires at least 2 years of hormone therapy to achieve end phenotypic results. While some patients remain on GnRHA until gonadectomy, many will transition off puberty blockers after adult hormone levels are attained. Upon cessation of GnRHA, patients may require higher doses of GAH therapy in order to both suppress natal endogenous hormone production and continue development of desired secondary sex characteristics.

Patients who are in Tanner Stage 3 or higher can start estradiol or testosterone GAH directly without the antecedent use of blockers. In order to reach desired gender-affirming masculinizing or feminizing effects and effectively shut down the HPG axis, these patients may require higher starting doses than those who have previously been on GnRHA. For patients who have already gone through endogenous puberty and developed secondary sex characteristics, neither blockers nor GAH will reverse the myriad skeletal, vocal, and genital changes already experienced (Table 14.3). For these patients, surgical interventions may become important goals of care if these physical attributes are causing dysphoria (see Chap. 16). Prior to initiating therapy, a standard medication consent should occur between provider, patient, and parent/guardian, and include a discussion of the reversible and irreversible changes associated with GAH to establish reasonable expectations. Tables 14.2 and 14.4 summarize information regarding the potential expected effects with GAH.

Post-puberty

Adolescents and young adults (AYA) may still meet their physical gender affirmation goals after having undergone endogenous puberty and the associated exposure to gonadal hormones, though achievement of these goals may become harder with time. GAH at this point will not reverse certain permanent physical body characteristics, and many TGD patients with fully developed secondary sex characteristics may require surgical intervention to support their goals. These patients will often have different goals or needs as they age, including regular age-appropriate healthcare maintenance. Providing GAH and information on surgical interventions to AYA 18 years or older does not require parental consent as it does in the pediatric TGD population, but it is still beneficial to assess for family, spouse, workplace, and community supports. See Chap. 16 for more information about surgical options.

Adjunctive Therapies

For transfeminine patients, there are additional medication options including spironolactone, finasteride, and progesterone that may support feminization alongside estradiol therapy. For transmasculine patients, presently testosterone is the sole masculinizing agent, primarily used in its injectable form. Topical testosterone can be used when there is an allergy to the suspension oil or a severe needle phobia, though these patients should be advised that topical application to the clitoral area has not been demonstrated to have significant effects on clitoral growth. Though finasteride is not considered a masculinizing agent, it may be used in transmasculine patients as well for treating male pattern baldness.

Spironolactone

Spironolactone, a potassium-sparing diuretic, is frequently used in conjunction with estradiol for feminizing hormone therapy. At higher doses, it may have minor effects on suppression of endogenous testosterone activity by directly inhibiting testosterone secretion and blocking androgen receptors [4]. It is most useful for blocking androgen receptors and continued testosterone effects on male pattern hair growth. It may also aid with breast development and reduce spontaneous erections. Following orchiectomy, transgender women will no longer require spironolactone.

In thc AYA population, spironolactone is generally well tolerated with minimal side effects. Side effects may include increased urinary frequency and dizziness secondary to its diuretic effects. Hyperkalemia is an unlikely but more serious side effect, and therefore spironolactone should be avoided in patients with renal insufficiency and used with caution in patients who also take an ACE inhibitor or angiotensin II receptor blocker [6]. Blood pressure and serum electrolytes (sodium and potassium) should be monitored during the first year and following medication or health changes, though parameters for how frequently to monitor levels and labs are under ongoing review [4]. The UCSF guideline recommends checking kidney markers (blood urea nitrogen and creatinine) and potassium every 3 months during the first year and then annually or as needed thereafter [6].

Finasteride

Finasteride is a 5α-reductase inhibitor that helps prevent the conversion of testosterone to dihydrotestosterone (DHT), a potent androgen, thus reducing male pattern body hair. It is an additional option for all TGD patients who have concerns regarding male pattern baldness and hair loss. Side effects of finasteride include decreased libido and erectile dysfunction, which also occur with estradiol therapy. As 5α-reductase inhibitors are less effective than spironolactone, finasteride may provide a reasonable option for patients with contraindications to spironolactone (i.e., renal dysfunction, potassium disorders, low blood pressure, and urinary frequency) or for those who continue to experience male pattern baldness after orchiectomy [6].

Progesterone

Progestins currently available in the USA include oral progesterone, oral medroxyprogesterone, and depo medroxyprogesterone (DMPA). For cisgender women, DMPA has been associated with weight gain and mood disturbances, while oral progesterone can have sedating side effects. The use of progestins in gender-affirming care remains controversial, with little or no evidence at present to document clinical effectiveness or harm. Anecdotally, progestins are associated with improved breast and areolar development [11]. There are, however, some concerns regarding the use of progestins based on the existing studies from the Women's Health Initiative, which have demonstrated an increase in cardiovascular disease and breast cancer in post-menopausal cisgender women [12]. However, it is unclear if these results are transferrable to the TGD population, because transgender woman are at much lower risk of breast cancer than their cisgender counterparts [6].

Long-Term Management

Titration and Monitoring

Once patients elect to begin GAH, their goals should direct hormone dosing. Since secondary sex characteristics are not linked to specific hormone levels, dosing should depend on desired effect. Some patients may seek maximum masculinization or feminization, while others may simply desire suppression of natal secondary sex characteristics [3]. Goals for patients on the nonbinary and genderqueer spectrum may also vary. To promote healthy and safe affirmation plans, alongside overall mental health and well-being, patient goals should be considered in the context of risks associated with hormone use as compared to risks of withholding them. In pediatric and AYA populations, GAH are considered to be safe, effective, and potentially lifesaving for patients experiencing suicidal ideation related to their GD.

The 2017 Endocrine Society Guidelines recommend laboratory monitoring of total testosterone or estradiol levels alongside a metabolic panel every 3 months during the first year of GAH therapy and every 6–12 months thereafter [4]. There is no clear literature to support best practices in obtaining hormonal levels, but many providers choose to reference average physiologic hormone ranges in cisgender individuals (testosterone 300–1000 ng/dL; estradiol 100–400 pg/mL) [5, 6]. Recommendations for lab monitoring frequency are rather conservative, and many practitioners will choose to reduce testing frequency when prior values have been consistent, GAH dosing is stable, and no additional medical concerns arise.

Long-Term Risks and Concerns

While there is limited data on the long-term risks of hormone therapy for TGD individuals, GAH therapy is generally considered safe when followed closely by a medical provider, with no documented increase in cancer prevalence or direct increase in mortality attributed to GAH [13].

Testosterone GAH

Current data is inconsistent regarding the use of exogenous testosterone and association with increased risk of cardiovascular disease in transgender men [13]. No studies have demonstrated an increase in myocardial infarctions, deep vein thrombosis, or cerebrovascular events [13–15]. It has been well demonstrated that testosterone therapy causes a clinically insignificant increase in hemoglobin and hematocrit levels during the first year of therapy; however, there is little data on the long-term hematopoietic effects [16].

Estradiol GAH

Hormones play an important role in bone health. Transgender women may be at higher risk for bone loss due to the use of estradiol. However, it is unclear whether decreased bone mineral density or osteoporosis can be attributed to GAH [5]. While the 2017 Endocrine Society Guidelines provide no specific recommendations, transgender female patients with risk factors for osteoporosis may need to be screened sooner and more frequently than the general population.

There has also been concern regarding increased risk of venous thromboembolisms (VTEs) in transgender females. Consistent with their cisgender peers in studies on contraception risks, pediatric and AYA transgender persons are typically at very low risks for VTE or related events. While several studies have found significantly increased risk of VTE events in transgender women overall, these studies did not account for pre-existing cardiovascular risk factors [14]. Ethinyl estradiol in particular has been demonstrated to increase VTE risk, and its use in GAH therapy has been discontinued [5]. A recent cohort study found that transfeminine adults were at slightly increased risk for VTE compared to cisgender men and women [17]. This increase in VTE risk is especially important to note for patients who may be self-medicating and taking higher-than-recommended doses of estradiol; however, data on supratherapeutic estradiol levels in transgender women is limited. Risks and benefits should be discussed prior to starting estrogen therapy. For transgender women with established cardiovascular risk factors or disease, transdermal estrogen is preferred for its lower rates of VTE and limited impact on lipid profile or coagulation [5, 18]. For transgender women who currently smoke or have a significant history of smoking, transdermal estrogen is also preferred in addition to smoking cessation counseling. See Table 14.5 for concerns and common misconceptions.

Table 14.5 Common misconceptions

Concerns and common misconceptions	
MYTH #1: GAH therapy must be lifelong and is irreversible	Many patients remain on hormone therapy for their entire lives, while others may discontinue hormones for short or long periods of time. For example, there is a short-term discontinuation for the purpose of pregnancy in transmasculine patients. Some GAH changes are reversible and others are not (see Tables 14.2 and 14.4). As our understanding of gender expands, we also understand there may be more patients who do not commit to a lifelong GAH plan.
MYTH #2: Transgender individuals often regret transitioning	While "desistance" or "transition regret" has been highlighted in the media, the literature suggests that this is exceedingly rare [19, 20]. In a recent cohort study by Olson-Kennedy et al., chest dysphoria was significantly higher in nonsurgical transmasculine youth compared to postsurgical patients. Ranging from 1 to 5 years after surgery with most respondents between 0 and 2 years, 67 of 68 subjects reported an absence of regret, further supporting the therapeutic benefit of gender-affirming care [21]. In a large longitudinal retrospective cohort study of transgender patients, only 0.6% of transwomen and 0.3% of transmen who underwent gonadectomy experienced regret [22].
MYTH #3: GAH therapy will help patients grow taller or change their underlying skeletal structure	See Table 14.3 for sources of distress and body parts that remain unaffected by hormones. Examples include the Adam's apple, significant body hair, or short/tall stature. Estradiol causes growth plates to close, so patients may consider waiting to initiate GAH until final height is achieved. It is important to counsel patients on what GAH therapy can and cannot do in order to establish realistic expectations.
MYTH #4: GAH therapy will cause infertility	The effects of hormones on fertility vary widely, therefore it is important to counsel patients on fertility preservation and contraception. Similar to their cisgender counterparts, transgender individuals can have biological children, and many pregnancies are actually unplanned.
MYTH #5: Being on GAH therapy for life is dangerous for one's health	Research suggests that GAH therapy for transgender individuals is generally safe. The significant psychosocial benefits of GAH therapy generally outweigh the risk of adverse events. It is recommended that patients receive screening and preventive care for both the body parts they maintain as well as the hormones they administer.

Conclusion

While GAH therapy is only one aspect of affirmative gender care, it is a powerful tool that can alleviate GD and help TGD individuals live as their authentic selves. With the significant increase in children and younger adolescents seeking gender-affirming therapy, early identification, support for authentic gender identity, effective management for sources of dysphoria, and GAH may offer improved long-term health outcomes for this new generation of TGD youth. In order to best support this patient population, it is important for providers across disciplines to understand the basics of GAH therapy, be able to help patients establish realistic expectations for gender-affirming care, and help patients identify means of achieving gender care goals.

Funding Source No funding was used for this review.

Financial Disclosures Michelle Forcier: Consultant Planned Parenthood League Massachusetts, author royalties Up To Date.

References

1. Fuss J, Auer MK, Briken P. Gender dysphoria in children and adolescents: a review of recent research. Curr Opin Psychiatry. 2015;28(6):430–4.
2. American Psychiatric Association. Diagnostic and statistical manual of mental disorders (DSM–5) [Internet]. DSM-5 [cited 7 Nov 2018]. Available from: https://www.psychiatry.org/psychiatrists/practice/dsm.
3. Rafferty J. Ensuring comprehensive care and support for transgender and gender-diverse children and adolescents. Pediatrics. 2018;142(4):e20182162.
4. Hembree WC, Cohen-Kettenis PT, Gooren L, et al. Endocrine treatment of gender-dysphoric/gender-incongruent persons: an endocrine society clinical practice guideline. J Clin Endocrinol Metab. 2017;102(11):3869–903. Available from: https://doi.org/10.1210/jc.2017-01658.
5. The World Professional Association for Transgender Health. Standards of care for the health of transsexual, transgender, and gender nonconforming people [Internet]. 2011 [cited 6 Nov 2018]. Available from: https://www.wpath.org/publications/soc.
6. Guidelines for the primary and gender-affirming care of transgender and gender nonbinary people [Internet]. [cited 6 Nov 2018]. Available from: https://transcare.ucsf.edu/guidelines.
7. Center for Disease Control MMWR. Youth risk behavior surveillance, 2017. Available from: https://www.cdc.gov/mmwr/volumes/67/ss/pdfs/ss6708a1-h.pdf.
8. Cabrera SM, Bright GM, Frane JW, et al. Age of thelarche and menarche in contemporary US females: a cross-sectional analysis. J Pediatr Endocrinol Metab. 2014;27:47–51. Available from: https://www.ncbi.nlm.nih.gov/pmc/articles/PMC4137967/.
9. Herman-Giddens M, Steffes J, Harris D, et al. Secondary sexual characteristics in boys: data from the Pediatric Research in Office Settings Network. Pediatrics. 2012;130(5):e1058–68. Available from: http://pediatrics.aappublications.org/content/130/5/e1058.
10. Rosenthal SM. Approach to the patient: transgender youth: endocrine considerations. J Clin Endocrinol Metab. 2014;99(12):4379–89.
11. Wierckx K, Gooren L, Tsjoen G. Clinical review: breast development in trans women receiving cross-sex hormones. J Sex Med. 2014;11(5):1240–7.

12. Writing Group for the Women's Health Initiative Investigators. Risks and benefits of estrogen plus progestin in healthy postmenopausal women principal results From the Women's Health Initiative Randomized Controlled Trial. JAMA. 2002;288(3):321–33. Available from: https://jamanetwork.com/journals/jama/fullarticle/195120.
13. Gooren LJ, Giltay EJ, Bunck MC. Long-term treatment of transsexuals with cross-sex hormones: extensive personal experience. J Clin Endocrinol Metab. 2008;93(1):19–25.
14. Weinand JD, Safer JD. Hormone therapy in transgender adults is safe with provider supervision; a review of hormone therapy sequelae for transgender individuals. J Clin Transl Endocrinol. 2015;2(2):55–60.
15. Gooren LJ, Giltay EJ. Men and women, so different, so similar: observations from cross-sex hormone treatment of transsexual subjects. Andrologia. 2013;46(5):570–5.
16. Jarin J, Pine-Twaddell E, Trotman G, et al. Cross-sex hormones and metabolic parameters in adolescents with gender dysphoria. Pediatrics. 2017;139(5):e20163173.
17. Getahun D, Nash R, Flanders W, Baird T, et al. Cross-sex hormones and acute cardiovascular events in transgender persons. Ann Intern Med. 2019;170(2):143.
18. Irwig MS. Cardiovascular health in transgender people. Rev Endocr Metab Disord. 2018;19(3):243–51.
19. Krege S, Bex A, Lummen G, et al. Male-to-female transsexualism: a technique, results and long-term follow-up in 66 patients. BJU Int. 2001;88(4):396–402.
20. Smith YLS, Goozen SHMV, Kuiper AJ, et al. Sex reassignment: outcomes and predictors of treatment for adolescent and adult transsexuals. Psychol Med. 2005;35(1):89–99.
21. Olson-Kennedy J, Warus J, Okonta V, et al. Chest reconstruction and chest dysphoria in transmasculine minors and young adults. JAMA Pediatr. 2018;172(5):431.
22. Wiepjes CM, Nota NM, Blok CJD, et al. The Amsterdam cohort of gender dysphoria study (1972–2015): trends in prevalence, treatment, and regrets. J Sex Med. 2018;15(4):582–90.

15 Fertility Considerations for Gender Diverse Youth

Leena Nahata, Anna Valentine, and Amy C. Tishelman

The number of transgender and gender diverse (TGD) youth presenting for both medical and surgical care related to gender dysphoria is steadily increasing [1, 2]. More attention is thus being paid to the potential for future treatment-related adverse effects including the potential for impaired fertility. The majority of fertility-related studies have been conducted in adolescents and young adults with cancer undergoing gonadotoxic chemotherapy and radiation [3, 4]. While less is known about fertility-related issues in non-oncologic populations, an expanding body of scholarship underscores the importance of considering fertility and reproductive health more broadly across pediatrics [5, 6]. We recognize that terminology continue to evolve over time, and will use "transgender and gender diverse (TGD)," "cisgender," and "birth assigned" for the purposes of this chapter.

The literature suggests that cancer survivors who declined or were not offered fertility preservation (FP) measures prior to initiating potentially gonadotoxic therapies later regretted their inability to have biologically related children [7, 8]. Recent studies in transgender adults also demonstrate a desire for biological children [9–13]. In this context, medical organizations such as the World Professional Association for Transgender Health (WPATH), the Endocrine Society, and the

L. Nahata (✉)
Department of Pediatrics, The Ohio State University College of Medicine/Nationwide Children's Hospital, Columbus, OH, USA

Center for Biobehavioral Health, The Research Institute at Nationwide Children's Hospital, Columbus, OH, USA
e-mail: leena.nahata@nationwidechildrens.org

A. Valentine
Department of Pediatrics, The Ohio State University College of Medicine/Nationwide Children's Hospital, Columbus, OH, USA

A. C. Tishelman
Departments of Endocrinology and Psychiatry, Harvard Medical School/Boston Children's Hospital, Boston, MA, USA

M. Forcier et al. (eds.), *Pediatric Gender Identity*,
https://doi.org/10.1007/978-3-030-38909-3_15

American Society for Reproductive Medicine have published guidelines recommending the discussion of FP options with TGD youth and their families prior to initiating any therapies, hormonal or surgical, that may have the potential to cause future impaired fertility [14–16].

This chapter will focus on potential risks of fertility impairment associated with the three most common hormonal therapies used in TGD youth (gonadotropin-releasing hormone agonists, estrogen, and testosterone), FP options related to pubertal stage and birth-assigned gender, attitudes toward FP in the TGD population, as well as both ethical and financial considerations related to FP.

Potential for Infertility Secondary to Hormonal Therapies

Gonadotropin-Releasing Hormone Agonists

Little is known about the impact of hormonal therapies on fertility; specifically no studies have been conducted to examine future fertility outcomes in individuals who began hormonal interventions in adolescence. TGD individuals may be candidates for gonadotropin-releasing hormone agonists (GnRHa), otherwise known as "puberty blockers," once they have begun endogenous puberty (Tanner stage 2). GnRHa are used to suppress the hypothalamic–pituitary–gonadal axis (the hormone cascade responsible for the production of sex steroids). They prevent germ cell maturation and both reversible and irreversible phenotypic changes of puberty. These agents are commonly used to treat precocious puberty (testicular enlargement prior to age 9 years in birth-assigned males, and breast development prior to age 8 years in birth-assigned females) and are not known to cause fertility impairment directly [17]. Historically, pediatric endocrinologists have reassured families about future fertility when pursuing GnRHa treatment in precocious puberty populations. One study that followed youth with central precocious puberty treated with GnRHa showed all patients over the age of 12 years achieved complete sexual maturity by 5 years post-treatment as defined by their hormone levels and clinical Tanner stages; no impairment of reproductive function was seen in adulthood [18]. However, given that GnRHa are used to suppress the hypothalamic–pituitary–gonadal axis, they prevent germ cell maturation and there have been reports of decreased testicular size in birth-assigned males [19]. Keeping this in mind, TGD youth on GnRHa would potentially require a period of time between the cessation of GnRHa and initiation of gender-affirming hormones to allow for further endogenous pubertal development if FP were desired. For TGD youth who want to continue GAH, this may be a barrier to FP as they began GnRHa for that express purpose of preventing permanent phenotypic changes of puberty. These changes would likely occur to some degree if this pause in GAH to allow FP was initiated.

Impact of Testosterone

Studies have shown inconsistent results about the impact of testosterone therapy on ovarian tissue removed from transgender men, partially associated with the duration of exposure. When used for shorter periods of time (~6–21 months), studies have shown little to no effect on the function and architecture of ovarian tissue [20]. Long-term testosterone use, however, can cause cystic follicles, collagenization, and stromal hyperplasia, much like what is seen in polycystic ovarian syndrome (PCOS), which is itself a hyperandrogenic state [21]. When considering the rates of fertility impairment in birth-assigned females with PCOS, exposure to higher levels of testosterone as the cause of these observed changes could serve as a potential mechanism to explain lower fertility rates [21]. Another theory suggests that follicular atresia is promoted by testosterone exposure, and can thereby negatively impact fertility [22]. One study assessing testosterone levels in birth-assigned females before and after starting exogenous testosterone therapy found that many of the individuals (40%) had pre-treatment testosterone levels consistent with those seen in PCOS, suggesting that this cohort may be at higher risk for infertility prior to initiating treatment with gender-affirming hormones [23]. Studies in individuals with PCOS who have higher than physiologic levels of circulating testosterone show the potential for fertility after ovarian stimulation, with successful pregnancies described in 30–40% who use clomiphene, and up to 82% in those who are treated with human menopausal gonadotropins [24].

Despite these reports of changed ovarian architecture, there have been documented pregnancies in transgender males who have previously been on testosterone therapy [25]. One study described pregnancies in most (88%) of their cohort that were achieved using their own oocytes, even after over half of them had taken exogenous testosterone prior to getting pregnant; age of testosterone initiation was 17–35 years and length of testosterone use ranged from <1 year (in 40% of patients) to >10 years (in 20% of patients) [25]. Of those who achieved pregnancy, 7% required fertility drugs and 12% used assisted reproductive technology including artificial insemination, in vitro fertilization, and gamete intrafallopian transfer [25]. Notably, however, this study only included individuals who had a live birth and the overall conception/miscarriage rates in this population remain unknown. There are also no data on the health outcomes of the neonates that resulted from these pregnancies. This study is also notable for the rates of unintended or unplanned pregnancies for TGD persons on testosterone that imitate rates (approximately half) in cisgender populations [26]. Counseling for TGD youth should thus highlight that even with cessation of menses and regular testosterone use, TGD engaged in sex that involves both sperm and oocytes need contraception to prevent unintended pregnancy.

Impact of Estrogen

Limited research has examined the impact of estrogen on sperm production, and again results have been variable. Men with a history of prolonged estrogen exposure secondary to estrogen secreting tumors have had evidence of spermatogenesis after tumor removal [27]. However, men treated with estrogen for prostate cancer have been shown to develop impaired spermatogenesis, which can lead to reduced fertility [28]. The extent to which these findings can be applied to clinical use of 17B estradiol used to create average cisgender physiologic levels in TGD feminized patients remains unclear.

Few studies have been conducted examining the effect of estrogen in TGD populations, and these are generally limited by small sample sizes. Some studies have shown architectural changes in testes examined microscopically after gonadectomy performed on transgender females exposed to estrogen, which have the potential to affect spermatogenesis, whereas others show less of an impact [29–32]. In one larger study of 108 gender diverse adults currently or previously treated with estrogen, results were heterogeneous. Normal spermatogenesis was found in 24% of individuals, with some level of impairment in spermatogenesis in the rest, including meiotic arrest in 24%, spermatogonial arrest in 35%, Sertoli-cell-only in 15% and tubular shadows in 2% [33]. Those who had been exposed to estrogen therapy up until gonadectomy had higher rates of these abnormalities as compared to those who had discontinued estrogen therapy weeks prior to the tissue collection [33]. Future research is needed to examine implications of these findings on actual fertility rates.

Fertility Preservation Options

TGD youth may seek hormonal interventions at various stages of pubertal development, impacting the availability of FP options. Youth in early stages of puberty may only have access to experimental options (which may or may not be appropriate or accessible), whereas those in later Tanner stages could consider established FP options [34].

Fertility Preservation for Birth-Assigned Females

In birth-assigned females who have achieved menarche, FP options include those commonly used in cisgender women who struggle with infertility. One technique commonly employed by reproductive endocrinologists is oocyte stimulation and retrieval, with subsequent cryopreservation. This process includes hormonal stimulation for 8–14 days, after which oocytes are retrieved trans-vaginally via needle aspiration with ultrasound guidance, and cryopreserved for future use [35]. Embryo cryopreservation is another option after oocyte retrieval, though less practical in pediatrics, as this technique requires a sperm donor [36]. While oocyte cryopreservation has been successfully described in adolescent birth-assigned females, it is important to remember that the injections and method of retrieval may be more difficult for TGD individuals; consideration of possible psychological ramifications (associated with invasiveness of procedures and hormonal stimulation) of pursuing this route is crucial. Procedural risks should also be discussed including ovarian hyperstimulation syndrome and intra-abdominal bleeding [37, 38]. The need to come off blockers to begin some degree of endogenous puberty and the resultant changes, or the delay in starting testosterone based GAH could be a barrier to considering FP [39].

Birth-assigned females in earlier stages of puberty do not have the same FP options as those having already achieved menarche; their gonadal tissue is less mature, so they can consider only the experimental option of ovarian tissue cryopreservation (OTC). This generally involves a laparoscopic unilateral oophorectomy, followed by cryopreservation of the retrieved ovarian tissue [40, 41]. This procedure is being increasingly utilized in oncology prior to chemotherapy and radiation known to be gonadotoxic, with promising data regarding live births in post-pubertal women [40, 41].

Several points should be discussed when considering OTC in TGD youth. First, while this method has now resulted in over 80–100 reported live births, the majority of cases were in women treated for cancer who underwent FP after menarche and opted for OTC (e.g., to avoid treatment delays required for oocyte retrieval and cryopreservation) [40, 41]. Less is known about the effectiveness of OTC in early stages of puberty, and thus it is still considered investigational [42, 43]. Second, live births have been reported only with tissue reimplanted into the donor (once they are cancer free), allowing for the tissue to mature via endogenous gonadotropin signaling. Reimplantation is not safe in some oncologic settings, such as in youth with malignant spread to their ovaries [43]. It may also be undesirable for individuals with gender dysphoria who may not want to experience the hormonal ramifications of reintroducing a natal ovary which may start to produce estrogen and progesterone in a cyclical manner, potentially leading to physical changes inconsistent with their gender identity [37]. Maturation of oocytes in vitro after prepubertal oophorectomy is currently being studied and refined as a technique that may be more viable in the future [44, 45]. Third, concerns have been raised that removal of an ovary could in itself negatively impact reproductive potential and it is thus only considered in patients with cancer at moderate-high risk of infertility; as described above, there is uncertainty as to whether or not exogenous testosterone administration will indeed lead to infertility in this cohort [39].

As referred to previously, pregnancies in transgender men assigned female at birth have also been described after the discontinuation of testosterone [25]. In this context, there are clinical and ethical dilemmas related to removing an ovary in a child in the early stages of puberty as this could theoretically decrease future endogenous fertility by decreasing ovarian reserve. Peripubertal TGD youth may not be able to fully understand the future implications of this decision, or be completely sure of the medical and surgical interventions they may opt for in the future. Thus, at this point, there is limited evidence to support offering OTC to TGD individuals, with the exception of adults who are planning to undergo gender-affirming gonadectomy [39]. When choosing the method that is best for each individual, it is important to consider medical risks and financial implications associated with general anesthesia and invasive procedures. As technology advances, new assisted reproductive technologies may become available.

Fertility Preservation for Birth-Assigned Males

For birth-assigned males who have achieved at least Tanner stage 2–3, the least invasive and cost-effective FP option is sperm cryopreservation from an ejaculated semen sample [34]. Once the sample is collected, a cryopreservation facility can store the sample until the individual is ready to use it. While this option may be feasible for some TGD adolescents, others may find the process of masturbation to supply a semen sample too psychologically difficult given their gender dysphoria. In addition, personal, cultural, and religious beliefs/teachings that discourage masturbation may also have a negative impact on an adolescent's ability to produce a sample for cryopreservation and/or pose additional challenges to communication between providers, patients, and families about FP [46].

The pediatric oncology community has described these barriers in cisgender males who are to undergo gonadotoxic chemotherapy or radiation, who are unable to comfortably use this method secondary to embarrassment, shame, and/or sexual inexperience making the process too difficult [46–50]. For peripubertal or post pubertal birth-assigned males, sperm extraction techniques may be employed in those still interested in FP by way of electroejaculation (EEJ), testicular/epididymal sperm extraction (TESE) or testicular/epididymal sperm aspiration (TESA) [51, 52]. For EEJ, a rectal probe is used to apply a gentle electrical current in order to stimulate ejaculation [51]. This procedure is usually performed under general anesthesia. TESE and TESA is usually done under anesthesia in the operating room, and involves either a biopsy or needle aspiration of semen from the testes/epididymis in order to isolate sperm for cryopreservation [52]. Spontaneous ejaculation for sperm cryopreservation has been described successfully in birth-assigned males as young as 13 years of age, and extraction techniques in those with testes measuring as small as 6 mL [53, 54]. When choosing the method that is best for each individual, it is important to consider medical risks and financial implications associated with general anesthesia and invasive procedures.

As is the case with birth-assigned females, FP options in prepubertal/early pubertal birth-assigned males are newer and less well described [55]. Due to the lack of mature sperm in prepubertal testes, any extraction techniques employed cannot guarantee viable sperm for future use for fertilization. Testicular tissue cryopreservation (TTC) is an investigational procedure in which tissue is extracted from prepubertal testes in the hope that immature gametes in the form of spermatogonial stem cells can be isolated and cryopreserved in either Sertoli cell containing tissue or in suspension [56]. The goal is to be able to induce these cells via tailored media to mature in vitro to produce viable sperm that may be used in intracytoplasmic sperm injection during in vitro fertilization in the future [57]. While there have been successful animal models described, no live human births have been reported using this technique, and the recommendation is to only pursue this option under an IRB-approved protocol [43].

Attitudes and Psychosocial Complexities

Research on attitudes toward fertility and parenthood goals in the transgender community is emerging. The literature to date portrays the adult transgender population as heterogeneous with regard to parenting goals and acceptance of reproductive technologies [13, 58], though significant percentages of transgender individuals do express a desire for biological children [9–13]. For instance, Wierckx and colleagues reported responses from a questionnaire completed by 50 transgender men (mean age = 37) who had undergone gender-affirming surgery [10]. Of the 39 participants who were not parents already, 54% reported wanting to have children; this study did not distinguish between ways of becoming a parent (biological children versus adoption, for example). Approximately 37.5% of respondents reported that they would have considered freezing their germ cells if that had been an option for them [10]. Another survey was conducted among 160 transgender or gender diverse adults (26.9% described their gender identity as male, 51.5% described their gender identity as female, and 21.6% characterized their gender in a variety of ways that were classified as gender diverse) [59]. Approximately 25% of respondents were already parents at the time of survey completion, with the majority having children prior to transitioning (59%) [59]. Eighteen percent of participants without children reported a desire to have children in the future (29% were unsure); of these, a higher percentage of identified males indicated a desire to have children (53%) than identified females (33%) or gender diverse (14%) participants. Younger respondents were more likely to express a desire for future parenthood and only 4 reported a desire to give birth [59]. In a recent survey of 99 transgender women and 90 transgender men, 70% of transgender women and 47% of transgender men wanted children in the future; 76% of each group said that they had thought about FP but less than 10% had completed FP [13].

Von Doussa and colleagues conducted qualitative interviews and found that prevailing notions of family and parenthood impacted respondents' own vision of options, and they tended to create families in less traditional ways (e.g., becoming step or foster parents) [12]. Some participant responses suggested misgivings about the lack of ability to be a biological parent, with one transgender man reporting feelings of "regret" about engaging in a physical transition without adequate counseling about fertility options [12]. Another recent study showed attitudinal differences between adult transgender men ($n = 24$) and women ($n = 8$), all childless but reporting a desire to become parents at a future point [11]. Transgender men more often reported a desire to become a parent by means of sexual intercourse or pregnancy (58.3%), while 75% of transgender women reported preferring to become a parent through adoption [11]. These results are noteworthy in light of the extra burden of cost, duration, and invasiveness associated with FP interventions for transgender men (birth-assigned females), which could conflict with their desires and parenthood goals.

In addition to this research involving transgender adults, recent studies have begun to investigate attitudes toward fertility in transgender youth. Consistent with adults, youth responses depict some attitudinal heterogeneity, with a subset of transgender youth expressing a desire for future biological children. For instance, Chen and colleagues conducted an online survey of sexual and gender minority teens aged 14–17 years, finding that 25% of transgender youth respondents expressed a desire for biological parenthood (as opposed to 43.8% of gender diverse or non-binary participants) [60]. Nevertheless, approximately 60% indicated a wish for more information related to fertility, with a minority of youth (13.5%) reporting having ever had a conversation with healthcare providers about the impact of hormones on fertility [60]. Strang and colleagues also examined transgender youth and parent attitudes toward fertility of those attending a gender clinic using a survey methodology [61]. Their results (similar to Chen et al.), indicated that about one quarter of transgender adolescents aspired to be a biological parent in the future, and slightly more than half expressed a wish to be a future parent through some means; one-third of respondents expressed uncertainty about parenthood goals [60, 61]. Notably, many of the TGD youth acknowledged that their parenthood goals may change in the future [61]. These attitudes are somewhat inconsistent with actual levels of FP utilization, with two recent retrospective reviews showing that less than 5% of youth receiving hormonal interventions opt for FP [62, 63].

As of yet, the factors that impact parenthood goals, and actual FP utilization, have not been systematically examined. Preliminary findings point to a number of barriers to FP, including social/cultural/family norms and expectations, inadequate counseling, desire to be a parent through alternate means (e.g., adoption), as well as cost, invasiveness, and gender dysphoria [12, 60, 62]. None of the studies on attitudes toward parenthood in youth or adults explored the possible interaction of mental health co-occurrences and parenthood desire; yet, numerous studies find the risks of a variety of psychological diagnoses, as well as suicidality, to be elevated in many transgender youth [64, 65]. Gender-affirming interventions are associated with alleviation of mental health morbidities [66], and therefore, delaying such intervention could be harmful to TGD youth and contraindicated in some circumstances when the anticipated negative ramifications of postponing intervention are significant. On the other hand, as Nahata et al. suggest, mental health concerns have the potential to impact perspectives, desires, goals, and future thinking [62]. For instance, youth with low self-worth may not have the ability to imagine being a competent parent, and thoughts of suicide may be inconsistent with contemplation of future desires. Research suggests that for many transgender individuals, gender dysphoria dissipates with gender-affirming medical treatments. As mental health status improves, perspectives on fertility and parenthood may evolve. In addition, normative perspectives on parenting likely modify with development from adolescence to young adulthood. However, as of yet, research has not examined stability and change in parenthood goals over time in transgender individuals, integrating developmental and psychosocial perspectives, which is an important priority for future research.

Ethical Considerations

Numerous ethical complexities are associated with medical treatments that have the potential to diminish fertility and/or cause infertility in TGD youth, and these issues are increasingly recognized [67–69]. These include the ability of youth to adequately engage in medical decision-making, parental legal rights to make decisions on behalf of their children's best interest, healthcare provider obligations to counsel about fertility even if they are aware that access to FP interventions may be blocked due to cost, the impact of mental-health distress and body dysphoria on decision-making, and cultural and parental wishes and values that may subtly or overtly impact adolescents beliefs and choices.

A significant body of literature addresses adolescent judgment and decision-making [70, 71]. Studies have examined adolescent cognitive capacities versus adult counterparts (how they think) as well as psychosocial differences between adolescents and adults. In general, findings suggest that logical abilities are generally mature by the age of 16 years. Reproductive health frameworks in the United States have recognized adolescents as competent to assent or consent to various important reproductive health decisions such as contraception, STI testing and treatment, as well as abortion and/or substance use [72]; although laws regarding confidentiality and consent with pediatric populations vary across states in the United States, in all states, minors are able to consent to sexually transmitted infection testing and interventions. The American Academy of Pediatrics (AAP) has also published guidelines on informed consent and decision-making in pediatrics, supporting appropriateness of providing care for a child's needs even if incompatible with parental desires [73]. This is important, as recent research suggests that TGD youth may feel pressured to have biological children and/or feel that they are disappointing their parents if they decide against this option [61]. It is important to ensure that parents remain focused on their youth's perspective and needs, while acknowledging their own concerns and sometimes grief about not having biological grandchildren, understanding that refusing GAH for a clearly asserted TGD individual is not a neutral option and can be associated with poorer mental health outcomes [61].

The AAP also provides a nuanced view of adolescent decision-making capacity, noting that the determination of maturity is not always straightforward, although capacity "is presumed but may be rebutted at age 14 or older" [73]. An element of reproductive decision-making and judgment involves non-cognitive abilities, and the broad characteristics of responsibility (self-reliance; independence), perspective (consideration of context), and temperance (thinking before acting), with researchers concluding that adolescents perform significantly worse than adults in these latter, non-cognitive realms, although there is variability within youth [71]. The AAP also notes that the prefrontal cortex, associated with executive function and risk-taking, is still developing in adolescents, possibly impacting decision-making. Normative decisional differences between adolescents and adults may be compounded by mental health distress and/or developmental differences, when present [74]. It is unclear as to how this might impact decision-making regarding fertility in TGD youth. As noted above, available research indicates that TGD youth receiving gender-affirming medical care experience improved mental health. Nevertheless, there is a disparity between reported low rates of FP utilization in youth [62, 63] and increased rates of reported desires for biological children reported among transgender adults [9–11, 13]. This highlights a need for further research into possible sources of this discrepancy. Given the potentially enduring implications of rejecting FP, decisional regret could result if counseling is inadequate or if youth are unable to anticipate their adult parenthood goals, issues that could equally apply to all adolescents with potentially fertility-impacting treatments (e.g., oncology patients), although more research is needed. Counseling may need to account for possible perspective limitations and the potential for impulsive responding, and both assess for and balance these concerns with the possible risks of delaying TGD youth gender-affirming medical care. As of yet, we lack a thorough understanding of best counseling practices for adolescents in the setting of desire for medical intervention and psychological distress of gender dysphoria, the benefits of affirming therapies and the unique perspectives that TGD youth may have in comparison to their cisgender counterparts. In addition, research thus far has examined decision-making and judgment in cisgender adolescents, but has yet to investigate whether similar impulsive tendencies are also found in TGD youth.

The ethical issues involving younger children in the early stages of puberty are no less profound. Puberty blockers enable youth to function in alignment with an affirmed gender, without progression through a distressing, biologically programmed puberty at odds with their gender identity. Nevertheless, because established FP options are unavailable at this stage, parents are in the position of needing to make a choice to support their child's gender identity and minimize dysphoria, or preserve fertility while possibly placing their child at psychological risk. In other instances, parent and child wishes may clash [69], and children may feel compelled to go along with parental desires to preserve fertility due to psychological factors such as guilt and desire to please, or more concrete factors such as financial dependence on parents for medical treatments. In other scenarios, youth who opt for expensive FP interventions may ultimately feel compelled to have a biological child, given the cost incurred to their families. A thorough understanding of ethical issues should help inform best practices so that, ultimately, TGD individuals feel comfortable with their choices and parents who are assisting them in this complex decision-making process feel supported.

Financial Considerations

Due to the wide range of FP options available, cost can vary greatly and potentially serve as a significant barrier for gender diverse youth and their families trying to access FP, especially given the fact that insurance coverage of FP in the United States is often lacking [75, 76]. FP and assisted reproductive technology costs may vary widely between centers and regions, so the following ranges are just estimates. Sperm cryopreservation is the least expensive option, generally ranging from $500 to $1500 for initial processing with yearly storage fees of $300–$500, assuming that a sample can be provided by masturbation [39]. If EEJ or TESE/TESA is required to retrieve a semen sample, procedural costs need to be considered; this can range from $1000 to $10,000. For birth-assigned females, the financial burden associated with oocyte retrieval is significantly higher, with the procedure costing anywhere from $5000 to $20,000 in addition to annual storage fees of $300–$500 for continued cryopreservation [39, 77]. The cost for future fertility therapeutics involving using preserved oocytes are estimated to cost approximately $10,000 [39]. The costs of experimental options vary between institutions and regions.

As science and technologies improve, it is hopeful that there will be more FP options that will be more easily integrated into gender-affirming care. Additionally, policy and insurers may adopt more trans-affirming policies that offer fertility coverage. In Rhode Island, legislation was signed that protects medically induced fertility. While this bill was passed with oncology patients in mind, this bill could also offer expanded insurance coverage and protections for TGD persons seeking fertility preservation.

It is important to remember that families of TGD youth, without even considering FP, are many times facing large out-of-pocket expenses for hormones, as coverage of these therapies is often denied or only partially paid for by insurance companies [65]. That being said, each patient and family deserves a comprehensive discussion surrounding FP. Informed consent to start GAH or surgery requires a thorough discussion about known and unknown fertility outcomes with TGD youth. Studies in oncology have shown higher overall satisfaction with care when FP is discussed and offered prior to starting gonadotoxic therapy [78]. Recently, several states have introduced legislature to mandate FP coverage for individuals undergoing gonadotoxic therapy [79].

Conclusions and Future Directions

The long-term impact of partially irreversible hormonal interventions, estradiol and testosterone, on future fertility remains poorly understood. As with patients using GnRHa for precocious puberty, there is no reason to suspect that TGD youth who start puberty blockers, but return to their endogenous hormones and birth-assigned gender would suffer any adverse or end effects of adult fertility.

For partially reversible GAH, research continues to grow that looks at FP options. At present, TGD youth and adults are generally limited to established methods that are low-risk and known to be effective [39]. Most of the current data guiding FP practices in TGD youth are derived from either studies in transgender adults or the pediatric oncology population, leaving many opportunities for research in gender diverse youth and how their needs and perspectives on FP may differ. Distress associated with gender dysphoria and other mental health comorbidities, urgency to start hormone therapy, and financial barriers could all play roles in lower FP utilization in this group [62, 63, 65], but there may be other factors specific to the transgender population that may influence their decision to forego FP prior to starting hormones.

Despite these knowledge gaps, clinical guidelines emphasize the importance of FP counseling for TGD youth prior to the partially irreversible medical and more permanent surgical interventions that may impact fertility [14, 15]. Counseling regarding parenthood goals can take place individually for each adolescent and young adult, including information about FP options as well as diverse ways to parent and build family over time for interested patients [60, 62]. Presenting current data and allowing adequate time for processing and decision-making could improve patient satisfaction and the quality of care being delivered. Physicians and mental health professionals involved in TGD patient care can offer counseling that incorporates decision-making about FP as they review both the benefits and risks of starting GAH. Mental health professionals experienced in working with TGD can also offer support, resources, and information for youth and parents to design a plan that best fits each individual. Gender-affirming consent-based care requires that we should offer a thorough explanation of FP options as a standard of care when starting gender-affirming therapies that may or may not impact future fertility. The benefits of GAH supporting more immediate and sometimes life-threatening gender needs can be incorporated as appropriate so that TGD youth and families understand that providers are working toward providing the fullest array of family-building options for the future.

References

1. Spack NP, Edwards-Leeper L, Feldman HA, Leibowitz S, Mandel F, Diamond DA, et al. Children and adolescents with gender identity disorder referred to a pediatric medical center. Pediatrics. 2012;129(3):418–25.
2. Aitken M, Steensma TD, Blanchard R, VanderLaan DP, Wood H, Fuentes A, et al. Evidence for an altered sex ratio in clinic-referred adolescents with gender dysphoria. J Sex Med. 2015;12(3):756–63.
3. Hudson MM, Ness KK, Gurney JG, Mulrooney DA, Chemaitilly W, Krull KR, et al. Clinical ascertainment of health outcomes among adults treated for childhood cancer. JAMA. 2013;309(22):2371–81.
4. Chow EJ, Stratton KL, Leisenring WM, Oeffinger KC, Sklar CA, Donaldson SS, et al. Pregnancy after chemotherapy in male and female survivors of childhood cancer treated between 1970 and 1999: a report from the childhood cancer survivor study cohort. Lancet Oncol. 2016;17(5):567–76.
5. Johnson EK, Finlayson C, Rowell EE, Gosiengfiao Y, Pavone ME, Lockart B, et al. Fertility preservation for pediatric patients: current state and future possibilities. J Urol. 2017;198:186.
6. Nahata L, Quinn GP, Tishelman AC, Section On E. Counseling in pediatric populations at risk for infertility and/or sexual function concerns. Pediatrics. 2018;142(2):pii: e20181435.
7. Stein DM, Victorson DE, Choy JT, Waimey KE, Pearman TP, Smith K, et al. Fertility preservation preferences and perspectives among adult male survivors of pediatric cancer and their parents. J Adolesc Young Adult Oncol. 2014;3(2):75–82.
8. Armuand GM, Wettergren L, Rodriguez-Wallberg KA, Lampic C. Desire for children, difficulties achieving a pregnancy, and infertility distress 3 to 7 years after cancer diagnosis. Support Care Cancer. 2014;22(10):2805–12.
9. De Sutter P, Kira K, Verschoor A, Hotimsky A. The desire to have children and the 101 preservation of fertility in transsexual women: a survey. Int J Transgenderism. 2002;6(3):97–03.
10. Wierckx K, Van Caenegem E, Pennings G, Elaut E, Dedecker D, Van de Peer F, et al. Reproductive wish in transsexual men. Hum Reprod. 2012;27(2):483–7.
11. Tornello SL, Bos H. Parenting intentions among transgender individuals. LGBT Health. 2017;4(2):115–20.
12. von Doussa H, Power J, Riggs D. Imagining parenthood: the possibilities and experiences of parenthood among transgender people. Cult Health Sex. 2015;17(9):1119–31.
13. Auer MK, Fuss J, Nieder TO, Briken P, Biedermann SV, Stalla GK, et al. Desire to have children among transgender people in Germany: a cross-sectional multi-center study. J Sex Med. 2018;15(5):757–67.
14. Coleman E, Bockting W, Botzer M, Cohen-Kettenis P, DeCuypere G, Feldman J, et al. Standards of care for the health of transsexual, transgender, and gender-nonconforming people, version 7. Int J Transgenderism. 2012;13(4):165–232.

15. Hembree WC, Cohen-Kettenis PT, Gooren L, Hannema SE, Meyer WJ, Murad MH, et al. Endocrine treatment of gender-dysphoric/gender-incongruent persons: an endocrine society clinical practice guideline. J Clin Endocrinol Metab. 2017;102(11):3869–903.
16. Ethics Committee of the American Society for Reproductive M. Access to fertility services by transgender persons: an ethics committee opinion. Fertil Steril. 2015;104(5):1111–5.
17. Chen M, Eugster EA. Central precocious puberty: update on diagnosis and treatment. Pediatr Drugs. 2015;17(4):273–81.
18. Neely EK, Lee PA, Bloch CA, Larsen L, Yang D, Mattia-Goldberg C, et al. Leuprolide acetate 1-month depot for central precocious puberty: hormonal suppression and recovery. Int J Pediatr Endocrinol. 2011;2010(1):398639.
19. Schagen SE, Cohen-Kettenis PT, Delemarre-van de Waal HA, Hannema SE. Efficacy and safety of gonadotropin-releasing hormone agonist treatment to suppress puberty in gender dysphoric adolescents. J Sex Med. 2016;13(7):1125–32.
20. De Roo C, Lierman S, Tilleman K, Peynshaert K, Braeckmans K, Caanen M, et al. Ovarian tissue cryopreservation in female-to-male transgender people: insights into ovarian histology and physiology after prolonged androgen treatment. Reprod Biomed Online. 2017;34(6):557–66.
21. Spinder T, Spijkstra JJ, van den Tweel JG, Burger CW, van Kessel H, Hompes PG, et al. The effects of long term testosterone administration on pulsatile luteinizing hormone secretion and on ovarian histology in eugonadal female to male transsexual subjects. J Clin Endocrinol Metab. 1989;69(1):151–7.
22. Ikeda K, Baba T, Noguchi H, Nagasawa K, Endo T, Kiya T, et al. Excessive androgen exposure in female-to-male transsexual persons of reproductive age induces hyperplasia of the ovarian cortex and stroma but not polycystic ovary morphology. Hum Reprod. 2013;28(2):453–61.
23. Baba T, Endo T, Honnma H, Kitajima Y, Hayashi T, Ikeda H, et al. Association between polycystic ovary syndrome and female-to-male transsexuality. Hum Reprod. 2007;22(4):1011–6.
24. Hunter MH, Sterrett JJ. Polycystic ovary syndrome: it's not just infertility. Am Fam Physician. 2000;62(5):1079–88.
25. Light AD, Obedin-Maliver J, Sevelius JM, Kerns JL. Transgender men who experienced pregnancy after female-to-male gender transitioning. Obstet Gynecol. 2014;124(6):1120–7.
26. Finer LB, Zolna MR. Declines in unintended pregnancy in the United States, 2008–2011. N Engl J Med. 2016;374(9):843–52.
27. Gabrilove JL, Nicolis GL, Mitty HA, Sohval AR. Feminizing interstitial cell tumor of the testis: personal observations and a review of the literature. Cancer. 1975;35(4):1184–202.
28. Oshima H, Sarada T, Ochiai K, Tamaoki B. Effects of a synthetic estrogen upon steroid bioconversion in vitro in testes of patients with prostatic cancer. Investig Urol. 1974;12(1):43–9.
29. Schneider F, Kliesch S, Schlatt S, Neuhaus N. Andrology of male-to-female transsexuals: influence of cross-sex hormone therapy on testicular function. Andrology. 2017;5(5):873–80.
30. Schulze C. Response of the human testis to long-term estrogen treatment: morphology of sertoli cells, leydig cells and spermatogonial stem cells. Cell Tissue Res. 1988;251(1):31–43.
31. Thiagaraj D, Gunasegaram R, Loganath A, Peh KL, Kottegoda SR, Ratnam SS. Histopathology of the testes from male transsexuals on oestrogen therapy. Ann Acad Med Singap. 1987;16(2):347–8.
32. Leavy M, Trottmann M, Liedl B, Reese S, Stief C, Freitag B, et al. Effects of elevated beta-estradiol levels on the functional morphology of the testis – new insights. Sci Rep. 2017;7:39931.
33. Schneider F, Neuhaus N, Wistuba J, Zitzmann M, Hess J, Mahler D, et al. Testicular functions and clinical characterization of patients with gender dysphoria (GD) undergoing sex reassignment surgery (SRS). J Sex Med. 2015;12(11):2190–200.
34. Ethics Committee of American Society for Reproductive Medicine. Fertility preservation and reproduction in patients facing gonadotoxic therapies: a committee opinion. Fertil Steril. 2013;100(5):1224–31.
35. Oktay K, Bedoschi G. Oocyte cryopreservation for fertility preservation in postpubertal female children at risk for premature ovarian failure due to accelerated follicle loss in turner syndrome or cancer treatments. J Pediatr Adolesc Gynecol. 2014;27(6):342–6.

36. Practice Committees of American Society for Reproductive M, Society for Assisted Reproductive T. Mature oocyte cryopreservation: a guideline. Fertil Steril. 2013;99(1):37–43.
37. Practice Committee of American Society for Reproductive M. Ovarian tissue cryopreservation: a committee opinion. Fertil Steril. 2014;101(5):1237–43.
38. McCracken K, Nahata L. Fertility preservation in children and adolescents: current options and considerations. Curr Opin Obstet Gynecol. 2017;29:283.
39. Nahata L, Chen D, Moravek MB, Quinn GP, Sutter ME, Taylor J, Tishelman AC, Gomez-Lobo V. Understudied and under-reported: fertility issues in transgender youth—a narrative review. J Pediatr. 2019;205:265–71.
40. Donnez J, Dolmans MM. Ovarian cortex transplantation: 60 reported live births brings the success and worldwide expansion of the technique towards routine clinical practice. J Assist Reprod Genet. 2015;32(8):1167–70.
41. Jensen AK, Macklon KT, Fedder J, Ernst E, Humaidan P, Andersen CY. 86 successful births and 9 ongoing pregnancies worldwide in women transplanted with frozen-thawed ovarian tissue: focus on birth and perinatal outcome in 40 of these children. J Assist Reprod Genet. 2017;34(3):325–36.
42. Donnelly L. Woman gives birth to baby using ovary frozen in her childhood in 'world first'. The Telegraph. 2016.
43. Oktay K, Harvey BE, Partridge AH, Quinn GP, Reinecke J, Taylor HS, et al. Fertility preservation in patients with cancer: ASCO clinical practice guideline update. J Clin Oncol. 2018;36:1994–2001. https://doi.org/10.1200/JCO.2018.78.1914.
44. Demeestere I, Simon P, Dedeken L, Moffa F, Tsépélidis S, Brachet C, et al. Live birth after autograft of ovarian tissue cryopreserved during childhood. Hum Reprod. 2015;30(9):2107–9.
45. Ladanyi C, Mor A, Christianson MS, Dhillon N, Segars JH. Recent advances in the field of ovarian tissue cryopreservation and opportunities for research. J Assist Reprod Genet. 2017;34(6):709–22.
46. Vadaparampil S, Quinn G, King L, Wilson C, Nieder M. Barriers to fertility preservation among pediatric oncologists. Patient Educ Couns. 2008;72(3):402–10.
47. Chapple A, Salinas M, Ziebland S, McPherson A, Macfarlane A. Fertility issues: the perceptions and experiences of young men recently diagnosed and treated for cancer. J Adolesc Health. 2007;40(1):69–75.
48. Crawshaw MA, Glaser AW, Hale JP, Sloper P. Young males' experiences of sperm banking following a cancer diagnosis – a qualitative study. Hum Fertil. 2008;11(4):238–45.
49. Crawshaw MA, Glaser AW, Pacey AA. The use of pornographic materials by adolescent male cancer patients when banking sperm in the UK: legal and ethical dilemmas. Hum Fertil. 2007;10(3):159–63.
50. Klosky JL, Wang F, Russell KM, Zhang H, Flynn JS, Huang L, et al. Prevalence and predictors of sperm banking in adolescents newly diagnosed with cancer: examination of adolescent, parent, and provider factors influencing fertility preservation outcomes. J Clin Oncol. 2017;35:3830–6. https://doi.org/10.1200/JCO.2016.70.4767.
51. Adank MC, van Dorp W, Smit M, van Casteren NJ, Laven JS, Pieters R, et al. Electroejaculation as a method of fertility preservation in boys diagnosed with cancer: a single-center experience and review of the literature. Fertil Steril. 2014;102(1):199–205.e1.
52. Moss JL, Choi AW, Fitzgerald Keeter MK, Brannigan RE. Male adolescent fertility preservation. Fertil Steril. 2016;105(2):267–73.
53. Keene DJ, Sajjad Y, Makin G, Cervellione RM. Sperm banking in the United Kingdom is feasible in patients 13 years old or older with cancer. J Urol. 2012;188(2):594–7.
54. Hagenas I, Jorgensen N, Rechnitzer C, Sommer P, Holm M, Schmiegelow K, et al. Clinical and biochemical correlates of successful semen collection for cryopreservation from 12-18-year-old patients: a single-center study of 86 adolescents. Hum Reprod. 2010;25(8):2031–8.
55. Wyns C, Collienne C, Shenfield F, Robert A, Laurent P, Roegiers L, et al. Fertility preservation in the male pediatric population: factors influencing the decision of parents and children. Hum Reprod. 2015;30(9):2022–30.
56. Wyns C, Curaba M, Vanabelle B, Van Langendonckt A, Donnez J. Options for fertility preservation in prepubertal boys. Hum Reprod Update. 2010;16(3):312–28.

57. Gassei K, Orwig KE. Experimental methods to preserve male fertility and treat male factor infertility. Fertil Steril. 2016;105(2):256–66.
58. M Russell A, Galvin KM, Harper MM, Clayman ML. A comparison of heterosexual and LGBTQ cancer survivors' outlooks on relationships, family building, possible infertility, and patient-doctor fertility risk communication. J Cancer Surviv. 2016;10(5):935–42.
59. Riggs DW, Power J, von Doussa H. Parenting and Australian trans and gender diverse people: an exploratory survey. Int J Transgenderism. 2016;17(2):59–65.
60. Chen D, Matson M, Macapagal K, Johnson EK, Rosoklija I, Finlayson C, et al. Attitudes toward fertility and reproductive health among transgender and gender-nonconforming adolescents. J Adolesc Health. 2018;63:62.
61. Strang JF, Jarin J, Call D, Clark B, Wallace GL, Anthony LG, et al. Transgender youth fertility attitudes questionnaire: measure development in nonautistic and autistic transgender youth and their parents. J Adolesc Health. 2018;62:128–35.
62. Nahata L, Tishelman AC, Caltabellotta NM, Quinn GP. Low fertility preservation utilization among transgender youth. J Adolesc Health. 2017;61:40.
63. Chen D, Simons L, Johnson EK, Lockart BA, Finlayson C. Fertility preservation for transgender adolescents. J Adolesc Health. 2017;61:120.
64. Reisner SL, Vetters R, Leclerc M, Zaslow S, Wolfrum S, Shumer D, et al. Mental health of transgender youth in care at an adolescent urban community health center: a matched retrospective cohort study. J Adolesc Health. 2015;56(3):274–9.
65. Nahata L, Quinn GP, Caltabellotta NM, Tishelman AC. Mental health concerns and insurance denials among transgender adolescents. LGBT Health. 2017;4:188–93.
66. de Vries AL, McGuire JK, Steensma TD, Wagenaar EC, Doreleijers TA, Cohen-Kettenis PT. Young adult psychological outcome after puberty suppression and gender reassignment. Pediatrics. 2014;134(4):696–704.
67. Hudson J, Nahata L, Dietz E, Quinn GP. Fertility counseling for transgender AYAs. Clin Pract Pediatr Psychol. 2018;6(1):84–92.
68. Chen D, Simons L. Ethical considerations in fertility preservation for transgender youth: a case illustration. Clin Pract Pediatr Psychol. 2018;6(1):93–100.
69. Nahata L, Campo-Engelstein LT, Tishelman A, Quinn GP, Lantos JD. Fertility preservation for a transgender teenager. Pediatrics. 2018;142:pii: e20173142.
70. Steinberg L, Cauffman E. Maturity of judgment in adolescence: psychosocial factors in adolescent decision making. Law Hum Behav. 1996;20(3):249–72.
71. Cauffman E, Steinberg L. (Im)maturity of judgment in adolescence: why adolescents may be less culpable than adults. Behav Sci Law. 2000;18(6):741–60.
72. Marcell AV, Burstein GR, Committee OA. Sexual and reproductive health care services in the pediatric setting. Pediatrics. 2017;140(5):e20172858.
73. Katz AL, Webb SA, Committee OB. Informed consent in decision-making in pediatric practice. Pediatrics. 2016;138(2):pii: e20161485.
74. Shumer DE, Reisner SL, Edwards-Leeper L, Tishelman A. Evaluation of asperger syndrome in youth presenting to a gender dysphoria clinic. LGBT Health. 2016;3(5):387–90.
75. Mersereau JE, Goodman LR, Deal AM, Gorman JR, Whitcomb BW, Su HI. To preserve or not to preserve: how difficult is the decision about fertility preservation? Cancer. 2013;119(22):4044–50.
76. Cardozo ER, Huber WJ, Stuckey AR, Alvero RJ. Mandating coverage for fertility preservation – a step in the right direction. N Engl J Med. 2017;377(17):1607–9.
77. Levine J, Stern CJ. Fertility preservation in adolescents and young adults with cancer. J Clin Oncol. 2010;28(32):4831–41.
78. Kelvin JF, Thom B, Benedict C, Carter J, Corcoran S, Dickler MN, et al. Cancer and fertility program improves patient satisfaction with information received. J Clin Oncol. 2016;34(15):1780–6.
79. Alliance for Fertility Preservation [cited 2017]. Available from: http://www.alliancefortertilitypreservation.org/advocacy/state-legislation.

16 Gender-Affirming Surgical Care

Vikram G. Mookerjee, Jonathan P. Brower, and Daniel Kwan

Transgender and gender diverse (TGD) individuals may pursue several gender-affirming therapies, including integrating changes in gender expression and role, individual and group-based psychotherapy and counseling, and hormone therapy. Gender-affirming surgery (GAS) often represents the final step in this spectrum, and even minor alterations can lead to profound improvements in patients' self-esteem and functioning [1]. It is difficult to accurately estimate the frequency of GAS prior to the passage of newer laws supporting insurance coverage for some of these procedures. Nevertheless, the number of patients seeking surgical intervention continues to increase dramatically every year, with prior investigations demonstrating a nearly three-fold increase over the past several decades [2, 3].

Recent groundbreaking research published by Canner et al. is the first of its kind to broadly evaluate national temporal trends in gender-affirming surgery in the United States [4]. Their findings demonstrate that among patients undergoing these procedures in the United States, an increasing proportion is pursuing genital surgery, which represents the most complex surgical treatment for gender dysphoria. Moreover, the percentage of patients who sought gender-affirming surgery covered by Medicare or Medicaid increased by threefold from 2012–2013 to 2014 [4]. As coverage for these procedures continues to increase, so too will demand for qualified surgeons to perform them. It is increasingly important for all members of a multidisciplinary care team to understand the indications, risks, and benefits of surgical intervention.

Surgery in the TGD youth population is a subject of great controversy. Most longitudinal studies of adult patients who have undergone gender-affirmation procedures have found high satisfaction rates with low rates of regret (1% or less) [5]. Initial studies evaluating gender-affirming surgery for TGD youth provide

V. G. Mookerjee (✉) · J. P. Brower · D. Kwan
Department of Plastic Surgery, Rhode Island Hospital, Alpert Medical School of Brown University, Providence, RI, USA

M. Forcier et al. (eds.), *Pediatric Gender Identity*,
https://doi.org/10.1007/978-3-030-38909-3_16

similarly high satisfaction and infrequent regret [6]. However, when regret does occur, it is surgically challenging and costly to address [7]. These considerations are magnified in a youth population, especially in the case of surgical procedures that limit future fertility or are technically irreversible. It is difficult to forecast future fertility goals, which are inherently stochastic, and many patients' goals will change from adolescence to adulthood. Further confounding the issue is the emerging concept of dynamic gender presentations, in which some transgender youth can experience both transition and subsequent "de-transition" from an affirmed gender identity [8]. Finally, these cautions must be balanced with patient-centered care that would necessarily incorporate means of relieving dysphoria, affirming bodily congruence and autonomy, and addressing health and safety risks inherent in untreated gender dysphoria. As with any medical care, declining to provide or consent to care by clinicians and parents is, in itself, a decision that may result in harm for certain TGD patients.

Figures 16.1 and 16.2 summarize the most common procedures available for patients seeking GAS. However, it is important to note that GAS is a dynamic space that continues to evolve, and there is significant heterogeneity across different surgeons, hospitals, and institutions with respect to how and when these procedures are performed. Many procedures, particularly those targeting the face and the urogenital system, are performed in coordination with other surgical teams, such as otolaryngology, urology, and obstetrics and gynecology. The specialties performing each surgical procedure can vary significantly based on local practice patterns within the health system through which care is provided.

From the patient's perspective, it can be difficult to learn about surgical options. There is a paucity of standardized literature for patient information and existing online resources for GAS lack readability and quality [9, 10]. Thus, primary care and mental health providers have the unique opportunity to interface between patients and surgeons available to participate in their care.

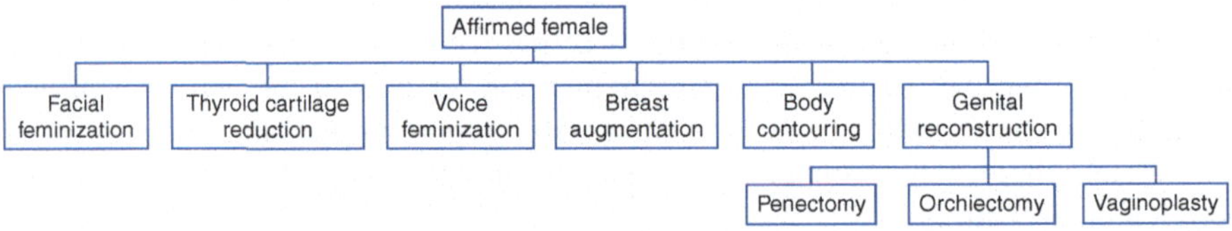

Fig. 16.1 Gender-affirming surgical options for asserted female patients

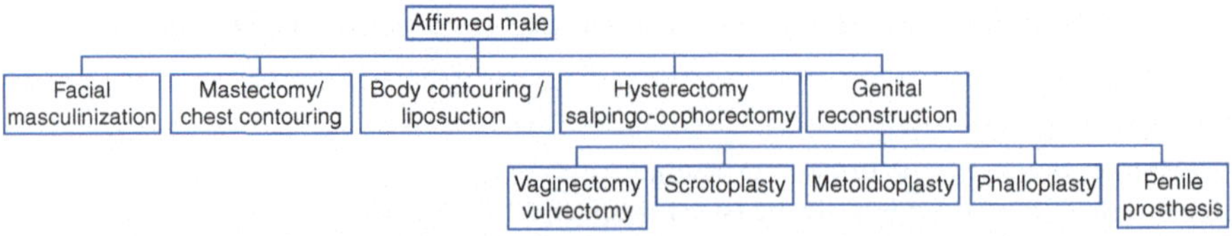

Fig. 16.2 Gender-affirming surgical options for asserted male patients

It is not the responsibility of primary care and mental health providers to understand the intricacies of each surgical procedure. Rather, these practitioners play the important role of providing accurate and reliable basic information regarding GAS and subsequently referring appropriate individuals to surgeons for more thorough discussion and rigorous evaluation. Primary care and mental health providers should also maintain an open and informed dialogue with patients not yet ready for surgery, such that a surgical referral is made at the appropriate time. It is important to note that patient selection for surgery is a shared responsibility of the entire multidisciplinary team, and communication among all team members is essential.

Surgical procedures can be broadly categorized into three domains:

1. Breast/chest or "top" surgery
2. Genital or "bottom" surgery
3. Non-breast/chest, non-genital surgery (such as facial feminization/masculinization, voice surgery, thyroid cartilage reduction, liposuction/lipoaugmentation, and various other aesthetic procedures)

Though there are no universal medical, legal, or ethical requirements for the performance of these procedures, the guidelines outlined in the World Professional Association for Transgender Health (WPATH) Standards of Care (Figs. 16.3 and 16.4) are often used as reference. These guidelines include the recommendation for 12 months of hormonal therapy prior to surgical intervention. This guideline is based on expert opinion; there are no data to suggest significant benefits or improved outcomes with the recommended 12-month waiting period of hormonal use prior to feminizing top surgery or feminizing/masculinizing bottom surgery. Additionally, there are a growing number of nonbinary patients who do not request or require gender-affirming hormones (GAH) to support their gender identity, but may request top surgery or suppression of menses as part of their unique gender expression.

For mastectomy and creation of a male chest in affirmed male patients, or for breast augmentation* (implants/lipoaugmentation) in affirmed female patients:

1. Persistent, well-documented gender dysphoria;
2. Capacity to make a fully informed decision and to consent for treatment;
3. Age of majority in a given country (if younger, follow the standard of care for children and adolescents);
4. If significant medical or mental health concerns are present, they must be reasonably well controlled.

*Recommended: minimum 12 months of feminizing hormone therapy prior to surgery (although some affirmed women seek breast implants prior to any hormone therapy).

Fig. 16.3 Criteria for top surgery (one referral). (Source: *The World Professional Association for Transgender Health, Standards of Care for the Health of Transsexual, Transgender, and Gender Nonconforming People, 7th version*)

For hysterectomy and oophorectomy in affirmed male patients and for orchiectomy in affirmed female patients:

1. Persistent, well-documented gender dysphoria
2. Capacity to make a fully informed decision and to consent for treatment;
3. Age of majority in a given country (if younger, follow the standard of care for children and adolescents);
4. If significant medical or mental health concerns are present, they must be reasonably well controlled.
5. 12 continuous months of hormone therapy as appropriate to the patient's gender goals (unless the patient has a medical contraindication or is otherwise unable or unwilling to take hormones).

For metoidioplasty or phalloplasty in affirmed male patients and for vaginoplasty in affirmed female patients:*

1. Persistent, well-documented gender dysphoria
2. Capacity to make a fully informed decision and to consent for treatment;
3. Age of majority in a given country (if younger, follow the standard of care for children and adolescents);
4. If significant medical or mental health concerns are present, they must be reasonably well controlled.
5. 12 continuous months of hormone therapy as appropriate to the patient's gender goals (unless the patient has a medical contraindication or is otherwise unable or unwilling to take hormones).
6. *12 continuous months of living in a gender role that is congruent with their gender identity.*

*Recommended: regular patient visits with a mental health or other medical professional.

Fig. 16.4 Criteria for genital surgery (two referrals). (Source: *The World Professional Association for Transgender Health, Standards of Care for the Health of Transsexual, Transgender, and Gender Nonconforming People, 7th version*)

Once considered rare, surgery among *post*pubescent TGD children is an area of rapid development, especially as related to breast and chest surgery. An important difference between gender dysphoric children and adolescents is in the proportion for whom dysphoria persists into adulthood. Gender dysphoria or a gender diverse presentation in childhood may not continue into adolescence or adulthood [11]. Many earlier studies attempting to measure persistence have methodological flaws that limit their validity. However, regardless of the unknown trajectory for some *pre*pubertal gender diverse children, current recommendations do not support surgical intervention, and in most cases, surgical intervention is not needed at this more androgynous age. Instead, *peri*pubertal patients may benefit from hormone treatments that block pubertal changes, leaving time for further gender exploration.

Early puberty blocking with gonadotropin-releasing hormone agonists (GnRH) is considered completely reversible and offers time to develop a gender identity, articulate dysphoria and/or goals, and establish a realistic and safe affirmation plan (see Chaps. 13 and 14). More importantly, blockers can halt the development of secondary gender phenotypic changes that are considered irreversible (male pattern hair, skeletal structure, cricoid cartilage, and voice changes) and prevent patients from undergoing a puberty that is not congruent with their internal gender identity.

Asserted females who have been taking puberty-blocking drugs such as gonadotropin-releasing hormone agonists (GnRH) and go on to gender-affirming estradiol will lack significant development of the penis, testes, and scrotal tissues. This lack of tissue development will affect construction of a neo-vulva and vagina. For youth who may one day desire bottom surgery, it is important to consider that results of a penile inversion vaginoplasty may be compromised by early puberty blocking, as less of the local donor tissue is developed during puberty.

However, puberty-blocking medicines remain preferable to patients who do not want to experience development discordant with their gender identity. Surgical options will continue to adapt as medical gender-affirming strategies become more common and sophisticated at an early age.

Patients who have advanced to GAH in addition to puberty blockers tend to have improved cosmetic outcomes after undergoing at least one year of GAH before any chest or body contouring procedures. The physiological changes associated with GAH administration, such as weight change, body fat redistribution, and change in muscle mass/gluteal shape, are helpful in achieving optimal long-term aesthetic outcomes from these interventions [12].

The persistence of gender dysphoria or TGD into adulthood appears to be much higher for patients whose symptoms present around the time of, or shortly after, puberty. A study of 70 adolescents who were diagnosed with gender dysphoria and given puberty suppressing hormones demonstrated that all continued into adulthood with the affirmed gender [13]. The Amsterdam cohort of adolescents followed for 30 years into adulthood estimates rates of regret for GAH and GAS to be less than 1% [6]. Although top surgery is classified as an "irreversible intervention" according to the WPATH Standards of Care, it can sometimes be classified as "partially reversible" from a surgical perspective. Asserted males who have had male chest reconstruction may undergo revision to restore female chest contour, albeit without ideal shape or erogenous sensation at the nipple. Similarly, adolescent asserted females can be offered removal of breast implants and re-contouring of the chest should they later desire a more masculine-appearing chest. Regardless, studies of both adults and adolescents continue to support satisfaction, benefit, and lack of regret following a well-considered approach and adequate preparation for GAS [5, 6].

The American Society of Plastic Surgeons recommends that routine cosmetic breast augmentation be performed in patients over the age of 18 [14]. However, there is a population of adolescents, primarily those with congenital or traumatic breast deformities, who undergo breast augmentation at a younger age. Despite the infrequency of aesthetic surgery in adolescents, there are data to suggest that these procedures may yield improvements in body satisfaction, bodily attitude, and appearance-related burdens [15]. When applied to the TGD youth population, the data cautiously support the use of reconstructive breast surgery like gender-affirming breast augmentation to improve body satisfaction among adolescents.

Accordingly, top surgery offered to select adolescent patients can be powerfully therapeutic during a critical period of development. The often-cited minimum age of 18 years is largely dictated by insurance policies and reimbursement requirements rather than outcomes-related data. For many affirmed male youth, maintaining a female chest from the time of breast bud development (average age 10 years) to age 18 may inflict significant harm during the preteen and teenage years. Therefore, adolescents who have thoughtfully and realistically explored their gender goals and affirmation, have persistent and severe dysphoria, demonstrate the maturity to participate in the informed consent process, and have family support are often considered excellent candidates for surgery earlier than age 18. As with all GAS, the decision to proceed with surgery is shared among the patient, family, surgeon, and primary care and mental health providers.

Vaginoplasty surgery in the United States is more uncommon, and it is not currently within the standard of care among youth TGD patients. It is, however, an option for those patients with severe dysphoria, the maturity to consent, and appropriate family support. Procedures that may affect fertility such as orchiectomy or hysterectomy/salpingo-oophorectomy are generally preferable in later adolescence and young adulthood according to current standards. In the Netherlands, where adolescents from age 16 are legally competent to make independent treatment choices, transgender clinics maintain a policy restricting genital surgery to patients age 18 and older [16]. Although Dutch clinicians agree that emotional maturity represents a better criterion than an enforced minimum age, they widely acknowledge that objective criteria do not exist in assessing readiness for genital surgery in adolescents [17]. Unlike chest contour, major genital alterations and the resulting consequences on fertility cannot be reversed.

Regarding surgery of the face, most plastic surgeons prefer waiting until age 18. As the facial skeleton is still developing in adolescence, procedures intended to alter facial features may have unpredictable results, necessitating further surgery with suboptimal aesthetic outcomes. Other nonbreast/chest, nongenital procedures such as liposuction or voice surgery can be judiciously considered in a select portion of the adolescent population whose dysphoria may be significantly alleviated as a result of the procedure. These determinations are to be made by the surgeon on a case-by-case basis to determine optimal timing for the desired result.

Patients receiving hormone therapy who wish to proceed to gender-affirming surgery should be evaluated to determine optimal timing and appropriate candidacy. Sometimes, hormone administration can cause changes in weight and fat distribution. Overweight and obese TGD youth and adults present unique surgical challenges, with worse aesthetic outcomes and higher complication rates. Though no studies have specifically examined overweight TGD surgical patients, there is sufficient evidence pertaining to patients in the general population undergoing body contouring procedures associating obese patients with worse outcomes. In particular, Rubin et al. have demonstrated a near-linear relationship between BMI and postoperative wound-healing complication rates [18].

Importantly, BMI is only one cardiometabolic risk factor and is actually more useful as a proxy for other comorbidities that can affect wound healing such as glucose intolerance and nutritional deficiencies. Surgeons typically prefer that obese patients lose some weight and maintain a lower BMI before undergoing surgery. Weight loss should always be pursued as part of an overall healthier lifestyle. Surgical goals need to be considered within the context of severity of dysphoria and anticipated benefit from removal of physical habitus incongruent with identified gender. It is critical that all providers maintain appropriate and consistent messaging about weight loss in a population that has a greater predisposition for eating disorders. Patients should be supervised by their physician to address and sustain long-term and stable improvements in weight. If a patient is already considering bariatric surgery to treat concomitant morbid obesity, it should be undertaken prior to gender-confirming surgeries if the severity of their dysphoria allows the time. Weight loss with maintenance of a lower BMI will decrease peri- and postoperative surgical risks and yield a superior aesthetic result.

For patients on GAH with a desirable bodyweight and ready for surgery, there are still no data guiding whether or not to hold hormones prior to GAS. Thus, perioperative hormone treatment practices are surgeon and institution specific. Various surgeons have reported continuing hormone therapy as usual, transitioning temporarily to a transdermal route, and holding hormone therapy altogether during the perioperative period. All these strategies are within the standard of care for surgical TGD patients. Exogenous estrogens present a well-known increased risk of perioperative venous thromboembolism (VTE), but the risk is lower now that most patients are no longer taking conjugated equine estrogen. Many surgeons will only restart hormones once patients are ambulating regularly, but these practices are largely enacted empirically.

There is less consensus regarding perioperative testosterone administration. Some centers similarly hold testosterone because of anecdotal associations with either thrombosis or increased bleeding risk. There are no studies to date evaluating clinical outcomes with existing perioperative hormone administration protocols in either cisgender or transgender patients. The decision to hold or continue hormone therapy at the time of surgery is ultimately made at the discretion of the surgeon and primary care provider, with insight from any additional medical providers caring for the patient.

Nicotine cessation is recommended before any surgery. It is well known that active smokers of cigarettes and vaporizers have higher complication rates, particularly in procedures performed by plastic surgeons, owing to the pharmacology of nicotine [19]. An analysis of over 40,000 plastic surgery patients showed that smokers had higher risk of complications, including impaired wound healing, superficial wound infection, and wound dehiscence [20]. For this reason, smoking cessation counseling is a central component of the informed consent process for smokers. The additional risk is so well documented that many plastic surgeons defer elective surgery entirely for active smokers. Nicotine cessation is especially crucial in penile inversion vaginoplasty, in which the large skin graft within the neovagina would likely fail in the setting of active nicotine consumption. At our center, we recommend 2 months nicotine free if the patient is planning to use surgery as an opportunity to quit nicotine use entirely. If the patient does not plan on nicotine cessation, we discuss the increased perioperative risks and weigh it against the benefits of expedited relief of symptoms related to their dysphoria. Though the surgical risks of nicotine exposure are well known, smoking history must be considered within the context of the greater clinical picture, and the overall surgical risks must be outweighed by the expected benefits of the procedure before proceeding with surgery.

It is equally important to ask young patients about marijuana, since more youth consume marijuana than tobacco; in fact, the Centers for Disease Control reports that at least 38% of high school students admit to using marijuana at some point [21]. Long-term marijuana use theoretically increases the risk of surgical complications, though no studies have formally quantified this risk. It is, however, known to increase the risk of respiratory compromise and impaired immune system functioning [22]. Accordingly, marijuana use is considered a relative, but not absolute contraindication to GAS. We prefer that patients attempt to reduce surgical risk by transitioning from smoking or vaping marijuana to edible or sublingual formulations. Consideration of substance use in the context of a patient's gender goals allows providers another opportunity to discuss healthy lifestyles and potentially improve long-term health outcomes.

Surgery is often planned to accommodate school, sports, employment, or other activities. Adolescents may be physically active and involved in team sports. Older teens and young adults who work have to factor finances and employment leave into their decision about timing of surgery. Surgery and adequate recovery time needs to be anticipated with appropriate time allocated for activity restrictions.

Gender-affirming mastectomy and breast augmentation are generally performed in an outpatient day-surgery setting. Chest/breast surgery is usually performed as a single-stage with the exception of breast augmentation, which may require placement of tissue expanders before a permanent breast implant can be safely accommodated. Though patients are usually discharged home shortly after surgery, they typically benefit from some assistance for immediate postoperative care. For example, mastectomies require a surgical drain for a short (1–2 weeks) period. Patients generally wear a compression garment after a mastectomy or a bandeau after breast augmentation. In addition, they are directed to limit athletic activity and perform incision care. These postoperative care plans are generally well tolerated by youth, who additionally benefit from family support.

Orchiectomy and hysterectomy/salpingo-oophorectomy may be undertaken as an outpatient or followed by a brief hospital stay, with postoperative care primarily consisting of activity limitations and incision care. Genital reconstruction, including vaginoplasty and phalloplasty, involves lengthier hospitalization with more demanding postoperative care requirements. For example, patients must perform vaginal dilations after vaginoplasty or maintain catheter care after phalloplasty. In these instances, patients significantly benefit from both the technical assistance and the emotional support provided by a family member.

Sexual function takes time to recover following bottom surgery. It is recommended that patients avoid receptive vaginal and penetrative penile intercourse with a partner for at least 12 weeks, until tissues have healed. Nevertheless, long-term sexual function following bottom surgery is generally satisfactory. Most patients who have undergone vaginoplasty are able to achieve orgasm after surgery and are satisfied with appearance and functionality. Patients who had undergone vaginoplasty are most commonly concerned with the overall frequency of sexual activity, as well as difficulty with lubrication and associated discomfort [23–25]. Similarly, most phalloplasty patients are able to achieve orgasm postoperatively and report overall satisfaction with the results of their surgery [26, 27]. Though a number of patients do report sexual activity prior to surgery, many patients defer becoming sexually active and using their genitals for sex until they achieve an anatomy that is congruent with their gender identity and sexuality. For many young adults, GAS can represent the first step in exploring their own sexuality and sexual development. Importantly, however, GAS does not completely eliminate the previous trauma of living in the wrong body or the impact of that prior experience.

Common complications following surgery are specific to the patient and procedure performed. A seroma or hematoma may develop after any of these procedures, but are more common in chest surgery which involve dissection of a large space. Patients continue to meet with their surgeon at scheduled follow-up appointments after surgery, but these fluid collections often occur in the interim, and patients may present to their surgeon or their primary care provider. Close monitoring around the time of surgery is needed, and if there is a significant collection, drainage in the operating room may be needed. Drains placed at the time of surgery decrease the risk of seroma, but seroma or hematoma can still occur. Other complications include hypertrophic or keloid scar formation. If patients have early signs of scar inflammation and irritation (itching and pain), surgeons may start intralesional steroid injections to help alleviate the inflammation. Any surgery can be complicated by infection, which often accompanies impaired wound healing.

Conclusion

Gender-affirmation surgery is increasingly requested by patients experiencing gender dysphoria or who present with diverse gender identities. GAS has demonstrated clear therapeutic benefit in appropriate surgical candidates. Although genital reconstruction is typically reserved for individuals over age 18, other procedures such as top surgery and body contouring can be appropriate in certain adolescents who meet established criteria, have already pursued psychological and medical treatment, and still experience persistent and significant dysphoria. Importantly, there is no discrete algorithm that can reliably identify gender diverse adolescents who are appropriate surgical candidates. Individualized treatment plans should incorporate established WPATH guidelines, but other patient-specific factors should be considered; patient maturity, family support, and availability of psychological and medical resources are essential determinants of a patient's fitness for surgery. As such, each patient must be considered individually to ensure informed consent and shared decision-making acknowledging the potential benefits and risks of these transformative surgical options.

References

1. Hage JJ, Karim RB. Ought GIDNOS get nought? Treatment options for nontranssexual gender dysphoria. Plast Reconstr Surg. 2000;105(3):1222–7.
2. Dhejne C, Öberg K, Arver S, Landén M. An analysis of all applications for sex reassignment surgery in Sweden, 1960–2010: prevalence, incidence, and regrets. Arch Sex Behav. 2014;43:1535–45.
3. Colebunders B, Brondeel S, D'Arpa S, Hoebeke P, Monstrey S. An update on the surgical treatment for transgender patients. Sex Med Rev. 2017;5:103–9.
4. Canner JK, Harfouch O, Kodadek LM, et al. Temporal trends in gender-affirming surgery among transgender patients in the United States. JAMA Surg. 2018;153(7):609–16.
5. Olson-kennedy J, Warus J, Okonta V, Belzer M, Clark LF. Chest reconstruction and chest dysphoria in transmasculine minors and young adults: comparisons of nonsurgical and postsurgical cohorts. JAMA Pediatr. 2018;172(5):431–6.
6. Wiepjes CM, Nota NM, de Blok CJM, et al. The Amsterdam cohort of gender dysphoria study (1972–2015): trends in prevalence, treatment, and regrets. J Sex Med. 2018;15(4):582–90.
7. Djordjevic ML, Bizic MR, Duisin D, Bouman MB, Buncamper M. Reversal surgery in regretful male-to-female transsexuals after sex reassignment surgery. J Sex Med. 2016;13(6):1000–7.
8. Turban JL, Keuroghlian AS. Dynamic gender presentations: understanding transition and "de-transition" among transgender youth. J Am Acad Child Adolesc Psychiatry. 2018;57(7):451–3.
9. Vargas CR, Ricci JA, Lee M, Tobias AM, Medalie DA, Lee BT. The accessibility, readability, and quality of online resources for gender affirming surgery. J Surg Res. 2017;217:198–206.
10. Kiwanuka E, Mehrzad R, Prsic A, Kwan D. Online patient resources for gender affirmation surgery: an analysis of readability. Ann Plast Surg. 2017;79(4):329–33.
11. Steensma TD, Mcguire JK, Kreukels BP, Beekman AJ, Cohen-kettenis PT. Factors associated with desistence and persistence of childhood gender dysphoria: a quantitative follow-up study. J Am Acad Child Adolesc Psychiatry. 2013;52(6):582–90.
12. Morrison SD, Wilson SC, Mosser SW. Breast and body contouring for transgender and gender nonconforming individuals. Clin Plast Surg. 2018;45(3):333–42. https://doi.org/10.1016/j.cps.2018.03.015.
13. De vries AL, Steensma TD, Doreleijers TA, Cohen-kettenis PT. Puberty suppression in adolescents with gender identity disorder: a prospective follow-up study. J Sex Med. 2011;8(8):2276–83.
14. American Society of Plastic Surgeons. Briefing paper: plastic surgery for teenagers. Available at: https://www.plasticsurgery.org/news/briefing-papers/briefing-paper-plastic-surgery-for-teenagers. Accessed 19 Oct 2018.
15. Simis KJ, Hovius SE, De beaufort ID, Verhulst FC, Koot HM. After plastic surgery: adolescent-reported appearance ratings and appearance-related burdens in patient and general population groups. Plast Reconstr Surg. 2002;109(1):9–17.
16. Cohen-Kettenis PT, Delemarre-van de Waal HA, Gooren LJ. The treatment of adolescent transsexuals: changing insights. J Sex Med. 2008;5(8):1892–7.
17. de Vries AL, Cohen-Kettenis PT. Clinical management of gender dysphoria in children and adolescents: the Dutch approach. J Homosex. 2012;59(3):301–20.
18. Bossert RP, Rubin JP. Evaluation of the weight loss patient presenting for plastic surgery consultation. Plast Reconstr Surg. 2012;130(6):1361–9.
19. Sørensen LT. Wound healing and infection in surgery. The clinical impact of smoking and smoking cessation: a systematic review and meta-analysis. Arch Surg. 2012;147(4):373–83.
20. Goltsman D, Munabi NC, Ascherman JA. The association between smoking and plastic surgery outcomes in 40,465 patients: an analysis of the American College of Surgeons National Surgical Quality Improvement Program Data Sets. Plast Reconstr Surg. 2017;139(2):503–11.
21. Centers for Disease Control and Prevention (CDC), High School Youth Risk Behavior Survey Data. 2016 [cited October 23, 2018]; Available from: http://nccd.cdc.gov/youthonline/.

22. Hall W, Degenhardt L. Adverse health effects of non-medical cannabis use. Lancet. 2009;374(9698):1383–91.
23. Buncamper ME, Honselaar JS, Bouman MB, Özer M, Kreukels BP, Mullender MG. Aesthetic and functional outcomes of Neovaginoplasty using penile skin in male-to-female transsexuals. J Sex Med. 2015;12(7):1626–34.
24. Bouman MB, van der Sluis WB, van Woudenberg Hamstra LE, et al. Patient-reported esthetic and functional outcomes of primary total laparoscopic intestinal vaginoplasty in transgender women with penoscrotal hypoplasia. J Sex Med. 2016;13(9):1438–44.
25. Sigurjónsson H, Möllermark C, Rinder J, Farnebo F, Lundgren TK. Long-term sensitivity and patient-reported functionality of the neoclitoris after gender reassignment surgery. J Sex Med. 2017;14(2):269–73.
26. Garcia MM, Christopher NA, De Luca F, Spilotros M, Ralph DJ. Overall satisfaction, sexual function, and the durability of neophallus dimensions following staged female to male genital gender confirming surgery: the Institute of Urology, London U.K. experience. Transl Androl Urol. 2014;3(2):156–62.
27. Wierckx K, Van caenegem E, Elaut E, et al. Quality of life and sexual health after sex reassignment surgery in transsexual men. J Sex Med. 2011;8(12):3379–88.

Late Adolescence to Early Adulthood

17

Naomi Libby and Maria Trumpler

Introduction

The period of transition from late adolescence to early adulthood is characterized by a number of important developmental tasks, including identity consolidation, commitment to intimate relationships, clarification of personal values and internal moral system, role exploration and the establishment of a career path and personal goals, and shifts in family relationships from dependence toward equality and mutual respect [1, 2]. Life context is critical in shaping this period of development, with marginalized groups facing additional challenges and at higher risk of certain medical, mental health, and social problems. Lesbian, gay, bisexual, transgender, queer, and questioning (LGBTQ) transitional age youth in particular face higher rates of sexual trauma, sexually transmitted infections, substance abuse, depression, suicide, and school and employment difficulties, likely linked to higher rates of discrimination, victimization, marginalization, and isolation [1]. These effects are especially pronounced for transgender and gender diverse (TGD) young adults [3]. There is good news as well: psychological distress and experiences of victimization decrease as LGBTQ youth enter adulthood, and there is often some improvement in health and wellness during this period [4]. Social support from family, peers, and significant others appears particularly important to reducing negative outcomes. Indeed, the presence of Gay-Straight Alliances in high schools is one of a few highly protective factors for transgender and LGB youth [5, 6].

The initial sections of this chapter will discuss challenges and outcomes for TGD people in late adolescence and early adulthood in relation to employment, access to

N. Libby (✉)
Yale Child Study Center, Yale University, New Haven, CT, USA
e-mail: naomi.libby@yale.edu

M. Trumpler (✉)
Office of LGBTQ Resources, Yale University, New Haven, CT, USA
e-mail: maria.trumpler@yale.edu

M. Forcier et al. (eds.), *Pediatric Gender Identity*,
https://doi.org/10.1007/978-3-030-38909-3_17

healthcare, and family relationships. The final section addresses issues pertinent to college-bound transgender youth, from the perspective of someone with experience working with LGBTQ youth in the university setting.

Employment

Economic security is critical to emotional well-being, and employment is often an important element of adult personal identity. In a survey of 350 self-identified transgender Virginians, 22.3% reported employment discrimination related to transgender identity [7]. According to the National Transgender Discrimination Survey (NTDS), of 6450 transgender-identified US-based respondents, 90% reported experiencing harassment, mistreatment, or discrimination in the workplace, 47% reported having experienced an adverse job outcome, and 26% reported losing a job due to being TGD. Transgender people of color in particular reported higher levels of job-related adversity as compared to white respondents. Unemployment is double the national average, and four times as high for trans people of color [8].

Workplace Protections

LGBTQ organizations have worked many years to pass the Employment Non-Discrimination Act (ENDA), a federal bill that would prohibit discrimination in hiring and employment on the basis of sexual orientation or gender identity. Most recently, the bill was introduced in the Senate by Sen. Jeff Merkley; it passed with a 64–32 vote, but died in the house [9]. Currently, there is no federal law that explicitly protects transgender employees, though there are a number of state and local laws prohibiting discrimination against transgender people [10].

In 2012, the Equal Employment Opportunity Commission (EEOC) ruled that Title VII of the 1964 Civil Rights Act covers discrimination against transgender people under the provisions concerning discrimination on the basis of sex, a decision ratified by the Department of Justice (DOJ) in 2013. In December 2014, Attorney General (AG) Eric Holder directed the DOJ to include gender identity under sex discrimination employment claims [11]. This direction was subsequently reversed in October 2017 by AG Jeff Sessions, who argued that "Title VII's prohibition on sex discrimination encompasses discrimination between men and women but does not encompass discrimination based on gender identity per se, including transgender status" [12]. Despite this, in March 2018 the United States Court of Appeals for the Sixth Circuit ruled in a case brought by the EEOC that job discrimination based on a person's transgender status violates Title VII of the Civil Rights Act of 1964, effectively rejecting the Trump administration's position [13].

Evidently, the landscape of federal protections for transgender individuals is dynamic and uncertain. Some state and local governments have enacted legislation protecting the rights of transgender individuals. See Chap. 20, Legal Considerations, for more information on legal workplace and hiring protections. Individual employers often have their own internal non-discrimination policies; these can usually be accessed through the Human Resources department.

Sex Work

In a survey of 27,715 transgender individuals in the United States, 12% reported participation in sex work at some point in their lives [14]. Given an unemployment rate that is double the national average, and four times as high for trans people of color, clinicians should be aware that TGD persons may engage in sex work at higher rates than cisgender patients and be open and non-judgmental in their approach to discussing this with their patients. Sex work comes in many forms, including pornography, exotic dancing, webcamming, and having sex in exchange for money, among others. There are many reasons that transgender people may turn to sex work, often related to survival and meeting basic needs such as food and shelter, though some may enter sex work as a matter of personal choice. Factors affecting LGBTQ youth entry into sex work include racism, family poverty, homelessness, inadequate safe housing options, lack of access to gender-affirming medical care, and rejection and discrimination from families, communities, and employers [15]. Sex work is particularly prevalent among trans-feminine individuals and in people of color [16].

Resources

There are a number of national resources that transgender young adults can take advantage of when setting out to enter the workforce. These include:

- Human Rights Campaign (HRC) Corporate Equality Index (CEI): Evaluates companies on policies and practices relevant to LGBTQ employees and produces a list of "Best Places to Work for LGBTQ Equality." Access at https://www.hrc.org/campaigns/corporate-equality-index.
- Transgender Employment Program (TEP): San Francisco-based organization providing a wealth of resources and services related to creating inclusive workplaces and finding jobs for transgender and gender diverse individuals. Access at http://transemploymentprogram.org/.
- TJobBank.com: Database of job listings posted by trans-friendly employers. Access at http://tjobbank.com/.
- Pride at Work: Non-profit labor organization through the American Federation of Labor and Congress of Industrial Organization (AFL–CIO) that represents LGBTQ union members and allies. Access at https://www.prideatwork.org/.
- OUT for Work: Holds a national career conference and helps prepare LGBTQ college students to enter the workforce. Access at https://www.outforwork.org/.

Healthcare

Access to healthcare is a common barrier for TGD individuals, including those in late adolescence and early adulthood. TGD youth face high rates of healthcare discrimination and inadequate access to routine healthcare services [8, 17]. In addition, they experience a dearth of safe spaces in which to access trans-specific healthcare needs, including hormones, gender-affirming surgery, fertility counseling and services, and cancer screening (e.g., pap smears for cervical cancer screening in natal females). In a series of focus groups of transgender youth aged 15–21, four areas of vulnerability were identified in relation to healthcare needs: lack of safe environments, poor access to physical health services, inadequate resources to address their mental health concerns, and a lack of continuity of caregiving by their families and communities [17].

Healthcare Disparities

According to the 2016 Minnesota Student Survey [18], 62.1% of TGD ninth and eleventh graders report poor, fair, or good general health, whereas 66.9% of their cisgender peers report very good or excellent general health. Significantly more TGD youth than cisgender youth report long-term physical disabilities or health problems, and 59.3% report long-term mental health problems, compared to 17.4% of cisgender youth. TGD ninth and eleventh graders also report more missed days of school due to illness, more frequent in-school nurse office visits, and lower rates of accessing preventive medical and dental care [18]. Transgender youth in late adolescence and young adulthood report higher rates of physical and sexual violence, human immunodeficiency virus (HIV) seropositivity, smoking, substance use, mental health concerns, and suicide attempts [7, 8, 19].

Recommendations

Healthcare providers can take many steps toward increasing safe and supportive access to care for TGD youth [20, 21].

- Update intake forms and other paperwork to be transgender-inclusive. Space should be provided for patients to indicate their preferred names and pronouns. When necessary to ask for patients' gender, answers should be left open-ended, or with multiple options beyond "male" and "female" (e.g., "transgender," "nonbinary," "intersex," "genderqueer," or "other, please specify"). Avoid having separate intake forms for males and females; office staff should not be in the position of guessing or assuming a patient's gender, nor should patients be required to divulge or explain this to staff.
- Include gender identity and expression in non-discrimination and other written policies, and clearly post these policies in your clinic or facility. Post materials in

the waiting room that demonstrate yours is an LGBTQ-friendly practice, such as pamphlets addressing LGBTQ health concerns and posters from LGBTQ organizations.
- Provide in-service training for clinicians and staff. This should include discussion of terminology and definitions (including the distinction between sexual orientation and gender identity), review of non-discrimination policies, identification of barriers to transgender-inclusive care and ways to address these, practical guidance for clinicians and staff on providing inclusive services (including educating about use of preferred names and pronouns), and opportunities for ongoing discussion and learning.
- Make and mark bathrooms as unisex or gender-inclusive. When it is not possible to eliminate gendered bathrooms (e.g., from the lobby, if you are renting space in a larger facility), ensure clear signage indicating where patients may access unisex or gender-inclusive bathrooms (most healthcare facilities have single-use bathrooms within their clinical spaces).

Family

For most transitional age youth, this period is marked by a shift in the family-youth dynamic. Youth move from being dependent on caregivers to increasing financial, social, and emotional independence. This developmental period is further complicated for TGD youth, who face high rates of family non-acceptance, as well as barriers to employment as discussed above. Fifty-seven percent of NTDS respondents reported experiencing family rejection, and 19% reported domestic violence from a family member related to their TGD status. Family rejection is strongly correlated with poorer physical and mental health outcomes as well as higher rates of homelessness, incarceration, and sex work among TGD individuals experiencing family rejection and/or domestic violence [8]. Indeed, family acceptance is among the strongest protective factors identified for TGD youth [5, 22].

Practical Steps

Healthcare providers working with TGD youth and their families are in an optimal position to assess and support family acceptance. Specific recommendations include:

- Ask youth about their family relationships, including whether they are out to their families, how their families reacted if/when they came out, and current levels of family support or rejection.
- Identify and refer youth and families to local and online resources, including parent support groups.
- Provide parents the opportunity to share their story and concerns in a supportive, non-judgmental manner.

- Educate parents on the impact of family non-acceptance on youth's physical and mental health.
- For parents and caregivers who are unable to accept their child's gender identity, educate them on ways in which they can still be supportive. The Family Acceptance Project® (familyproject.sfsu.edu) is an excellent resource for families and providers, with a number of educational publications geared toward parents and families of LGBT youth.

Additional Resources

- Gender Spectrum Education and Training (www.genderspectrum.org).
- National LGBT Health Education Center (www.lgbthealtheducation.org).
- Family Acceptance Project® (https://familyproject.sfsu.edu).
- National Transgender Discrimination Survey, Executive Summary (https://transequality.org/issues/resources/national-transgender-discrimination-survey-executive-summary).
- American Academy of Pediatrics (AAP) Policy Statement: Ensuring Comprehensive Care and Support for Transgender and Gender diverse Children and Adolescents (http://pediatrics.aappublications.org/content/142/4/e20182162).

College

For a young person who has begun to explore their gender identity in high school, but who feels they are in an unsupportive family or community environment, attending a residential college can be deeply transformative. They may find a community of people in various stages of transition as well as those that are embracing a variety of non-binary identities. They may encounter professors who are attentive to their pronouns and who teach classes that explore the history and cultures of people resisting binary genders. Based on a 15-year experience of directing Yale's Office of LGBTQ Resources, this part of the chapter will talk about the expectations a student could have of inclusive practices by their University. This should apply to four-year public and private colleges in the United States and Canada that are not closely affiliated with a religious organization.

College Choice

Choosing a college is especially important if transitioning or fully expressing a non-binary gender identity will be an essential part of those years. Searching the website for "LGBTQ" should yield a page of resources and some of those should specifically be for transgender and non-binary students. Look for a non-discrimination policy that includes gender identity and gender expression. Colleges that have at least one student group with "trans" in their name, gender neutral housing available to students in all years, and at least one all-gender restroom in all of the main classroom and student activities buildings are indicators of some measure of support. Considering the larger, social context (east/west coast versus central USA, larger urban area versus smaller town or rural locations, and the individual culture of the institution) may factor into issues of convenience and access to gender-related mental health, hormonal, primary, and surgical care.

Starting college away from home can be a moment to socially establish a name and gender identity different from those used in high school. Most schools will allow students to use a "lived" or "preferred" name different from a legal name. Usually, this lived name can be added easily via an online form. This name can then be on the University ID card and on professor's class lists and in the directory. Many universities also have more than binary gender options and this change can also be made with an online form. "All Gender" or "Gender Neutral" housing allows students to be assigned roommates without regard to gender. This allows non-binary or transitioning students (and others) to avoid being assigned to single sex suites or floors. It also allows for shared experiences and support of hallmates – a new experience for many young people who may not have had a sense of community before. LGBTQ persons have adapted over many years in the construction of unique chosen families when biological family members cannot offer support.

A Non-binary Student Community

Having a critical mass of non-binary students who are willing to be public about their experiences may provide an environment in which new students entering this community may feel comfortable identifying outside of a "master narrative" – specifically, a common, socially reinforced gender narrative. This was exemplified at a recent Trans Awareness week at Yale University, where there was a robust discussion around the comfort of students identifying as "trans" who embraced non-binary identities. Since then, there has been a significant number of students from this community who are more outspoken around their identity. Their conversations, spoken word performances, paintings, and social activism give all students a chance to think deeply about the social dynamics of gender. Theater has always been particularly welcoming to LGBTQ students, and the recent mainstage performance of the play "Men in a Boat" in which all characters are played by non-binary actors also led to deep discussions on the performativity of traditional white masculinity.

The transgender and non-binary student community at Yale is large enough that there are visible members in long-term relationships and in short-term ones as well. At Yale, alums have gone on to careers in consulting, engineering, and the Episcopal priesthood and are willing to Skype into conversations with current students. We have also created a regular dinner that includes trans and non-binary faculty and staff, so that students can connect across generations and imagine the details and pleasures of an adult life. These activities that focus on inclusion and mentorship help students understand the issues relative to professional development and may fight against the doubts that may be strongly articulated by families about their future jobs or relationships. Families and prospective students are encouraged to seek which universities offer such programs. Universities hoping to foster a more supportive environment may add these programs to their existing initiatives to support TGD students.

Academic Engagement

Universities also offer courses and majors that look at gender historically and regionally, exploring questions such as the origins of scientific and medical ideas about gender binaries, and the cultures and practices of people outside those binaries. To be able to take classes and do research on a topic that is also of deep personal interest is transformative for many students. Some are drawn to queer theory, others to international human rights activism.

Athletic Engagement

Sports play a significant role in many campuses, and varsity teams remain male or female. For TGD athletes, the National Collegiate Athletic Association (NCAA) has eligibility rules based on testosterone levels. Club sports are usually more flexible. Intramurals may offer gender-neutral options for athletic participation each semester. Students who are TGD or transitioning may be self-conscious about changing in locker rooms and about wearing form-fitting clothing or gendered clothing such as bathing suits. Colleges have opportunities to encourage lifelong fitness and good health habits by offering their TGD students recreational opportunities that explicitly support TGD students in nongendered activities or mixed gender activities such as queer yoga or weight training, special pool hours, and gender-neutral areas or specific locker rooms.

Considering Family

Conflict with families often arises when students share their TGD identities or plans to socially or medically transition. Many families are completely unfamiliar with these identities and do not know anyone personally who shares this identity with them. Particularly if the family has made sacrifices to send the student to college, they may be very worried that this gender identity may negate the professional and social advantages the college degree can confer. Some worry that they did something wrong, and some simply cannot conceive of their daughter or son as being anything other than female or male. In practice, it is impressive and positive to see how many families do indeed come around to supporting their offspring over the course of a year or two. They become accustomed to the student's new appearance and name, and see how much happier they are and how much energy they now have for other pursuits. In the United States, educational privacy laws prohibit University officials from communicating with parents without the student's permission, but students may ask faculty or staff to facilitate disclosure regarding their TGD identity and help talk with a parent(s) by phone or in person. Institutions of higher education may offer resources to bridge this time of change, such as appropriate online resources and local experts who may provide support.

Box 17.1 Checklist for a Gender-Inclusive College or University

- Non-discrimination statement that includes gender identity and gender expression.
- Lived name on class lists and ID cards.
- All-gender housing options.
- All-gender restrooms in every building.
- Gender studies courses.
- Healthcare coverage and support for gender affirmation.

Conclusion

TGD youth face a number of challenges during the transition from late adolescence to young adulthood, as they navigate developmental tasks including increasing autonomy from family, assuming responsibility for their own healthcare needs, attending college, or finding a job. This period may also present new opportunities for TGD youth, particularly for those distancing themselves from non-affirming or rejecting families and searching for supportive peer communities. Healthcare providers can support TGD youth as they bridge the divide between adolescence and adulthood by providing affirmative care in safe, welcoming environments, educating themselves about the unique challenges faced by this population, and supporting their patients in identifying appropriate resources, such as those provided in this chapter.

References

1. Leebens PK, Williamson ED. Developmental psychopathology: risk and resilience in the transition to young adulthood. Child Adolesc Psychiatr Clin N Am. 2017;26(2):143–56.
2. Gilmore KJ, Meersand P. Normal child and adolescent development: a psychodynamic primer. Arlington: American Psychiatric Publishing; 2014.
3. Rieger G, Savin-Williams RC. Gender nonconformity, sexual orientation, and psychological well-being. Arch Sex Behav. 2012;41(3):611–21.
4. Birkett M, Newcomb ME, Mustanski B. Does it get better? A longitudinal analysis of psychological distress and victimization in lesbian, gay, bisexual, transgender, and questioning youth. J Adolesc Health. 2015;56(3):280–5.
5. Johns MM, Beltran O, Armstrong HL, Jayne PE, Barrios LC. Protective factors among transgender and gender variant youth: a systematic review by socioecological level. J Prim Prev. 2018;39(3):263–301.

6. Protective Factors for LGBT Youth: Information for Health and Education Professionals. https://www.cdc.gov/healthyyouth/disparities/lgbtprotectivefactors.htm. Accessed 2 Nov 2018.
7. Bradford J, Reisner SL, Honnold JA, Xavier J. Experiences of transgender-related discrimination and implications for health: results from the Virginia Transgender Health Initiative Study. Am J Public Health. 2013;103(10):1820–9.
8. Grant JM, Mottet LA, Tanis J, Harrison J, Herman JL, Keisling M. Injustice at every turn: a report of the National Transgender Discrimination Survey, Executive Summary. Washington, DC; 2011.
9. Senate Bill 815 – Employment Non-Discrimination Act of 2013. 113th Congress (2013–2014).
10. Know Your Rights: Transgender People and the Law. American Civil Liberties Union. https://www.aclu.org/know-your-rights/transgender-people-and-law. Accessed 2 Nov 2018.
11. Attorney General Holder Directs Departments to Include Gender Identity Under Sex Discrimination Employment Claims [press release]. United States Department of Justice, Office of Public Affairs, 2014.
12. Revised Treatment of Transgender Employment Discrimination Claims Under Title VII of the Civil Rights Act of 1964 [memorandum]. United States Office of the Attorney General, 2017.
13. Equal Employment Opportunity Commission, Aimee Stephens, vs. R.G. & G.R. Harris Funeral Homes, Inc. United States Court of Appeals for the Sixth Circuit, 2018.
14. James SE, Herman JL, Rankin S, Keisling M, Mottet L, Anafi M. Executive Summary of the Report of the 2015 U.S. Transgender Survey. Washington, DC; 2016.
15. Dank M, Yahner J, Madden K, Banuelos I, Yu L, Ritchie A, et al. Surviving the streets of New York: Experiences of LGBTQ Youth, YMSM, and YWSW Engaged in Survival Sex. 2015.
16. Fitzgerald E, Patterson SE, Hickey D, Biko C, Tobin HJ. Meaningful work: transgender experiences in the sex trade. 2015. https://www.transequality.org/sites/default/files/Meaningful%20Work-Full%20Report_FINAL_3.pdf.
17. Grossman AH, D'Augelli AR. Transgender youth: invisible and vulnerable. J Homosex. 2006;51(1):111–28.
18. Rider GN, McMorris BJ, Gower AL, Coleman E, Eisenberg ME. Health and care utilization of transgender and gender nonconforming youth: a population-based study. Pediatrics. 2018;141(3):e20171683.
19. Harrison J, Grant J, Herman JL. A gender not listed Here: genderqueers, gender rebels, and otherwise in the national transgender discrimination survey. LGBTQ Policy J Harvard Kennedy School. 2012;2(2011–2012):13–24.
20. Rodgers SM. Transitional age lesbian, gay, bisexual, transgender, and questioning youth: issues of diversity, integrated identities, and mental health. Child Adolesc Psychiatr Clin N Am. 2017;26(2):297–309.
21. Providing Transgender-Inclusive Healthcare Services. Planned Parenthood of the Southern Finger Lakes, 2006.
22. Health Risks Among Sexual Minority Youth. Centers for Disease Control and Prevention. https://www.cdc.gov/healthyyouth/disparities/smy.htm; 2018.

Cultural Considerations in the United States

18

Cecil R. Webster Jr. and Cynthia J. Telingator

Introduction

America's youth is an increasingly diverse group racially and ethnically. It is projected that while the United States as a whole will become a plurality nation in 2045, the US child population is projected to become majority-minority as soon as 2020 [1]. Additionally, transgender youth are not a monolithic group, having a great diversity of identities and experiences. Reflective of this heterogeneity, terminology in the field, as discussed in other chapters, is ever evolving [2]. As such, the terms of transgender or gender diverse (TGD) in this chapter are meant as umbrella terms to encompass those individuals who understand or express their gender in a way that crosses, transcends, conflicts with, or enlarges upon culturally defined categories of gender [3–5].

It should be noted that these young people are seeking health care in a variety of geographic and sociocultural settings and have a wide array of clinical needs. The National Academy of Medicine (formerly the Institute of Medicine) has identified provider clinical knowledge about gender and sexual minority patients and the impact of stigma on sexual minorities' health as areas requiring further attention [6]. They identify a need for more cross-sectional and longitudinal research related to demographic and intersectional realities of gender and sexual minority youth in general and to elucidate the risk and resilience mechanisms of these subgroups of sexual minority youth [6] (Table 18.1).

C. R. Webster Jr. (✉)
Harvard Medical School, Department of Psychiatry, McLean Hospital, Boston, MA, USA
e-mail: mail@cecilwebstermd.com

C. J. Telingator
Harvard Medical School, Department of Psychiatry, Cambridge Health Alliance, Cambridge, MA, USA
e-mail: cindy_telingator@hms.harvard.edu

M. Forcier et al. (eds.), *Pediatric Gender Identity*,
https://doi.org/10.1007/978-3-030-38909-3_18

Table 18.1 Sample initial identity questions and statements

Framing the discussion:
Tell me about yourself.
What is important to know about you in addition to what we've discussed?
Gender identity questions:
How do you feel regarding your gender? What is your relationship to your gender? How would you describe it?
How did your ideas and feelings about gender change as you were growing up?
How did you learn about gender? When did you first begin to explore gender and/or sexuality?
What was puberty like for you? What aspects of puberty were easier, what aspects were more difficult?
For younger children: How do you feel when you think about being a boy, girl, or some other way of being a kid? Do you like your body? What parts of your body do you like? What parts of your body do you like less?
How has your family/community/school reacted to your relationship with gender?
Exploring intersectional identities:
What are other important identities for you?
What other racial, ethnic, religious, and sexual identities resonate with you in addition to gender?
When do you first feel that identity described an aspect of who you are?
How did you begin to realize that you were that identity?
What does your family say about your identities? Think of your identities? Do they know about all of your identities? If not, what's behind that decision?
Some kids find that different parts of their identity compete with others. What has your experience been?
What is it like to be both [identity A] and [identity B]?
Where do you feel most comfortable expressing all of the identities you've described? Where do you feel least comfortable with [identity A]?; [identity B]?; [identity C]?
What messages do you get about your identities from your family? From your school? From your neighborhood? From media (e.g., television, film, social media)?
Which parts about your identity are you most proud? Least comfortable with? Most unclear about?
If you could let others know, what would you like them to know about your identity?
Sample questions regarding safety and rejection:
Where do you feel supported? Who do you feel supported by?
Do you have any role models for being [identity]?
Do you have places where you are open and able to discuss different aspects of your identity?
Have you felt that you've been endangered because of your identity?
Who do you imagine in your family/community/school may have the hardest time understanding your gender? How come?
Some kids wonder if people who love or care about them may stop if they knew about their gender. Are there some you worry about in that way?
Sample questions and statements about the clinician–patient relationship:
Some kids feel uncomfortable at first talking about what it is like to be a certain race in here at first. I hope you will know that I'm curious about all parts of you to include your family, culture, and race.
What is it like to have a clinician who is [obvious identity, e.g., white, female, Muslim]? For some that may make them feel it is easier or more difficult to talk about these important experiences.

About 0.7% of youth aged 13–17, or roughly 150,000 children, identify as transgender in the United States [7]. Data about the racial or ethnic composition of transgender youth populations in the United States are scant [6]. Transgender *adult* populations are more likely to be ethnically and racially diverse than the general population. The authors of a Williams Institute study found that adults who are African-American or Black (0.8%), Latino or Hispanic (0.8%), and of another race or ethnicity (0.6%) are more likely than White adults (0.5%) to identify as transgender [7]. As US children are a group projected to be majority nonwhite by 2020 [1], one may, therefore, infer that *transgender* children are a diverse group reflecting a wide spectrum of ethnicities, races, and cultures.

While gender identity terminology attempts to capture all those individuals who transcend the social norms associated with their gender assigned at birth (e.g., transgender, queer, gender diverse), more detailed demographic and related research is required to accurately characterize this population (e.g., race, ethnicity, socioeconomic level, religion). Available research most often explores identity (e.g., ethnic identity and gender identity) as a singular aspect rather than a component of one's identity (e.g., ethnic and gender identity) [8]. As such, many of those with intersected identities are obscured in academic discourse and thus are made largely invisible in research, theory, and clinical interventions [8]. Intersecting identities combine to create unique oppression and marginalization and conversely may offer potential for resilience in the face of challenges [6, 9]. Lastly, data for those with intersected identities from a specific adolescent or developmental lens are scarcer still [6].

It is the goal of this chapter to help clinicians consider relevant issues for these populations. With the above important caveats in mind, it is the task of the authors to exemplify the complexity of these issues utilizing a fictional clinical case.

Isaac is an artistically skilled 14-year-old multiracial birth-assigned male who comes to his pediatrician accompanied by his father, Daniel, an Ethiopian-American post office worker, and mother, Sara, a white American technician at a telephone company. Both parents have grown up with and maintain strong religious and cultural traditions in Judaism. Daniel was raised in his community of Jewish-Ethiopians in Gondar, Ethiopia, and Sara in small Jewish family in the mid-Atlantic region. Isaac's parents have been amicably divorced since he was 4 years old. In describing Isaac, they reveal that they had felt that his interests, expression, and social interactions were different from what they had observed in his older brother. Isaac rejected the hand-me-down "masculine" toys and clothing of his 16-year-old brother Abe, maintained primary relationships with females, and enjoyed having long, dark, and loosely curled hair that consistently has strangers gender Isaac as female. They emphasized that they have always affirmed Isaac's choices in play, clothing, and friendships, and lightly joked that Isaac had been a sweet relief as compared to Isaac's rough and tumble older brother.

Isaac's parents stated that they are, however, concerned about his drop in grades, his increased irritability at home, and a few previously unknown school absences revealed on his most recent report card. Most importantly, they sought a consultation because Isaac's close friend and schoolmate called last week to tell Sara that she has been worried about the harassment Isaac has faced by his male peers at his high school relating to his feminine behavior. This friend also expressed alarm about Isaac's recent social media posts. Those posts had been uncharacteristically dark and alluded to his wishes that he had not been born. Daniel and Sara, who worked closely together with Abe's developmental challenges, are eager to address these troubling events *with Isaac*.

A critical prelude to adulthood, adolescence is both a time of tremendous expectations for normative gender expression and sexuality and a time when gender identities are highly salient in social interactions [10]. During adolescence, challenges of integrating the development of secondary sexual characteristics and the psychological responses to these developments are unique. Sexual orientation and gender identity (discussed in greater detail in Chap. 1) encompass wide aspects of our identity. Gender identity includes one's journey toward what it means to experience and identify one's gender, what roles are expected of us or performed according to these expectations, and what roles one assumes considering these social frameworks [11]. These overlaying social frameworks may include cultural expectations. Some cultural groups may have expectations from within or outside about ideals of masculinity or femininity. Family loyalty and social conformity may be prioritized over individualism. Also, children and adolescents may be sanctioned or rejected for going against social mores [8].

Youth may, therefore, be hyperaware of potential or perceived rejection within their social frameworks as they search for these identities. Adolescents may align themselves with behaviors and activities which are culturally congruent with peers, parents, communities, other individuals, and spaces. They may also begin to express themselves in ways that are not congruent with their authentic selves.

Prior research has outlined that LGBTQ+ youth may be poorly equipped to buffer against invalidating experiences during family or peer interactions. Understanding their own experiences is complicated by their vulnerability toward internalizing homophobic or transphobic attitudes [12, 13]. Isaac's pediatrician may consider if Isaac's rejection of more "masculine" toys and clothing was affirmed, supported, or spurned in a variety of settings including his home, school, neighborhood, and religious organizations. How does Isaac's racial or religious identity influence perceived expectations of gender? Where is there space enough to explore gender?

The Clinical Disclosure Environment and Risk Assessment

A sense of safety, privacy, and validation are paramount in creating a clinical alliance with these individuals. Reviewing confidentiality in a developmentally appropriate way (with attention to legal parameters) is a vital step toward comprehensive evaluative discussions [14]. Youth have likely experienced hostility and bias leading them to remain vigilant about whether they can safely disclose information regarding their gender in the clinical space. As cultural pressures encourage a shift toward more inclusive gender-neutral language, there may also be an increasing stigmatization, discrimination, and aggression that may include overt hostility [15].

This is an important consideration as the American Academy of Child and Adolescent Psychiatry outlines that diagnostic evaluations of all youth should include assessment of gender role behavior and gender identity [14]. As a matter of course, care should be taken to inquire about the names and pronouns patients use or prefer to use [16]. In a community cohort study of 129 transgender and gender diverse

(TGD) youth, researchers asked participants if they were able to use a name that they preferred versus the one they were conferred at birth at home, school, work, or with friends and measured depression, suicidal ideation, and suicidal behavior with a number of scales. They found that TGD youth who were able to use a name they preferred across multiple contexts reported fewer depressive symptoms, less suicidal ideation, and less suicidal behavior. The authors hypothesize that use of a chosen name in multiple contexts may affirm gender identity and thus lower mental health risks in this group [17]. For the clinician, in addition to utilizing gender-affirming language, correcting previous, incorrect gendered language and following relevant interview openings regarding gender may greatly aid one's efforts.

In the clinical sphere, having visible cues of nondiscriminatory practices both online and in the office may also convey that the clinician's office is a safe environment for disclosure. Depending on the setting, having LGBT-affirming symbols (e.g., "rainbow" or "safe space" symbols, appropriate waiting room information, and literature) may be constructive [18].

After inviting Isaac into the room, the clinician stated, "As a matter of routine, I'd like to check in with you about which pronouns or names you'd like to use here." Isaac sheepishly stated that they would prefer gender-neutral pronouns and "Isaac" in the office. They reported that they have only sporadically experimented with gender-neutral pronouns with some close friends at temple.

"My parents don't know yet," Isaac said. "Could you use he/him/his when they are around?" The clinician acknowledged this request and stated that she had previously used masculine pronouns in the office with them, and apologized. Isaac nods with a faint smile.

Gender exploration necessitates privacy; however, this may present some practical clinical dilemmas. The clinician may be asked to hold details of the patient's gender identity exploration in confidence. This may include the use of names or pronouns, details of novel gender expression, or other feelings and experiences of one's own gender of which the patient's family or others may be unaware. Placing this potential dilemma in a cultural context with the child or adolescent may elucidate matters. For example, Isaac's clinician may broadly inquire why it may be important she hold Isaac's exploration in confidence. In a narrower lens, she may ask how Isaac's line of identity exploration fits with their cultural identities? Is there concern for physical safety and homelessness or embarrassment and doubt? These questions are unlikely to be answered all at once. Consistent, routine inquiry about gender identity using a fluid style in a welcoming physical space may effectively illuminate the sensitive details and challenges of the youth's environment.

Some clinicians, however, may inadvertently fail to routinely inquire about gender identity, may be unaware of the standards of care, or may underestimate the impact of being a gender minority on health. There is little data about how often clinicians include gender identity inquiries in their clinical interviews or their relative comfort with doing so. One study conducted in Washington DC showed that 68% of pediatricians and adolescent medicine specialists did not include *sexual orientation* or *sexual histories* in clinical visits (is this 19 as well?). Ninety percent of respondents reported having reservations about discussing sexual orientation during their clinical visit with youth. The mostly commonly selected reservations were not knowing enough about sexual minority youth's health needs (33%); not knowing how to ask relevant questions about sexuality (35%); and the worry it may offend young patients to ask questions related to sexuality (37%) [19].

While there is scant data specifically concerning gender disclosure during clinic visits in gender diverse pediatric populations, one may infer that it is challenging for young patients to talk with their clinician about gender identity and that clinicians may not feel equipped enough to inquire about these areas.

The pediatrician asked, "Your parents sound quite alarmed by some changes they've noted. How do you make sense of their concerns?"

Isaac quickly pointed out that his parents are supportive but overreact to things at times. Isaac was not sure why they are so concerned, but noted that they told Isaac of their receiving concerning communication from Isaac's friend and had felt that Isaac was more isolated and withdrawn. Isaac did endorse feeling more down and irritable, but not to the point of suicide. "I would never do that to my family," Isaac insisted. Isaac shared with some hesitation that kids in their ninth grade class have not been welcoming, and verbally taunt them in the locker room after gym class. Isaac emphasized they have found great support in family and in their boyfriend of several months.

"He's at my temple, but I don't get to see him at school," Isaac explained after the clinician followed up on their first mention of a boyfriend. Isaac adds that the two have had relative secrecy of their romantic, nonsexual relationship as they are unsure how their temple members or parents will react. Isaac emphasized they are not worried about their safety there or at home. "I think my parents are cool and love me a lot, but they may not totally get it."

When asked more about school, Isaac added that they have explored changing their name and school email address but remains reluctant given their current isolation at school. They increasingly opt to eat alone in spite of invitations to sit with art class classmates. Isaac revealed that they, in general, have had a greater sense of anxiety in recent months.

Gender and sexual minority youth must contend with stigma and shame, and the repercussions of this on their well-being should not be overlooked. Minority stress theory (see Chap. 5) suggests that persistent stigma such as social exclusion, victimization, and discrimination may lead to greater risk of mental illness. Importantly, it highlights that social support may mitigate the effects of these chronic or singular stigmatizing events [20]. The minority stress theory was originally developed to understand the impact of the stresses that sexual minorities endure. However, the minority stress theory has found wider application in TGD populations [21]. It is worth noting that due to this marginalization, the stress they endure may impact critical aspects of adolescence, such as developing a growing connection and community with peers, school and career exploration, and romantic/sexual relationships.

A narrative study of 30 TGD participants outlined consistent themes of expectations of rejection that were highly salient for these populations and for participants of color in particular [22]. Participants of color noted that they felt more prepared to anticipate *gender*-based rejection based on their previous experiences of *race/ethnicity*-based rejection. The authors also postulate that this preparedness may indicate either a mechanism of resilience or an effect of habitual discrimination.

Similar series of studies show that for *sexual* minorities, acceptance by families confers greater physical and mental well-being, while family rejection increases risk of mental illness, risky sexual behavior, and substance use [23, 24]. We can infer that the mechanisms (e.g., social supports such as family acceptance) that confer protection against negative mental and physical health outcomes in *sexual* minorities may also confer protections to *gender* minority individuals although further specific research is needed.

Psychological effects of family rejection and other stigmatizing experiences are more thoroughly outlined in Chap. 9. There is a greater degree of internalizing psychopathologies in these populations related to negative cultural messages about transgender identities (e.g., depression and anxiety). This may be congruent with transgender adults having more internalizing disorders than youth, and adolescents more than children [25, 26]. In addition to these important mental health concerns, risk of suicide should be a part of any clinical evaluation of youth but particularly for gender and sexual minority individuals [14].

A recent large-scale analysis of a sample of 120,617 adolescents aged 11–19 years has given a more detailed look at suicide behavior in transgender youth with intersecting identities [27]. Suicide behavior was assessed using a self-reported single question, "Have you ever tried to kill yourself?" Of all adolescents in the sample, regardless of gender or sexual identity, 14.1% reported that they had attempted suicide one or more times. Transgender, asserted male adolescents reported the highest rates of suicide behaviors (50.9%), and nonbinary adolescents reporting the next-highest rate (41.8%). Interestingly, the authors point out that this study, while relatively underrepresented for youth of color, did *not* reveal a compounding effect of identifying as a person of color in comparison to previous research of sexual minorities of color. They posit that there should be greater consideration of uniquely protective factors that may emerge with intersecting ethnic and gender identities.

One school-based study found that 80% of transgender youth were the victims of bullying [28]. An analysis of the Minnesota Student Survey, a survey of nearly 82,000 public high school students in the state, reveals that sexual minority adolescents and those adolescents with higher degrees of "gender nonconformity" have greater degrees of victimization [29]. Further, transgender people of color are more likely than their white counterparts to be victims of violence or discrimination as the Report of the 2015 U.S. Transgender Survey outlines [30]. Inquiries around bullying should be a part of discussions with youth [6, 14, 31].

It is important to inquire about the child/adolescents' experiences of the multiple settings in which they live and interact with others of all ages. In addition to emotional functioning, peer/social relationships and school experience should be at the center of any evaluation of gender diverse youth [32].

Race and Culture in the Office

It may remain a difficult task to create a therapeutic relationship in which the role of race and ethnicity and its intersection with gender is included in the dialogue. Avoidance of the discussion of race and ethnicity may occur due to discomfort in how to broach these subjects. Psychoanalyst Kimberlyn Leary, PhD, offers the clinical concept of "racial enactments," or sequences of our cultural attitudes and actions toward race and racial differences. She postulates that America's most significant racial enactment has been its relative silence about racial issues [33].

Other authors, drawing on a psychoanalytic perspective, suggest clinicians are not apart *from* but *of* the society where they are raised and thus may unconsciously offer culturally informed racial slights and oversights (read racial enactments) [34]. Isaac's clinician may have missed opportunities to directly inquire about Isaac's unique cultural history as they discussed their uncertainties for acceptance by their synagogue, school, and family. These inquiries might have led to discussions with Isaac about places where they experienced support and/or rejection and places where they experienced validation and/or invalidation, stigma, and discrimination.

If not specifically attended to by the clinician, the clinician may inadvertently subject our patients to fresh, subtle, and commonplace verbal, behavioral, and environmental indignities described frequently as micro-aggressions and inadvertently induce feelings of shame the patient may already have experienced both consciously and subconsciously [35]. Conversely, a deeply observant clinician may find themselves preoccupied by guilt arising out of their participation in a seemingly intractable system and may lose sight of the very indignities they sought to outline. Lastly, some clinicians may fear that questions regarding race or ethnicity, even clinical, may simply be experienced negatively for a variety of reasons.

In each of the scenarios, the clinician may unintentionally and implicitly suggest to patients that their identities, nascent or central, are linked to apprehension in the clinician or shame in general. Further still, a relative lack of these questions may convey that the clinician is not interested and/or has a limited capacity to observe, elicit, or process major elements of their worldview.

It may be wise to acknowledge our relative discomfort with these themes and ask families about how their race/ethnicities, cultures, and national origins affect their relationship with schools, family, and larger community [18].

The clinician stated, "Isaac, some feel it can be hard to talk about things like race or religion in the clinical office, but I want to emphasize that I am interested in learning about you and your life. Could you tell me about how you see yourself and your identity across race, religion, ethnicity, gender, and sexuality? I am also curious about how your parents' cultural backgrounds and values have impacted you. What concerns do you have about your parents learning more about parts of your gender and sexual identity exploration?"

Isaac described feeling really connected to their Jewish faith and culture as both Isaac's Ethiopian father and Jewish-American mother share this identity. Although Isaac's father's uniquely Ethiopian Jewish traditions are quite different from Isaac's mother's American Jewish customs, Isaac feels quite comfortable at each of their parents' houses at major holidays and family gatherings. "I like hanging out with my cousins," Isaac concluded, "but my mom's sisters don't always invite us. I don't think they get my dad's traditions and I'm not sure they think we are all that Jewish. I mean, I guess we didn't always practice so much, and Abe and I look really different than them, but it makes me feel really connected to my family."

Isaac chuckled that many of the teachers and classmates gave him skeptical looks when they said they'd need to be absent for Rosh Hashanah. "There aren't many Jewish people in my school, much less Black Jewish people." Isaac continued, "Sometimes I just don't know where I fit. I feel like my brother and I look more Black but I don't feel very connected to the few Black kids in my high school. At the same time, I know I'm not white. I'm reminded

> of that all the time. I know I don't have many friends, especially guys, because I'm not very 'boy.' I worry that if more people knew I was queer though, maybe I would have even fewer friends. I think my parents would be cool, but what if I lost them too? I can't lose them too."

From a developmental lens, children prior to middle school generally adapt to US social norms that avoid discussion of race and ethnicity. However, their need to adhere to social norms that ignore discussions of race may conflict with the need to process racialized experiences. Research has shown that parents of color typically discuss race and ethnicity with their children in contrast to white parents [36]. Integration of the multiple aspects of one's identity may be impeded by the inability to explore them with others including the clinician.

Another overlooked component a clinician should consider is religion and spirituality, which may influence youths' expectations for gender and identity. Some may experience rejection, a lack of acknowledgment, or poor representation within their religious community or organizations. An individual may experience being a member of a spiritual community and embracing nontraditional gender expression as mutually exclusive.

A small Ohio study surveyed 115 adolescents and their caregivers at a transgender clinic to identify if a measure was suitable for measuring "spiritual struggle," or the tensions that may arise when basic tenets of spiritual beliefs, practices, and strivings are threatened [37]. The measure asked questions such as, "Is spirituality or religion important to you as you think about your transgender issues?" and "How much strength or comfort do you get from your religion/spirituality right now?" The written measure was found to have acceptable specificity and sensitivity as compared to previously validated oral measures. More germane to spirituality in transgender adolescent populations, however, the authors note that one-third of adolescents and 47% of caregivers screened positive for spiritual struggle utilizing the measure. With Isaac, one may observe an early reluctance to discuss these areas, and possible tension between race, religion, culture, and family. Isaac, like many youth, may be searching for how to make sense of seemingly conflicting identities.

There are many faith communities that embrace LGBTQ+ participants; it would be inaccurate to assume that religion cannot serve a positive role. For example, a small study of young transgender women mostly of color demonstrated protective effects of religiosity [38]. This has been at the heart of some national spiritual organizations, such as Dignity USA (Catholic), Keshet (Jewish), and the Muslim Alliance for Sexual and Gender Diversity. They outline similar missions to help individuals integrate both gender diverse and spiritual identities. Referral to similar groups as a part of a larger treatment plan may be integral to alleviating the potential for a fractured sense of self and internal struggle. Many of these organizations are based in large metropolitan centers and, therefore, may be at an inaccessible distance for many youth populations who live outside of cities or for whom transportation is an issue.

Recognition that aspects of one's identity may feel mutually exclusive from one another may also serve as a useful framework. If there are family members or spiritual community traditions that reject or fail to observe major aspects of an individual, it may prove difficult for that individual to articulate negative feelings toward those family members or spiritual community traditions and not feel at risk of losing them [8]. It may be terrifying to be marginalized and targeted as a member of a sexual or gender minority group and imagine not having the support of one's racial, family, or spiritual community that might have provided resilience in the past. Exploring these aspects of loss and fear and how these may interact with changing needs are an important concept to consider.

What is essential is understanding how individuals with marginalized identities interact with and understand their social world, and appreciating what their identities elicit within themselves and in others [16]. A clinician must continually offer invitations to keenly identify all environments our patients move within and their potential invisibility.

Interviewing Considerations

Isaac, like many young persons exploring important aspects of their identity, presents a complex field of intersecting identities. It may require careful attention to accomplish the task of understanding potentially marginalized identities and what these identities bring out in others and themselves. This task may be accomplished in a number of ways.

A key interviewing framework includes continually exploring and assessing social identities that may be important to the individual, while not assuming the centrality of these identities [8]. A second key is considering how these multiple social identities (e.g., race, religion, sexual orientation, and gender) may affect a person independently and within their various individual and group relationships. Assumptions and projections by others can deeply impact one's sense of self as one tries to make sense of those assumptions and their own unique, developing identities. Intersecting identities may combine not only to create unique challenges (where most of our research and therapeutic interventions focus) but may also offer mechanisms for resilience (where more research is needed) [6, 9]. It is especially important to consider that exploration into certain identities may offer the threat that the patient may lose family and community support [8]. This may prove especially resonant for developing children tasked with making sense of themselves and their world.

To aid clinicians, the authors have collected a number of example questions that do not assume the centrality of these multiple lines of identities and allow for discussions about their intersections (Table 18.1).

Summary

Gender identity is a wide-ranging and difficult to define term that eludes research precision at times. Further, much research has focused on single aspects of gender rather than where gender may intersect with a myriad of other identities [3–5].

Much remains to be discovered about mechanisms of risk and resilience in gender diverse youth and their intersecting identities [6, 9]. While there are infinite possible lines of identities that develop alongside gender, there are some dominant themes to integrate in clinical practice.

Youth in the United States are increasingly racially and ethnically diverse, and gender diverse populations are more likely to be racially and ethnically diverse as compared to the general population [1, 7]. Clinicians may approach topics of race and ethnicity with some trepidation. Health-care clinicians, providing both medical and mental health, are also a part of a culture that generally avoids directly addressing many sensitive topics to the detriment of their patients [34]. TGD individuals of color may be more poised to expect rejection generally, and our relative lack of inclusion of these topics may mirror similar experiences of rejection they may face outside of the clinical office [22]. For younger children, America's lack of discussion of these subjects may suggest to children that this should be normative [36]. This may further impede our ability to explore these lines of identity with children and preclude children's ability to make sense of racialized experiences in a healthy way.

Similarly, spirituality represents another underappreciated area that presents some dilemmas when considering culture. Some youth may see their exploration of gender expression and identity as mutually exclusive to their membership to religious or spiritual organizations [37]. Others may engage in faith communities that are open and accepting of all gender and sexual identities. Poor processing of racial and spiritual identity (as well as other untold albeit important areas) and where they intersect gender may lead to a fractured sense of self. Clinicians may offer benefit when working with youth who prioritize their religious identity to explore gender-affirming faith communities as a positive way to engage this intersectionality.

Families are often a place where children get early messages about who they are, what is acceptable and valued, and who parents imagine them to be in their adult future. Decreased familial rejection may offer protection from the ill effects of an external environment that offers stigmatizing messages. In line with the minority stress model, family acceptance has been shown to positively influence mental and physical health and promote long-term improved health outcomes [23, 24]. Understanding families and their unique cultural perspectives is critical to assessing risk-mitigating influences and strength building opportunities in the lives of gender diverse youth.

Youth may rely on family, community, and spirituality for safety, sustenance, and survival. Clinicians may find it helpful to acknowledge a young person's fear of losing these supports and hold this concern while exploring visible and invisible identities. Cultivating a safe space with an emphasis on privacy is vital although may present dilemmas while holding in confidence a young person's exploration of gender, and the impact of this on their family and community. A comfort with using gender-neutral language, asserted name, correct pronouns, and avoiding misgendering will help to create a gender-affirming environment where these topics may be discussed comprehensively. Clinicians may find it prudent to acknowledge unintentional misgendering or lack of knowledge about the variety of patients' intersecting identities. This direct communication may lend authenticity to the clinician's work with the patient, and more in-depth conversations may occur as a consequence of validating vulnerabilities.

Physical spaces that reflect nondiscrimination and gender affirmation may also support the patients' experience that the clinical space is a safe space to talk about matters of gender, sexuality, race, and ethnicity [18]. Clinicians who remain open, respectful, and curious about every patient's unique gender and sexual development can both elicit important information and help to provide them with critical resources. Clinicians who inquire about rather than assume the centrality of any given identity, remain patient and supportive, and encourage exploration across identities and identifications will foster a sense of connection and understanding which will allow for the integration of the whole person during adolescence and beyond.

References

1. Vespa J, Armstrong DM, Medina L. Demographic turning points for the United States: population projections for 2020 to 2060. Current Population Reports, p. 25–1144, U.S. Census Bureau, Washington, DC, 2018.
2. Turban J, Zucker K, DeVries A. Gender dysphoria and gender incongruence. In: Martin A, Bloch M, Volkmar F, editors. Lewis's child and adolescent psychiatry: a comprehensive textbook. 5th ed. New York: Wolters Kluwer; 2018. p. 632–43.
3. Bockting WO. From construction to context: gender through the eyes of the transgendered. SIECUS Rep. 1999;28:3–7.
4. Davidson M. Seeking refuge under the umbrella: inclusion, exclusion, and organizing within the category of transgender. Sex Res Soc Policy. 2007;4:60. https://doi.org/10.1525/srsp.2007.4.4.60.
5. White-Hughto JM, Reisner SL, Pachankis JE. Transgender stigma and health: a critical review of stigma determinants, mechanisms, and interventions. Soc Sci Med. 2015;147:222–31. https://doi.org/10.1016/j.socscimed.2015.11.010.
6. Institute of Medicine. The health of lesbian, gay, bisexual, and transgender people: building a foundation for better understanding. Washington, DC: The National Academies Press; 2011.
7. Herman JL, Flores AR, Brown TN, Wilson BD, Conroe KJ. Age of individuals who identify as transgender in the United States. Los Angeles: The Williams Institute; 2017.
8. Ferguson AD, Miville BL. It's complicated: navigating multiple identities in small town America. J Clin Psychol. 2017;73:975–84. https://doi.org/10.1002/jclp.22507.
9. Hatchel T, Marx R. Understanding intersectionality and resiliency among transgender adolescents: exploring pathways among peer victimization, school belonging, and drug use. Int J Environ Res Public Health. 2018;15:1289. https://doi.org/10.3390/ijerph15061289.
10. Pascoe CJ. Dude, you're a fag: masculinity and sexuality in high school. Berkeley: University of California Press; 2007.
11. Williams R. The new gay teenager. Cambridge, MA: Harvard University Press; 2005.
12. Grossman AH, D'Augelli AR. Transgender youth: invisible and vulnerable. J Homosex. 2006;51:111–28. https://doi.org/10.1300/J082v51n01_06.
13. Mustanski BS, Garofalo R, Emerson EM. Mental health disorders, psychological distress, and suicidality in a diverse sample of lesbian, gay, bisexual, and transgender youths. Am J Public Health. 2010;100:2426–32. https://doi.org/10.2105/AJPH.2009.178319.
14. Adelson S, Walter H, Bukstein O, et al. Practice parameter on gay, lesbian, or bisexual sexual orientation, gender nonconformity, and gender discordance in children and adolescents. J Am Acad Child Adolesc Psychiatry. 2010;51:957–74. https://doi.org/10.1016/j.jaac.2012.07.004.

15. Sendén MG, Bäck EA, Lindqvist A. Introducing a gender-neutral pronoun in a natural gender language: the influence of time on attitudes and behavior. Front Psychol. 2015;6:893. https://doi.org/10.3389/fpsyg.2015.00893.
16. Greene B. African-American lesbians and gay men in psychodynamic psychotherapies? In: Moodley R, Palmer S, editors. Race culture and psychotherapy. New York: Routledge; 2006. p. 163–76.
17. Russell ST, Pollitt AM, Li G, Grossman AH. Chosen name use is linked to reduced depressive symptoms, suicidal ideation, and suicidal behavior among transgender youth. J Adolesc Health. 2018;63:503. https://doi.org/10.1016/j.jadohealth.2018.02.003.
18. Webster CR, Telingator CJ. Lesbian, gay, bisexual, and transgender families. Pediatr Clin N Am. 2016;63:1107–19. https://doi.org/10.1016/j.pcl.2016.07.010.
19. East JA, El Rayess F. Pediatricians' approach to the health care of lesbian, gay, and bisexual youth. J Adolesc Health. 1998;23:191–3. https://doi.org/10.1016/S1054-139X(97)00164-X.
20. Meyer IH. Prejudice social stress, and mental health in lesbian, gay, and bisexual populations: conceptual issues and research evidence. Psychol Bull. 2003;129:674–97. https://doi.org/10.1037/0033-2909.129.5.674.
21. Hendricks ML, Testa RJ. A conceptual framework for clinical work with transgender and gender nonconforming clients: an adaptation of the minority stress model. Prof Psychol Res Pract. 2012;43:460–7. https://doi.org/10.1037/a0029597.
22. Rood BA, Reisner SL, Surace FI, Puckett JA, Maroney MR, Pantalone DW. Expecting rejection: understanding the minority stress experiences of transgender and gender nonconforming individuals. Transgend Health. 2016;1:151–64. https://doi.org/10.1089/trgh.2016.0012.
23. Ryan C, Huebner D, Diaz RM, Sanchez J. Family rejection as a predictor of negative health outcomes in white and Latino lesbian, gay, and bisexual young adults. Pediatrics. 2009;123:346–52. https://doi.org/10.1542/peds.2007-3524.
24. Ryan C, Russell ST, Huebner D, Diaz R, Sanchez J. Family acceptance in adolescence and the health of LGBT young adults. J Child Adolesc Psychiatr Nurs. 2010;23:205–13. https://doi.org/10.1111/j.1744-6171.2010.00246.x.
25. Steensma T, Zucker K, Kreukels B, VanderLaan D, Wood H, Fuentes A, Cohen-Kettenis P. Behavioral and emotional problems on the teacher's report form: a cross-national, cross-clinic comparative analysis of gender dysphoric children and adolescents. J Abnorm Child Psychol. 2014;42:635–47. https://doi.org/10.1007/s10802-013-9804-2.
26. de Vries AL, Kreukels BP, Steensma TD, Doreleijers TA, Cohen-Kettenis PT. Comparing adult and adolescent transsexuals: an MMPI-2 and MMPI-A study. Psychiatry Res. 2011;2011(186):414–8. https://doi.org/10.1016/j.psychres.2010.07.033.
27. Toomey R, Syverten A, Shramko M. Transgender adolescent suicide behavior. Pediatrics. 2018;142:e20174218. https://doi.org/10.1542/peds.2017-4218.
28. McGuire J, Anderson C, Toomey R, Russell S. School climate for transgender youth: a mixed method investigation of student experiences and school responses. J Youth Adolesc. 2010;39:1175–88. https://doi.org/10.1007/s10964-010-9540-7.
29. Baams L. Disparities for LGBTQ and gender nonconforming adolescents. Pediatrics. 2018;141:e20173004. https://doi.org/10.1542/peds.2017-3004.
30. James S, Herman J, Rankin S, Keisling M, Mottet L, Anafi M. The report of the 2015 U.S. transgender survey. Washington, DC: National Center for Transgender Equality; 2016.
31. Jamil OB, Harper GW, Fernandez MI. Sexual and ethnic identity development among gay/bisexual/questioning (GBQ) male ethnic minority adolescents. Cultur Divers Ethnic Minor Psychol. 2009;15:203–14. https://doi.org/10.1037/a0014795.
32. WPATH. Standards of care for the health of transsexual, transgender, and gender nonconforming people. 7th ed. 2011. https://www.wpath.org/media/cms/Documents/SOC%20v7/SOC%20V7_English.pdf. Accessed 29 Sept 2018.
33. Leary K. Racial enactments in dynamic treatment. Psychoanalytic Dialogues. 2000;10:639–53.
34. Cisz, J. White privilege and the therapist's subjectivity. Race and subjectivity: the politics of interracial and therapeutic and supervisory interactions. Panel presented at the convention of the American Psychological Association, San Francisco. 1998.

35. Farr RH, Crain EE, Oakley MK, Cashen KK, Garber KJ. Microaggressions, feelings of difference, and resilience among adopted children with sexual minority parents. J Youth Adolesc. 2016;45:85–104. https://doi.org/10.1007/s10964-015-0353-6.
36. Pauker K, Apfelbaum E, Spitzer B. When societal norms and social identity collide: the race talk dilemma for racial minority children. Soc Psychol Personal Sci. 2015;6:887–95. https://doi.org/10.1177/1948550615598379.
37. Grossoehme DH, Teeters A, Jelinek SM, Dimitriou S, Conard LA. Screening for spiritual struggle in an adolescent transgender clinic: feasibility and acceptability. J Health Care Chaplain. 2016;22:54–66. https://doi.org/10.1080/08854726.2015.1123004.
38. Dowshen N, Forke CM, Johnson AK, Kuhns LM, Rubin D, Garofalo R. Religiosity as a protective factor against HIV risk among young transgender women. J Adolesc Health. 2011;48:410–4. https://doi.org/10.1016/j.jadohealth.2010.07.021.

International Considerations & Variations in Practice: An African Perspective

19

Anusha Lachman

Introduction

Despite the socio-economic and geopolitical differences across continents, there is an accelerating awareness and recognition of the natural variations of an individual's sexual orientation, gender identity and sexuality. However, states and governments, especially in Africa, may not offer gender diverse individuals protection and freedom of expression. Thirty-eight of fifty-three African nations criminalize homosexuality and impose varying degrees of legislative restrictions on sexual desires and practices. They also restrict the fulfilment of human rights of individuals. On the other hand, South Africa serves as a model of one of the few African countries where human rights, gender equality and freedom of expression are legally and constitutionally protected. This chapter draws on these basic tenets of this model and presents a case study on the protection, challenges and cultural development of gender identity, specifically in the context of children and adolescents in Africa. In this chapter, we will begin by describing some common perspectives on gender and sexuality that have existed in the African continent over time. We will then discuss the influence of the international scientific and advocacy community in shaping this view in more recent years. Subsequently, the case of South Africa will be used to provide a more specific example of the experiences of gender diverse youth outside a major European or North American country, and describe the nature and structure of available services.

A. Lachman (✉)
Department of Psychiatry, Stellenbosch University, Cape Town, South Africa
e-mail: anusha@sun.ac.za

M. Forcier et al. (eds.), *Pediatric Gender Identity*,
https://doi.org/10.1007/978-3-030-38909-3_19

African Perspectives on Gender and Sexuality

As social constructs, the concepts of sexuality, sexual orientation and categories of gender identity mean different things in different societies at different times. Generally, however, sexuality is a more commonly discussed and understood concept than gender identity. Most African cultures have traditionally accommodated this diversity and recognized people with a wide range of sexual orientations, identities and practices as members of the community whose well-being is a part of the communal well-being [1, 2]. African societies of the past, although regulated by traditional communities, were, with some exceptions, much more tolerant and accepting of non-normative sexualities and behaviours than the people who colonized them.

Homosexuality was already a known behaviour across much of the African continent before colonialism. Social anthropologists [3, 4] suggest that the intolerance of homosexuality, and systems of surveillance and regulation of sexual expression were introduced by the colonial invaders. In addition to political and economic changes, colonialism challenged indigenous religious and social practices to the extent that the conquered peoples often embraced a traditional Christianity that did not see a religious role for people with non-normative sexualities. A number of colonial era laws that criminalized sexual diversity and behaviours are still upheld, perpetuating the belief that homosexuality is a modern development [5].

Traditional societies in Africa developed ways of ordering same-sex attractions and behaviour, and it was during the height of imperialism that more precise 'definitions' of sexual orientations and gender identity were developed. It was also at this time that the punishment, both legal and extra-juridical, of non-normative behaviour started to occur in earnest [6]. Countries such as Cameroon, Burundi, Uganda and Nigeria criminalize and prohibit relationships and freedom of expression for individuals within the Lesbian Gay Bisexual Transgender and Queer/Questioning (LGBTQ+) community, as well as those with Intersex conditions. Legal punishments may include extensive periods of imprisonment or even the death penalty (Sudan, Nigeria, Mauritania, South Somalia).

Many African countries do not just implement legal sanctions against lesbian, gay, bisexual, transgender, queer and intersex (LGBTQI) populations, but may impose additional hardships and barriers to care that affect long-term health outcomes. Many communities do not have easy access to healthcare providers and services that are knowledgeable and offer culturally sensitive LGBTQI preventive health. Even in places with accessible healthcare systems, many intersex individuals face harmful practices including involuntary or coercive treatment, while in places without such systems, infanticide, abandonment and mutilation may occur. These practices can result in the reversal of key public health gains in terms of sexual health education, HIV/AIDS programs and addressing increasing levels of social violence, particularly against women and children [7].

Impact of Science and Global Discussions on LGBTQI Human Rights

There is global consensus among scientists that variation in sexual orientation and practices, including same sex relationship and pansexual orientations, is a normal and natural variation of human sexuality without any inherently detrimental health consequences. Scientific understanding of gender beyond binary concepts is additionally becoming a part of the health and social conversation. More and more transgender and gender diverse (TGD) persons, as well as persons born with disorders of sexual development (i.e., intersex) experience and live a gender identity that varies from that assigned at birth. As a result of this global shift in attitudes and perspectives, there has been an expansion of activity in both legal and social sectors of some African nations to ensure the protection of human rights amongst sexual and gender minoritized groups. The African Commission on Human and People's Rights (ACHPR) adopted a resolution in 2014 calling '*for an end to all acts of violence and abuse, whether committed by State or non-state actors, including by enacting and effectively applying appropriate laws prohibiting and punishing all forms of violence including those targeting persons on the basis of their imputed or real sexual orientation or gender identities, ensuring proper investigation and diligent prosecution of perpetrators, and establishing judicial procedures responsive to the needs of victims*' [8].

In November 2017, the first African Intersex Meeting took place in South Africa bringing together representatives of Intersex organizations from seven African countries. This meeting reaffirmed the principles of the International Intersex Forum which demands the abolition of discrimination against people with Intersex in Africa, and fights to ensure the rights of bodily integrity, autonomy and self-determination. Iranti-org (https://www.iranti-org.co.za/), an NGO that advocates for Intersex awareness in Africa, drives political and social legislative changes that aim to end the societal misinformation and stigma that perpetuate the violence and killing (often infanticide) of intersex people. In late 2018, Iranti-org ran workshops for school children and their families to increase awareness and provide support for trans- and gender diverse learners in Johannesburg, South Africa. In August of that year, the South African Department of Higher Education and training together with the University of Witwatersrand held a Critical Thinking Forum to focus on gender identity and diverse sexual orientation in tertiary learning institutions. These and similar efforts assure civil rights and protection is particularly important in the context of extending these rights and decreasing ongoing risk of violence targeting persons on the basis of their sexual orientation or gender identities.

The South African Example

The South African post-apartheid state enacted a multitude of laws and policies to prevent discrimination and ensure the health of its people, including support for gender-affirming care (GAC) including access to legal, ethical and medical practice which theoretically is available in both public and private health sectors in the country. South Africa subscribes to the rights contained in the Sexual Health Charter (Constitution of the Republic of South Africa) and is, therefore, obliged to ensure that the sexual rights of all persons are respected and protected [9]. Sexual and reproductive rights are included as human rights such as the right to expression of sexual orientation without interference, equality and equity, freedom to make choices free from gender-based discrimination, and freedom from sexual violence or coercion. Despite legislation and freedom of expression, actual access to GAC remains severely limited. As in other countries, the access to GAC that is available is often unequal, can be extremely protracted and is out of reach for all but the wealthiest in society [10].

Gender Narratives in South African Youth

A study assessing the lived experiences of individuals within the transgender community in South Africa reported that many transgender youth were able to recall 'knowing from an early age' that they were different, resulting in a dissonance that most often was only defined in adulthood [11]. Reflecting on their childhood, participants shared their difficulty and sadness with the early awareness of the socially enforced rules relating to gender and the sense of confusion and distress as this dissonance between their assigned sex and their sense of gender identity grew. Discrimination and risks resulting from sexual or gender minoritized status is particularly relevant to adolescents who often face intense pressure to conform to gender roles and identities in multiple domains – with peers in school, at home and in religious circles. In addition, poorer health outcomes are known to be related to stress caused by high levels of social alienation, bullying and violence and potential rejection by family and community.

Many young TGD persons seek family and community support, but may in turn find themselves rejected by families who do not understand or are unsupportive as their children explore diverse gender or sexual identities. The resulting alienation and absence of social support may affect adolescent self-image, peer mastery and the innate sense of community belonging which increases the vulnerability for mental health disorders in adolescence. In addition, sexual and gender minoritized youth are at risk for sexual assault [13, 14]. A study by the Academy of Science in South Africa (ASSAf) found no evidence to corroborate the cultural belief that LGBTQI identification is a result of sexual abuse or that the LTGBQI community 'recruits' members in this fashion. This myth is routinely used to justify the marginalization of LGBTI persons in many communities. The ASSAf study interestingly also found evidence that more repressive environments may increase stress and negatively impact priority health outcomes in Africa, specifically with reference to HIV/AIDS and sexually transmitted infection reduction efforts.

Medical and Affirming Care for Gender diverse Youth

There are currently no Department of Health–issued policies or guidelines on transgender health or GAC. This has implications for care provision and attitudes of healthcare professionals [10]. Urban centre public hospitals provide some aspects of GAC (including hormone treatments and surgical intervention), but there after often long waiting lists for these services. Private practice medical care physicians can provide GAC, although many procedures are not covered under 'essential' private medical insurance benefits by the top five medical insurance providers in South Africa. 'Essential benefits' covered by private insurance in South Africa does not include any non-emergency or elective gender-related surgery or chronic hormone replacement for persons seeking GAC. Gender identity and sexual orientation, like other social determinants of health, can lead to health disparities if not supported or assured of access to care. Compared to their non-transgender socio-economically matched peers, LGBTQI youth are more likely to face barriers accessing appropriate health care [10]. At present, mental health professionals have a role as gatekeepers to transition services for transgender people [12]. However, when mental health workers act in this role, it can lead to the assumption that those seeking transition invariably have mental health issues or require psychiatric review [12]. Furthermore, mental health providers do not necessarily receive adequate training which creates additional barrier to both access and quality of GAC. In addition, having mental health providers in the role of gatekeepers, perpetuates stigma and associations of diversity as deviance for those LGBTQI patients who do not otherwise have mental health needs.

South Africa has come a long way with regards to the biomedical and legal treatment of variations of gender identity and variations of sexual development, with many activists considering the country to be among the most progressive worldwide. Nevertheless, people with variations of gender identity and/or sex development, still face an array of obstacles. The economic divide plays an important role concerning access to information, access to health care and body alteration.

Despite the progressive standing, there are very few dedicated clinical services that operate specifically for LGBTQI children and adolescents in South African health care settings including primary health clinics or academic hospitals. Services for TGD youth are especially limited. In urban communities, multidisciplinary services do exist and are typically based at tertiary academic training hospitals. Patients are primarily referred by local community service organizations such as Gender Dynamix (https://www.genderdynamix.org.za/) and the Triangle Project (a LGBTI service organization), community health clinics, district and regional hospitals, as well as general practitioners from rural areas or from neighbouring African countries. Organizations such as Gender DynamiX, Iranti-org and Intersex South Africa (ISSA) focus on eradicating discrimination against and within the LGBT community [15]. These organizations maintain diversity within their staff, broker information to diverse socio-economic groups and have a strong advocacy role in the community.

At Cape Town's Red Cross Children's Hospital, the Gender Identity Development Service is run by a child psychiatrist, with additional support from a psychologist, nurse therapist and a pediatric endocrinologist. The service straddles two areas – supervision for professionals working with gender diverse children and the facilitation of family and adolescent groups for TGD adolescents. The adolescents have an additional social media support group and online platform to interact with other youth across the country. (Personal communication by Dr S Pickstone-Taylor, Red Cross Gender Identity Development Service, 2018.) Although less than ideal, the gender identity development clinic at Red Cross Hospital serves as a prototype for how mental health professionals may play an integral role in the multidisciplinary assessment, ongoing support and treatment of many transgender children and adolescents as they move through their transition process [12].

Youth with Disorders of Sexual Development (DSD)

Although clearly distinct from Gender Diversity, DSD have a more established history of treatment in South Africa, and are informative as an example of how gender may be managed within the healthcare system. In South Africa, for ethical and legal reasons, the decision regarding DSD care, including surgery, is made by a team of healthcare professionals. The team in most cases consists of a psychologist, an endocrinologist, the parents and the surgeon. These multidisciplinary teams are a necessary resource for training, research and follow-up, even in economically challenged African countries. However, if these centres are not available, the current South African recommendations are that medical providers should refrain from any potentially harmful practices and postpone surgery until the onset of puberty, or until the child is old enough to make their own decision [16, 17].

Parents, guardians and the medical team supporting them make decisions on behalf of the infant with the goal of promoting a well-adjusted adult. Delaying genital surgery may be satisfactory in cases where the family and social dynamics are supportive of anatomical ambiguity, but in some cases indeterminate genital anatomy causes such distress to the family unit that early surgical intervention is requested by parents [18]. It should be noted that what is in the best interest of the family might not be in the best interest of the child. The evolving autonomy of the child must be balanced with the child's need for parental support and guidance. Care must be integrated across medical, cultural, social and psychological realms [19].

A controversial area of gender diversity involves the international incident in 2009, when a South African adolescent had an unexpected victory in the women's 800 m final of the International Association of Athletic Federations (IAAF) World Championships in Berlin. This athlete recorded the world's fastest time of the year for the 800 m race. The race result fuelled concerns about the athlete's 'masculine' features, including her deep voice, her muscular build and facial features. Speculation was raised regarding her gender from her competitors.

Despite a history of gender verification policies and practices, and the stakes involved in adjudicating on the gender of a female athlete, no sports governing bodies could supply clear guidelines as to what makes a female athlete 'female' [20]. In 2010, reacting to the gender verification controversy, the International Olympics Committee (IOC) announced that gender verification tests would no longer be done in the service of competitive fairness, but in the service of health. Gender verification technologies have revealed a broad diversity of anatomical, genetic and hormonal conditions that challenge the gender binary codified in sport and make eligibility rulings on the basis of anatomical or chromosomally assigned sex impossible. Current medical technology has made it possible to diagnose DSDs more accurately than ever before. Children and youth have more opportunities for genital surgery to 'correct' abnormalities once detected. But science cannot create a binary where there is not one – and so athletics societies cannot determine the 'real' sex of an intersex athlete, nor can these technologies address the philosophical problem of what constitutes an 'unfair advantage' for the IOC's purposes. It is suggested that the long-term well-being of patients with DSDs is best accomplished by aligning with medical standards that protect a patient's right to privacy regarding their medical information.

Conclusion

Africa as a continent reveals a diversity of attitudes, legal constructs and socio-economic disadvantages facing LGBTQI and TGD youth. This brief overview of the current available information on practices in South Africa and highlights the ongoing challenges in terms of availability of guidelines, state protections and the accessing of evidence-based health care for TGD and DSD children, along with the additional cultural, socio-economic, and other obstacles these children and families face.

References

1. Cantu L. Boy-wives and female husbands: studies of African homosexualities. Contemp Sociol. 1999;28(5):554.
2. Herdt G. Third sex, third gender: beyond sexual dimorphism in culture and history. New York: Zone Books; 1996.
3. De Vos P. On the legal construction of gay and lesbian identity and South Africa's transitional constitution. S Afr J Hum Rights. 1996;12:256–89.
4. Kendall K. Lesbian expression in Lesotho: homophobia is the white Folk's disease. Pietermaritzburg: University of Natal; 1996.
5. Foucault M. The history of sexuality: volume 1: an introduction. Knopf Doubleday Publishing Group; 1990.
6. Amnesty International. Making love a crime. Criminalisation of same-sex conduct in sub-Saharan Africa. UK: Amnesty International Publications; 2013. [Online]. Available from: https://www.amnestyusa.org/wp-content/uploads/2017/04/making_love_a_crime_-_africa_lgbti_report_emb_6.24.13_0.pdf [cited 20 Novemnber 2018].

7. Academy of Science of South Africa. Diversity in human sexuality: implications for policy in Africa 2015 [Online]. Available at: https://doi.org/10.17159/assaf/0022
8. African Commission on Human and Peoples' Rights. Resolution on protection against violence and other human rights violations against persons on the basis of their real or imputed sexual orientation or gender [Online]. ACHPR 2018. Available at: http://www.achpr.org/sessions/55th/resolutions/275/ [cited 20 November 2018].
9. The constitution of the republic of South Africa. 5th ed. Cape Town: Juta & Co Ltd; 1996.
10. Spencer S, Meer T, Müller A. "The care is the best you can give at the time": health care professionals' experiences in providing gender affirming care in South Africa. PLoS One. 2017;12(7):e0181132.
11. Ashwal JE. "Lived experiences of gender identity and expression within the South African transgender community" [Doctoral dissertation]. Faculty of Humanities, University of the Witwatersrand, Johannesburg; 2017.
12. Wilson D, Marais A, De Villiers A, Addinall R, Campbell MM. Transgender issues in South Africa, with particular reference to the Groote Schuur Hospital Transgender Unit. S Afr Med J. 2014;104(6):448–9.
13. Lehavot K, Molina Y, Simoni JM. Childhood trauma, adult sexual assault, and adult gender expression among lesbian and bisexual women. Sex Roles. 2012;67(5–6):272–84.
14. Roberts AL, Glymour MM, Koenen KC. Does maltreatment in childhood affect sexual orientation in adulthood? Arch Sex Behav. 2013;42(2):161–71.
15. Klein T. Intersex and transgender activism in South Africa. Liminalis. 2009;3:15–41.
16. Ganie Y, Aldous C, Balakrishna Y, Wiersma R. The spectrum of ovotesticular disorders of sex development in South Africa: a single-centre experience. Horm Res Paediatr. 2017;87(5):307–14.
17. Wiersma R. True hermaphroditism in southern Africa: the clinical picture. Pediatr Surg Int. 2004;20(5):363–8.
18. Rebelo E, Szabo CP, Pitcher G. Gender assignment surgery on children with disorders of sex development: a case report and discussion from South Africa. J Child Health Care. 2008;12(1):49–59.
19. Turban JL, Ehrensaft D. Research review: gender identity in youth: treatment paradigms and controversies. J Child Psychol Psychiatry. 2018;59(12):1228–43.
20. Wells C, Darnell SC. Caster Semenya, gender verification and the politics of fairness in an online track & field community. Sociol Sport J. 2014;31(1):44–65.

Legal Considerations for Transgender and Gender Diverse Youth

20

Ryan Thoreson

Introduction

Practitioners working with transgender and gender diverse (TGD) youth are guided in their practice by a variety of considerations, ranging from the general edict to do no harm to more detailed ethical guidelines issued by professional bodies. The treatment of TGD youth should also be informed by relevant federal and state laws, including laws related to discrimination, privacy, informed consent, children's rights, and parental rights. As transgender rights become increasingly salient in the public sphere, law in this area has evolved rapidly and created a patchwork of protections that can vary considerably from state to state. While healthcare providers should be attentive to legal developments as they occur, it is helpful also to think of some of the general considerations that might arise in the course of working with TGD youth.

This chapter reviews some of the main legal guideposts for treating TGD youth. It provides an overview of relevant federal law, with a special focus on the Patient Protection and Affordable Care Act (ACA), the Health Insurance Portability and Accountability Act (HIPAA), Title IX of the Education Amendments of 1972, and the Family Educational Rights and Privacy Act (FERPA). It also takes stock of various state laws, and relevant requirements regarding informed consent, parental notification, and name and gender marker changes. It finally addresses emerging questions around religious or moral objections to providing transition-related care. In this dynamic landscape, the chapter identifies some guiding legal principles that can act as dependable lodestars for practitioners seeking to provide sensitive, compassionate, and effective care.

R. Thoreson (✉)
Yale Law School, New Haven, CT, USA

M. Forcier et al. (eds.), *Pediatric Gender Identity*,
https://doi.org/10.1007/978-3-030-38909-3_20

Federal Law

As of 2019, there were very few federal laws that explicitly prohibited discrimination based on gender identity.[1] Nonetheless, practitioners should be aware that there is considerable authority establishing that discrimination based on gender identity constitutes a form of discrimination based on sex. Discrimination on the basis of sex is prohibited under a much wider range of federal statutes, including those related to health care, which extend important protections to TGD youth.

In 2010, the Congress enacted, and President Obama signed, the Patient Protection and Affordable Care Act (ACA). The ACA includes a nondiscrimination provision, Section 1557, which prohibits discrimination based on race, color, national origin, sex, age, and disability in any health programs or activities that are funded or administered by the US Department of Health and Human Services (HHS) [1]. It also prohibits discrimination in insurance plans offered by health insurance issuers who participate in the Health Insurance Marketplaces [1]. Since its enactment in 2010, Section 1557 has been enforced by the Office of Civil Rights at HHS, and has helped protect the rights of patients who might otherwise face discrimination in health care on one of these protected grounds.

In 2016, HHS promulgated a rule that clarified the scope of Section 1557. The rule clarified that discrimination based on "sex" not only includes discrimination against men and women because they are men or women, but also discrimination based on pregnancy status, sex stereotyping, and gender identity [2]. While the rule primarily uses the term "gender identity," it defines the concept expansively to include a person's gender expression and transgender status. It also expressly states that it aims to protect nonbinary individuals from sex discrimination, and therefore defines "gender identity" as an internal sense of one's gender which "may be male, female, neither, or a combination of male and female" [2].

Recognizing that Section 1557 prohibits discrimination against TGD patients has practical repercussions for providers offering care. Under the rule, for example, providers cannot refuse to treat patients because of their gender identity or expression, deny TGD patients the services that they offer to cisgender patients, or harass or mistreat patients because of their gender identity or expression [3]. Insurers are also obligated to comply with Section 1557 and cannot refuse to insure a person or increase their rates because of their transgender status, categorically exclude transition-related care from the plans they offer, or deny transgender people coverage for services that are typically associated with their sex assigned at birth [3].

Shortly after the Obama Administration issued the rule implementing Section 1557, eight states and religiously affiliated healthcare providers challenged it in court, arguing that its interpretation would violate the religious exercise of providers who assert objections to offering reproductive and transition-related care [4]. A federal judge in Texas responded by issuing a preliminary injunction, preventing

---

[1] Statutes that expressly use the term "gender identity" include the Matthew Shepard and James Byrd Jr. Hate Crimes Prevention Act of 2009 and the reauthorization of the Violence Against Women Act in 2013 [34, 35].

HHS from enforcing its interpretation as the case proceeded [5]. In May 2017, HHS – now under the Trump Administration – notified the court that it planned to roll back the rule's language clarifying that discrimination based on sex includes discrimination based on gender identity [6]. In April 2018, HHS informed the court that such a revision had been submitted to the White House for review [7]. In May of 2019, the administration released the proposed rule, and opened it for public comment shortly thereafter.

Practitioners should be aware that the Trump Administration's roll back only affects how HHS interprets Section 1557. It does not (and cannot) alter the statutory text of Section 1557 itself, in which Congress prohibits healthcare providers and insurers from discriminating on the basis of sex. As of July 2019, six federal appellate courts – collectively covering Alabama, Alaska, Arizona, California, Delaware, Florida, Georgia, Hawaii, Idaho, Illinois, Indiana, Kentucky, Maine, Massachusetts, Michigan, Montana, Nevada, New Hampshire, New Jersey, Ohio, Oregon, Pennsylvania, Rhode Island, Tennessee, Washington, and Wisconsin – have issued rulings indicating that statutory language prohibiting discrimination based on sex covers discrimination based on gender identity [8–13]. Thus, some courts may interpret Section 1557 to prohibit discrimination based on gender identity and enforce it accordingly even if the Trump Administration formally adopts a narrower understanding of the statute's scope.

The Trump Administration's decision to roll back the rule is nevertheless dangerous. It is likely to sow confusion among providers and insurers about what their obligations are under federal law, making it more likely that TGD individuals will face discrimination and be denied care to which they are entitled. It also means that HHS will not proactively enforce Section 1557 in an inclusive way. Such a move puts the onus on TGD patients who experience discrimination to bring suit and assert their rights in court, a remedy that may be functionally inaccessible for those without the means or desire to litigate.

In addition to Section 1557, federal privacy laws provide protections that are relevant to TGD people, including TGD youth. In healthcare settings, the Health Insurance Portability and Accountability Act (HIPAA) protects patient privacy, including a person's transgender status and information about their transition related care [3]. In order to avoid disclosing protected information, providers should consider adopting record-keeping systems that recognize a patient's gender identity in addition to their sex assigned at birth, appropriately integrate use of patient asserted names and pronouns in medical interactions, and respect patient autonomy regarding disclosure of their transgender status. Efforts to educate and support administrative staff can help ensure protection of TGD patients and their right to privacy and quality care.

Providers working in schools or advising TGD youth on social transition should also be aware of federal protections in educational settings. Title IX of the Education Amendments of 1972 prohibits sex discrimination in all schools that receive federal assistance. In May 2016, the Obama Administration's Department of Education and Department of Justice issued guidance affirming that discrimination based on gender identity constitutes discrimination based on sex and is therefore impermissible under Title IX. The guidance noted that, where schools provide sex-segregated activities and facilities, "transgender students must be allowed to participate in such activities and access such facilities consistent with their gender identity" [14]. A handful of states challenged the guidance in court and a federal judge enjoined it from taking effect as the case proceeded. In February 2017, the Department of Education and Department of Justice – now under the Trump Administration – rescinded the guidance and stopped actively enforcing Title IX in cases of discrimination based on gender identity in schools [15].

Even in the absence of guidance, however, Title IX continues to provide protection for TGD youth. Like Section 1557 of the ACA, Title IX is a federal statute that has meaning independent of the executive branch's interpretation of its provisions. Since the guidance was withdrawn, at least two federal courts of appeals have indicated that Title IX prohibits discrimination on the basis of gender identity in schools [8, 9]. The withdrawal of the guidance also does not prevent schools from enacting strong and affirming policies of their own. Providers working with TGD youth, their parents, and their school administrators should be mindful of the ways that explicit protections can contribute to positive physical and mental health outcomes. Research shows that school policies that affirm and respect gender identity can alleviate bullying and harassment, ameliorate health concerns, protect privacy, and improve TGD students' ability to learn [16].

Providers working in educational settings should also be aware of the Family Educational Rights and Privacy Act (FERPA), which permits students to request a change to their school records if they are "inaccurate, misleading, or in violation of the student's rights of privacy" [17]. Students considering a request to have their name and/or gender marker changed at school should note that, at present, FERPA gives parents rights over some school records until the minor is 18 or enrolls in postsecondary education. TGD youth who are under 18 and enrolled in junior high or high school will typically need a parent or guardian's approval to request these formal name and gender marker changes. It is important to note, however, that nothing in FERPA prevents school personnel, including providers, from respecting students' gender identity, using gender-affirming names and pronouns, and providing access to appropriate facilities on school grounds.

While explicit protections for gender identity are scarce in federal law, these nondiscrimination and privacy protections offer important safeguards for TGD youth. As discussed below, the legal landscape around treatment of TGD youth can vary somewhat from state to state. Even given a wide variation in state laws and protections, providers should continue to ensure that their conduct does not violate essential professional standards, including the right for all minors, including TGD youth, to obtain treatment free from discrimination, and to ensure that their legal rights to privacy are respected at all times in healthcare and educational settings.

State Law

Beyond federal protections, state law also offers guidance for providers to follow in treating TGD youth. Providers should be particularly aware of state laws related to trans-inclusive nondiscrimination protections, consent to medical care, and name and gender marker changes.

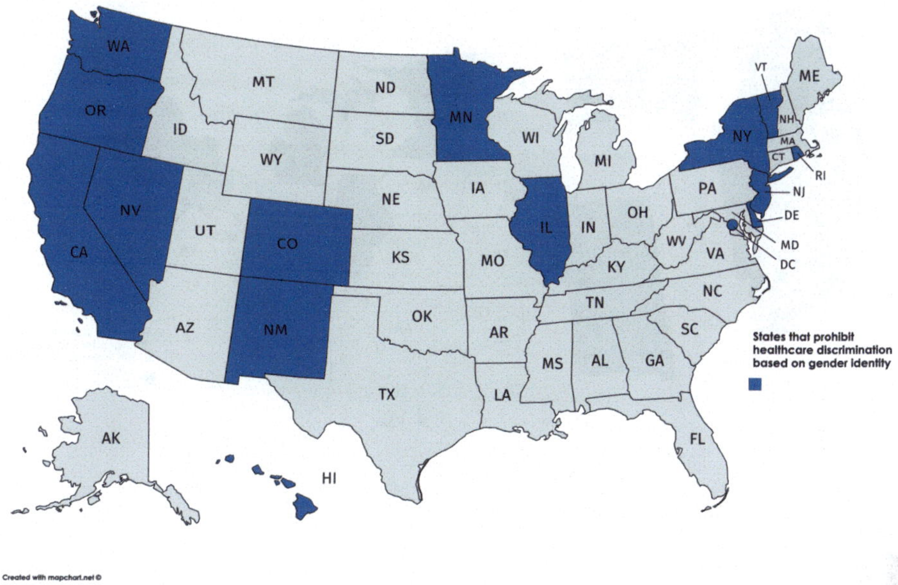

Fig. 20.1 States that prohibit healthcare discrimination based on gender identity, July 2019

Section 1557 prohibits sex discrimination in health care nationwide, but until HHS interprets and enforces the sex discrimination provision in a trans-inclusive way, state protections remain vitally important. Unfortunately, relatively few states have expressly prohibited discrimination against TGD people in healthcare. As of July 2019, a mere 14 states and the District of Columbia prohibit private insurers from discriminating on the basis of gender identity [18]. Only 20 states and the District of Columbia prohibit private insurers from offering plans with "transgender exclusions," or provisions that categorically deny coverage for any services related to gender transition [18].[2] States are similarly divided in terms of the coverage they provide for TGD individuals under state Medicaid policies (Figs. 20.1, 20.2, and 20.3). Medicaid expressly covers transition-related care in 18 states and the District of Columbia, is unclear on the question of transition-related care in 24 states, and expressly excludes transition-related care in 8 states [18].

In 2018, courts in two states that explicitly exclude transition-related care issued rulings against such exclusions. In Iowa, the court ruled that the exclusion violated the Iowa Civil Rights Act and the Iowa Constitution, and in Wisconsin, the court found the exclusion likely constitutes sex discrimination and violates Section 1557 of the ACA and the Equal Protection Clause of the US Constitution [19, 20]. In 2019, Iowa revised its law to again allow Medicaid to opt out of providing transition-related care, prompting a new legal challenge. Although these types of cases are still working their way through the system, they illustrate that courts may be receptive to trans-inclusive understandings of sex discrimination provisions, and that states that maintain these exclusions may be vulnerable to judicial challenges.

[2] At the federal level, Medicare eliminated its "transgender exclusion" in 2014 [36].

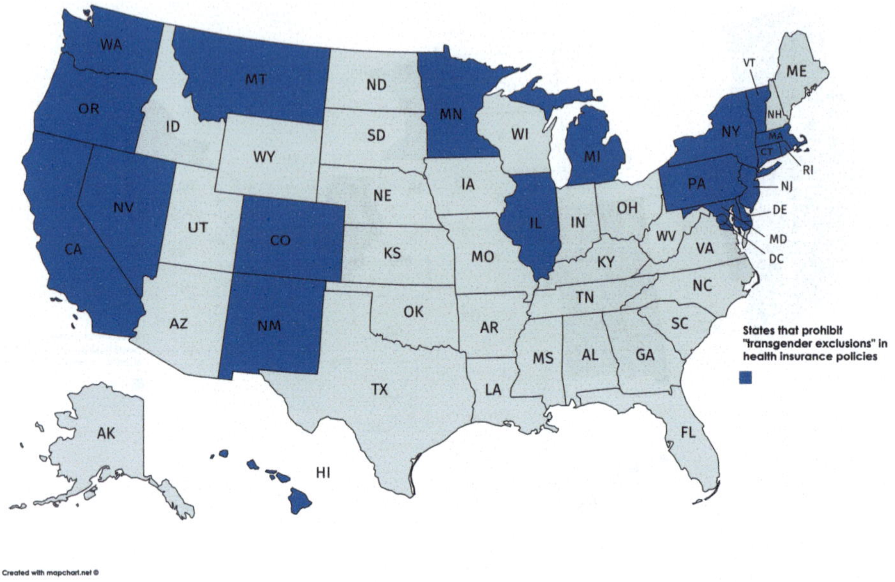

Fig. 20.2 States that prohibit "transgender exclusions"in healthcare policies, July 2019

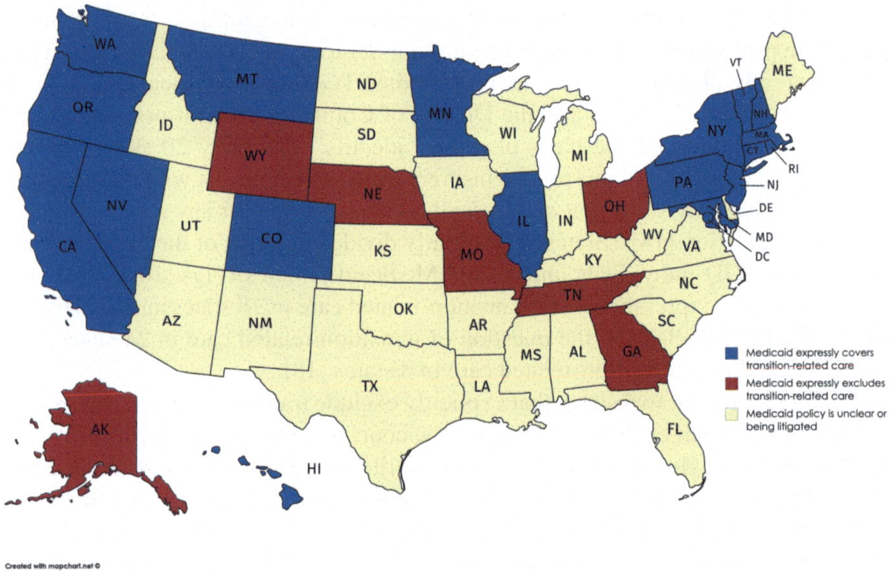

Fig. 20.3 State policies related to transgender health and Medicaid, July 2019

For TGD youth, however, other considerations also come into play. Practitioners should be mindful of the conditions under which young people can consent to general medical care, which can vary from state to state. In every US state, there is a general requirement that parents or guardians must consent to medical care administered to minors, with some limited exceptions.[3] Providers may be held legally liable if they administer medical care in the absence of required parental consent; at the same time, providers may feel they are ethically or professionally required to provide gender-affirming care to a TGD youth who would experience harm without it.

Minors' access to confidential care, and protections that assure this care, have long been an issue for providers of adolescent medicine. Historically, as with issues of sexual activity, contraception, and sexually transmitted infection prevention, adolescent healthcare providers have had to operate at the edges of legal requirements that vary by state, when these and parental wishes are in conflict with medically necessary standards of care. Helping parents understand their own personal feelings and issues that may conflict with medical science is a part of working with families. Including a harm reduction perspective as well as a careful weighing of risks and benefits is critical to help parents who are struggling to understand why certain medical recommendations are in the best interest of their child's health and safety. In most states, medical consent laws do not require dual parent consent, but generally require that at least one parent or guardian with legal custody consent to care. If the child's parents are married, they typically both have legal custody over the child. If the child's parents are divorced or separated, legal custody may be more complicated, and providers should determine who is in a position to access records and make decisions regarding the child's care. While having all parents or guardians consent to care and affirm their child's TGD identity is optimal, it is not necessary or possible in many cases. Ensuring that a single primary caregiver understands the issues and is willing to support their TGD child may be the best that can be achieved in certain situations. When presented with documentation about legally required dual parent consent for medical decision making in the case of divorced parents or a legal cease and desist notification, the medical provider must act in accordance with the law. However, many providers work with youth, supportive family members, and the legal system and go to court to work around issues of medical neglect, verbal or emotional child abuse, and the imperative of extending medically necessary care to their minor patients.

Complications may thus be created when one or more legal guardians of a child object to a particular course of treatment. One consideration for providers to keep in mind, however, is whether a state has adopted or rejected the mature minor doctrine, which recognizes that sufficiently informed and mature youth may be equipped to consent to a course of treatment without parental consent. Generally, the mature minor doctrine applies to youth who are at least 16 years old, although some states allow practitioners and courts to extend the designation to younger individuals. The

[3] Exceptions exist, for example, when youth are legally emancipated or in life-threatening emergencies.

doctrine varies in its existence and applicability from state to state. In some jurisdictions, it has been codified into law; in others, it has been developed in the courts; and in others, it does not exist. Practitioners faced with parental disapproval of a course of treatment for a TGD minor should consult the laws of their state, legal counsel, or professional associations in their state and consider whether the mature minor doctrine would apply.

A final consideration that practitioners should keep in mind are the requirements for changing a person's name and gender marker under state law. Obtaining legal recognition of one's name and gender can be an important part of social transition with benefits for a person's health and well-being. While all US states generally allow individuals to change their names, the requirements for documents like driver's licenses and birth certificates differ from state to state [21].

The requirements to change gender markers on driver's licenses vary widely. In 22 states and the District of Columbia, the state will change a person's gender marker without any documentation or with documentation from a wide range of professionals. In 14 states, a person must meet a slightly higher burden by providing proof of clinical treatment or updated documentation. In 9 states, a person must meet far more stringent requirements by providing proof of gender confirmation surgery, a court order, or an updated birth certificate to change the gender marker on their driver's license. In the final 5 states, the policy remains somewhat unclear (Fig. 20.4). Notably, 12 states – Arkansas, California, Colorado, Hawaii, Indiana, Maine, Maryland, Minnesota, Nevada, Oregon, Utah, and Vermont – and the District of Columbia allow people to select a nonbinary gender marker on their driver's license [21].

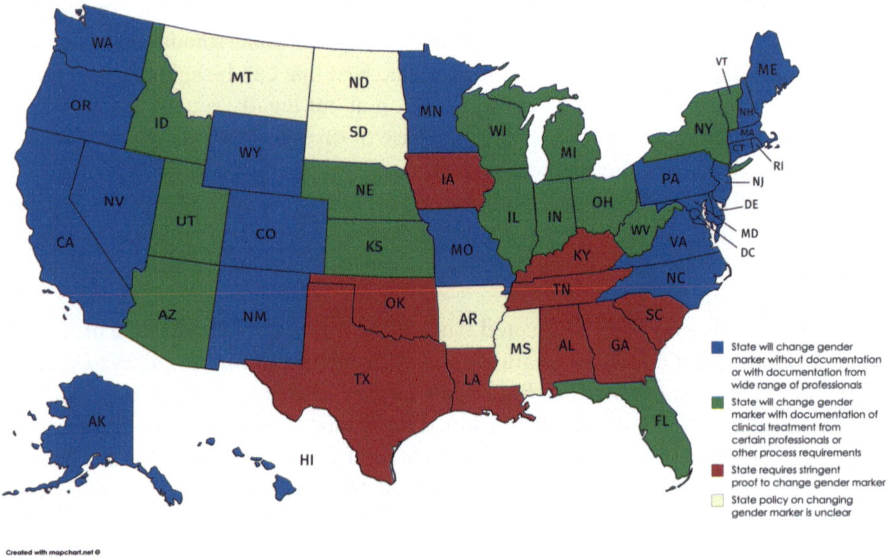

Fig. 20.4 State policies on changing gender markers on identification, July 2019

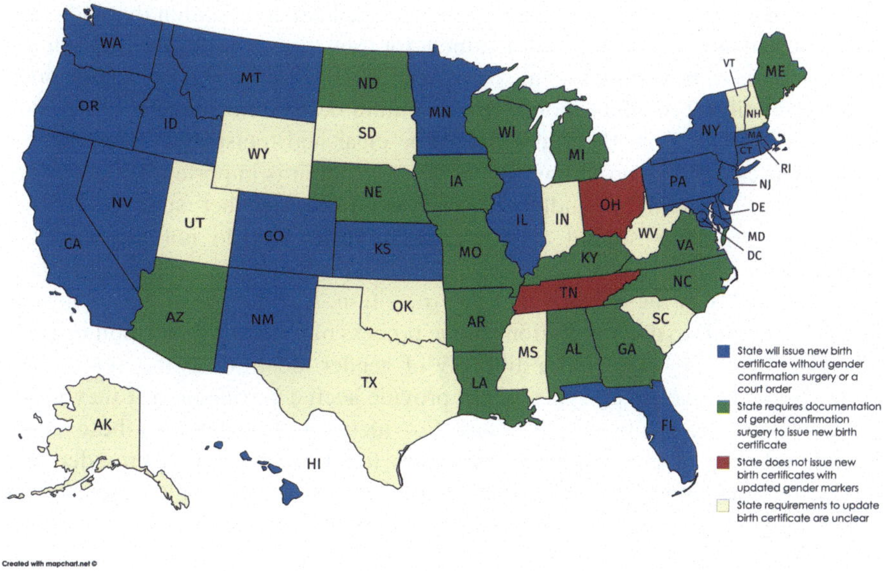

Fig. 20.5 State policies on amending birth certificates, July 2019

The requirements to change gender markers on birth certificates are generally more stringent. In two states – Ohio and Tennessee – state law does not permit an individual to change their gender marker on their birth certificate. In another 15 states, individuals can only change their gender marker if they have undergone gender confirmation surgery, which may create a particularly high barrier for TGD youth. In yet another 12 states, the medical requirements for a gender marker change are unclear and/or require a court order (Fig. 20.5). In the remaining 21 states and the District of Columbia, the state does not require gender confirmation surgery or a court order to issue a revised birth certificate, and in 7 of these states – California, Colorado, New Jersey, New Mexico, Oregon, Utah, and Washington – individuals have the option to select a nonbinary designation rather than identifying as male or female [21].

Input from medical providers can be a critical component of these gender marker changes on driver's licenses and birth certificates. Understanding a state's specific requirements and providing easy to use resource materials to help patients and parents begin these legal processes is another important aspect of trans-affirmative care. There are a number of online resources that keep up to date with current state-by-state regulations.[4]

In some instances, practitioners may be asked to certify that an individual is undergoing transition [22, 23]. To change a person's sex on their passport, for

[4] https://transequality.org/documents and https://transgenderlawcenter.org/resources/id/state-by-state-overview-changing-gender-markers-on-birth-certificates

example, the US State Department requires "a medical certification that indicates you have had appropriate clinical treatment for transition to male or female, or are in the process of transition to male or female" [24]. What this means can be open to interpretation. Providers should at a minimum be aware that such certification may be requested from them and should be clear and transparent with patients about their criteria for providing such a letter. While it is important for providers to use their professional judgment in determining whether such a letter is warranted, providers should also be mindful that they do not impose rigid expectations about what a transgender person should look or act like or place undue obstacles in the way of patients' transition. As understandings of gender diversity expand, so do expectations in the process of transition, variation in goals of gender-affirming care, and a diversity of gender identities as the outcome of such care. Providers of all types might provide such a certification if they know the patient and are involved in their care. Providers should ensure that these letters include relevant facts or language necessary for it to be valid. If providers are unsure about what information to include, they may wish to consult sample letters that transgender organizations and experienced providers have composed (Fig. 20.6) [25].

Licensed Physician's Letterhead
(including address and telephone number)

I, [PHYSICIAN'S FULL NAME], [PHYSICIAN'S MEDICAL LICENSE OR CERTIFICATE NUMBER], [ISSUING STATE OR COUNTRY OF MEDICAL LICENSE/CERTIFICATE], [DEA REGISTRATION NUMBER OR COMPARABLE FOREIGN DESIGNATION], am the physician of [NAME OF PATIENT], with whom I have a doctor/patient relationship and [WHOM I HAVE TREATED OR WHOSE MEDICAL HISTORY I HAVE REVIEWED AND EVALUATED].

[NAME OF PATIENT] has had appropriate clinical treatment for gender transition to the new gender [MALE OR FEMALE].

[INCLUSION OF ADDITIONAL INFORMATION IS NOT REQUIRED OR RECOMMENDED].

I declare under penalty of perjury under the laws of the United States that the foregoing is true and correct.

Signature of Physician

Typed Name of Physician

Date

Fig. 20.6 Sample provider letter from Transgender Legal Defense and Education Fund

In these different areas, state law is highly relevant to what providers are able to offer and what requirements they must meet to offer it freely. Where state law protections are lacking, practitioners may also wish to consult municipal nondiscrimination ordinances to see if gender identity is protected locally.

Frontiers in Law

In recent years, litigants and lawmakers have argued for an expansion of exemptions that permit medical providers to decline to provide services based on their religious or moral beliefs. Such challenges were raised in court, for example, in response to the preventive care and nondiscrimination provisions of the ACA. Under the leadership of Attorney General Jeff Sessions and Secretaries of Health and Human Services Tom Price and Alex Azar, federal agencies have promulgated rules that aim to expand the grounds under which medical providers can legally refuse to provide services. It is important for providers to understand what these rules do and do not permit, and for hospitals and other medical institutions to take steps to ensure that any objections do not interfere with a patient's ability to obtain accessible, timely, effective health services without discrimination.

On October 6, 2017, Attorney General Sessions released new guidance aimed at summarizing and clarifying existing protections for religious objectors under US law [26]. On January 18, 2018, HHS announced it would be creating a new division within its Office of Civil Rights to pursue claims related to conscience protections in health care [27]. On January 26, 2018, HHS proposed a new rule that would expand the circumstances under which individuals and institutions can deny care to patients on the basis of the entities' moral or religious beliefs [28]. The rule identified ten statutes that contain conscience protections, mainly for providers who may be in a position to perform abortions but have moral or religious reservations about doing so. While it purported to clarify and streamline existing protections, it would functionally expand them by redefining key terms used in the statutes, broadening what constitutes a "health care entity," expanding what it means to "assist in the performance of" a healthcare service, and purporting to exempt providers from a wide range of referral requirements [29].

The final rule was released in May 2019 but its implementation was delayed by a legal challenge, and it is not yet clear how HHS intends to enforce conscience claims with regard to gender-affirming care. The rule interprets statutes that, by their own terms, are limited to abortion; sterilization; assisted suicide; euthanasia or mercy killing; counseling and referrals under Medicare and Medicaid; foreign assistance for HIV/AIDS; certain compulsory medical tests or immunizations; and religious nonmedical health care institutions [28]. In the text of the proposed rule, however, HHS offered examples of instances where it felt that conscience had been insufficiently protected in the past; one of these examples was *Minton v. Dignity Health*, in which a transgender man is suing a provider who canceled his hysterectomy after being informed that he is transgender [28]. The inclusion of this specific example in the proposed rule suggests that HHS regards the enforcement of nondiscrimination protections as a threat to religious freedom, and intends to use its authority expansively to back providers who decline to provide to TGD people services that they would provide to their cisgender patients. One way that HHS may do so is by adopting an expansive vision of what "sterilization" entails to include procedures that only incidentally affect a person's reproductive capacity – a shift that would broaden the term far beyond its statutory meaning and jeopardize various forms of transition-related care. In the final rule, HHS indicated that objections to treatment for gender dysphoria would be evaluated on a case-by-case basis.

While much attention has been paid to possible federal regulatory shifts, states have enacted sweeping exemption laws as well. The most expansive is in Mississippi, which licenses discriminatory conduct that is grounded in any of three beliefs: that marriage should be between a man and a woman, that sex outside of marriage is improper, and that "biological sex" is immutable and fixed at birth. It protects these beliefs in a range of areas, including when a medical provider "declines to participate in the provision of treatments, counseling, or surgeries related to sex reassignment or gender identity transitioning or declines to participate in the provision of psychological, counseling, or fertility services" [30].

While Mississippi's law directly targets TGD patients, other states have laws that may also be used to deny patients care. For years, Illinois has had an expansive law that protects a provider's "conscientious refusal to receive, obtain, accept, perform, assist, counsel, suggest, recommend, refer or participate in any way in any particular form of health care services contrary to his or her conscience" [31]. Tennessee has a narrower law stating that "[n]o counselor or therapist providing counseling or therapy services shall be required to counsel or serve a client as to goals, outcomes, or behaviors that conflict with a sincerely held religious belief of the counselor or therapist" [32]. Both of these laws contain some protections for patients; Tennessee requires the objecting mental health professional to facilitate a referral [32], while Illinois requires that objectors refer the patient, notify the patient about other providers, or have a non-objecting provider perform the service in their stead [31]. Research suggests that providers may not be aware of or complying with the referral provisions, however, and the patient protections in Illinois are being challenged in court by religious providers who feel that facilitating a referral would also violate their religious beliefs.

When discussing religious exemptions in healthcare, it is important for hospitals to stay appraised of what these laws actually cover and what they do not protect. Some advocates, for example, argue that Alabama law also addresses religious refusals targeting TGD people. The relevant statute states: "A health care provider has the right not to participate, and no health care provider shall be required to participate, in a health care service that violates his or her conscience when the health care provider has objected in writing prior to being asked to provide such health care services" [33]. The statute narrowly defines "health care service," however, to include only "medical care, treatment or procedure that is limited to abortion, human cloning, human embryonic stem cell research, and sterilization" [33]. While some transition-related care may have the functional effect of rendering a person sterile, that is not the primary purpose of transition-related care, and other procedures that have that incidental effect are generally not regarded as "sterilization." Providers should construe these laws narrowly, and to err on the side of ensuring that patients are provided with affirming and nondiscriminatory care.

Providers should also be conscious of the changing legal landscape regarding "conversion therapy," or efforts to change the sexual orientation or gender identity of youth. The practice of conversion therapy has been roundly rejected by a wide range of professional associations in medicine and is increasingly prohibited by law. As of July 2019, eighteen states – California, Colorado, Connecticut, Delaware, Hawaii, Illinois, Maine, Maryland, Massachusetts, Nevada, New Hampshire, New Jersey, New Mexico, New York, Oregon, Rhode Island, Vermont, and Washington – and the District of Columbia had banned the practice, as have many municipalities in other states. Providers should ensure they are equipped to provide parents and guardians with medical guidance about the inefficacy and harmfulness of conversion therapy and should intervene in the event they learn that it is being performed (Fig. 20.7).

Providers can play an important role in opposing conversion therapy and countering the adverse effects of refusal laws. When legislation on these issues is proposed, providers can be a valuable source of information for legislators and can help articulate why these laws might affect the ability of TGD youth to access needed care. Where conversion therapy bans are proposed, providers can share their professional judgment about the harmful effects of seeking to change a TGD youth's sexual orientation or gender identity, and the benefits of providing trans-affirmative care. Where refusal laws have been enacted, providers should work to develop

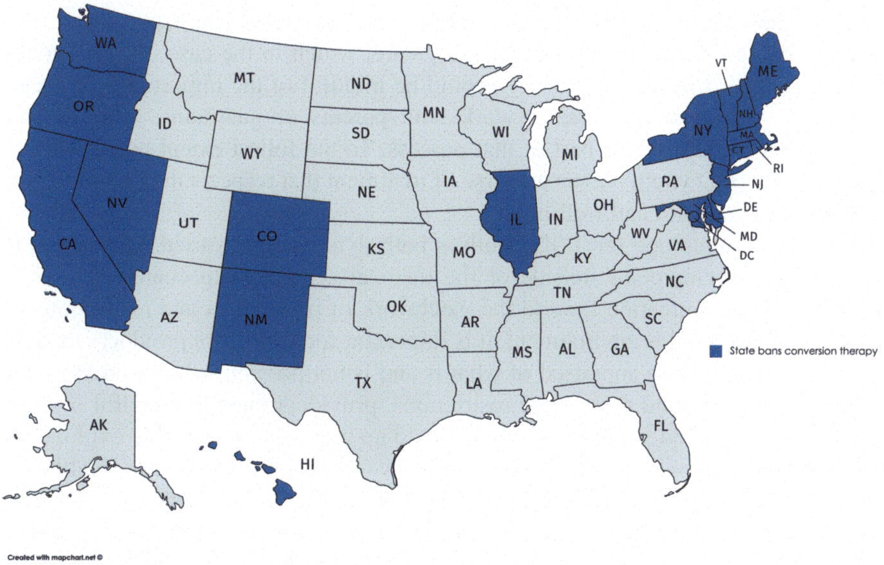

Fig. 20.7 State policies on conversion therapy, July 2019

institutional protocols to minimize disruptions in care. Such protocols might, for example, require that providers register religious or moral objections in advance, ensure that willing providers are in place to step in and deliver care without disruption or embarrassment to the patient, provide referrals so patients can obtain any services that are not offered at all, and make exceptions in the event of a medical emergency. Research also suggests that refusal laws may make TGD people less likely to seek care for fear of facing discrimination in healthcare [29]. In states where such laws have been enacted, providers may wish to affirmatively advertise their willingness to work with TGD youth and provide gender-affirming care.

Conclusion

As the above examples illustrate, many of the political and legal battles being fought over transgender rights have profound effects, both direct and incidental, on the provision of care to TGD youth. At times, political attempts to restrict transgender rights may run counter to professional standards, and pose an immediate dilemma for providers balancing their ethical and legal commitments. As bills related to transgender rights are being debated, providers who are committed to working with TGD youth should consider participating in public deliberations and sharing their professional perspectives with lawmakers and the public.

In this dynamic context, however, providers are not without guideposts. A wide range of medical professional organizations have emphasized the importance of providing affirming care for TGD youth. Providers who are unsure of the laws in their jurisdiction should clarify potential restrictions and inquire into workarounds that are legal and move affirmative care forward. Seeking out legal counsel or professional organizations can be helpful for this. As with all youth, providers must ensure they provide respectful and quality care, which in the case of TGD youth means gender-affirming care. They should be mindful of the importance of social transition, and take the time to work with parents or guardians, schools, and institutions who may be a part of that process. To the fullest extent possible, they should help TGD youth pursue a course of treatment that respects their identity and promotes their health and well-being.

The legal landscape for TGD youth is both dynamic and varied. Often, this is because of developments outside of the medical setting, from contestation over federal nondiscrimination laws to the patchwork of protections and restrictions in different states. In this environment, it is important for healthcare providers to keep up to date and remain appraised of what is and is not possible when working with TGD youth. But amid these legal restrictions, providers must be mindful of their own professional judgment and the edict to do no harm, and thoroughly explore the possibilities for providing care for TGD youth even in restrictive contexts. Healthcare professionals may participate in improving both education and services related to gender-affirming care, and in this professional capacity, work toward trans-affirmative laws and cultural environments. Healthcare professionals, with the privilege of education and information, not only have opportunities to provide TGD youth and families with support and resources, but have some obligation to work toward health equity and human rights for a population that often faces medical and legal barriers.

References

1. Department of Health and Human Services: Section 1557 of the Patient Protection and Affordable Care Act. https://www.hhs.gov/civil-rights/for-individuals/section-1557/index.html. Accessed 13 Nov 2018.
2. Office for Civil Rights, Department of Health and Human Services: non-discrimination in health programs and activities. 2016. https://www.federalregister.gov/documents/2016/05/18/2016-11458/nondiscrimination-in-health-programs-and-activities?utm_campaign=subscription+mailing+list&utm_medium=email&utm_source=federalregister.gov. Accessed 13 Nov 2018.
3. National Center for Transgender Equality: know your rights: healthcare. https://transequality.org/know-your-rights/healthcare. Accessed 13 Nov 2018.
4. U.S. District Court for the Northern District of Texas: complaint in *Franciscan Alliance v. Burwell*, No. 7:16-cv-00108. 2016. https://www.aclu.org/legal-document/franciscan-alliance-v-burwell-complaint. Accessed 13 Nov 2018.
5. U.S. District Court for the Northern District of Texas: order in *Franciscan Alliance v. Burwell*, No. 7:16-cv-00108. 2016. https://www.aclu.org/legal-document/franciscan-alliance-v-burwell-order-motions-preliminary-injunction. Accessed 13 Nov 2018.
6. U.S. District Court for the Northern District of Texas: defendants' motion for voluntary remand and stay in *Franciscan Alliance, Inc. v. Price*, No. 7:16-cv-00108. 2017. https://transequality.org/sites/default/files/docs/releases/1557%20motion%20for%20remand.pdf. Accessed 13 Nov 2018.
7. Pear R. Trump plan would cut back health care protections for transgender people. New York Times. 2018. https://www.nytimes.com/2018/04/21/us/politics/trump-transgender-health-care.html. Accessed 13 Nov 2018.
8. U.S. Court of Appeals for the Third Circuit: Doe v. Boyertown area School District, 2018 WL 3016864. 2018.
9. U.S. Court of Appeals for the Seventh Circuit: *Whitaker v. Kenosha Unified School District*, 858 F.3d 1034. 2017.
10. U.S. Court of Appeals for the Eleventh Circuit: *Glenn v. Brumby*, 663 F.3d 1312. 2011.
11. U.S. Court of Appeals for the Sixth Circuit: *Smith v. City of Salem*, 378 F.3d 566. 2004.
12. U.S. Court of Appeals for the First Circuit: *Rosa v. Park West Bank & Trust Co.*, 214 F.3d 213. 2000.
13. U.S. Court of Appeals for the Ninth Circuit. *Schwenk v. Hartford*, 204 F.3d 1187. 2000.
14. US Department of Justice & US Department of Education: Dear colleague letter on transgender Students. 2016. http://www2.ed.gov/about/offices/list/ocr/letters/colleague-201605-title-ix-transgender.pdf. Accessed 13 Nov 2018.
15. Peters JW, Becker J, Hirschfeld Davis J. Trump rescinds rules on bathrooms for transgender students. New York Times; 2017. https://www.nytimes.com/2017/02/22/us/politics/devos-sessions-transgender-students-rights.html. Accessed 13 Nov 2018.
16. Human Rights Watch: Shut out: Restrictions on bathroom and locker room access for transgender youth in US schools. 2016. https://www.hrw.org/report/2016/09/14/shut-out/restrictions-bathroom-and-locker-room-access-transgender-youth-us-schools. Accessed 13 Nov 2018.
17. Lambda Legal: a transgender advocate's guide to updating and amending school records. https://www.lambdalegal.org/know-your-rights/article/youth-ferpa-faq. Accessed 13 Nov 2018.

18. Movement Advancement Project: Healthcare laws and policies. http://www.lgbtmap.org/equality-maps/healthcare_laws_and_policies. Accessed 13 Nov 2018.
19. Crowder C. A judge has struck down Iowa's Medicaid ban on transgender transition-related care. Here's why. Des Moines Register. 2018. https://www.desmoinesregister.com/story/news/investigations/2018/06/07/iowas-medicaid-ban-transgender-transition-care-struck-down/682175002. Accessed 13 Nov 2018.
20. Mills S. Judge deems state health policy denying treatment for transgender Medicaid recipients unlawful. Wisconsin Public Radio 2018. https://www.wpr.org/judge-deems-state-health-policy-denying-treatment-transgender-medicaid-recipients-unlawful. Accessed 13 Nov 2018.
21. Movement Advancement Project: Identity document laws and policies. http://www.lgbtmap.org/equality-maps/identity_document_laws. Accessed 13 Nov 2018.
22. National Center for Transgender Equality: how trans-friendly is the driver's license gender change policy in your state? https://transequality.org/sites/default/files/docs/id/Drivers%20License%20Grades%20June%202018.docx. Accessed 13 Nov 2018.
23. Lambda Legal: changing birth certificate sex designations: state-by-state guidelines. 2018. https://www.lambdalegal.org/know-your-rights/article/trans-changing-birth-certificate-sex-designations. Accessed 13 Nov 2018.
24. US Department of State: change of sex marker. https://travel.state.gov/content/travel/en/passports/apply-renew-passport/gender.html. Accessed 13 Nov 2018.
25. Transgender Legal Defense and Education Fund: model doctor's letter certifying applicant's gender change (for U.S. passport or consular report of birth abroad. http://transgenderlegal.org/page.php?id=91. Accessed 13 Nov 2018.
26. US Department of Justice: attorney general sessions issues guidance on federal law protections for religious liberty. 2017. https://www.justice.gov/opa/pr/attorney-general-sessions-issues-guidance-federal-law-protections-religious-liberty. Accessed 13 Nov 2018.
27. US Department of Health and Human Services: HHS announces new conscience and religious freedom division. 2018. https://www.hhs.gov/about/news/2018/01/18/hhs-ocr-announces-new-conscience-and-religious-freedom-division.html. Accessed 13 Nov 2018.
28. US Department of Health and Human Services: protecting statutory conscience rights in health care; delegations of authority. 2018. https://www.federalregister.gov/documents/2018/01/26/2018-01226/protecting-statutory-conscience-rights-in-health-care-delegations-of-authority. Accessed 13 Nov 2018.
29. Human Rights Watch, You don't want second best: anti-LGBT discrimination in US health care, 2018, https://www.hrw.org/report/2018/07/23/you-dont-want-second-best/anti-lgbt-discrimination-us-health-care. Accessed 13 Nov 2018.
30. Mississippi House Bill 1523. 2016. http://billstatus.ls.state.ms.us/documents/2016/html/HB/1500-1599/HB1523SG.htm. Accessed 13 Nov 2018.
31. Illinois Health Care Right of Conscience Act, 745 Ill. Comp. Stat. Ann. 70/5. http://www.ilga.gov/legislation/ilcs/ilcs3.asp?ActID=2082&ChapterID=58. Accessed 13 Nov 2018.
32. Tennessee Senate Bill 1556. 2016. https://legiscan.com/TN/text/SB1556/id/1319613/Tennessee-2015-SB1556-Draft.pdf. Accessed 13 Nov 2018.
33. Alabama House Bill 95. 2017. https://legiscan.com/AL/text/HB95/2017. Accessed 13 Nov 2018.
34. Matthew Shepard and James Byrd Jr. Hate Crimes Prevention Act of 2009, codified at 18 U.S.C. § 249.
35. Violence Against Women Reauthorization Act of 2013, codified in part at 42 U.S.C. § 13701 et seq.
36. Cha AE. Ban lifted on Medicare coverage for sex change surgery. Washington Post 2014. https://www.washingtonpost.com/national/health-science/ban-lifted-on-medicare-coverage-for-sex-change-surgery/2014/05/30/28bcd122-e818-11e3-a86b-362fd5443d19_story.html. Accessed 13 Nov 2018.

Index

M. Forcier et al. (eds.), *Pediatric Gender Identity*,
https://doi.org/10.1007/978-3-030-38909-3

The manufacturer's authorised representative in the EU is Springer
Nature Customer Service Centre GmbH, Europaplatz 3, 69115 Heidelberg,
Germany. If you have any concerns regarding our products, please
contact ProductSafety@springernature.com

Printed and bound by CPI Group (UK) Ltd, Croydon, CR0 4YY
05/10/2026
02228122-0008